Supportive Care in Cancer Therapy

Cancer Treatment and Research

WILLIAM L. MCGUIRE, *series editor*

R.B. Livingston, ed., Lung Cancer 1, 1981, ISBN 90-247-2394-9.
G. Bennett Humphrey, Louis P. Dehner, Gerald B, Grindey and Ronald T, Acton, eds., Pediatric Oncology 1, 1981, ISBN 90-247-2408-2.
Jerome J, DeCosse and Paul Sherlock, eds., Gastrointestinal Cancer 1, 1981, ISBN 90-247-2461-9.
John M. Bennett, ed., Lymphomas 1, including Hodgkin's Disease, 1981, ISBN 90-247-2479-1.
C.D. Bloomfield, ed., Adult Leukemias 1, 1982, ISBN 90-247-2478-3.
David F. Paulson, ed., Genitourinary Cancer 1, 1982, ISBN 90-247-2480-5.
F. M. Muggia, ed., Cancer Chemotherapy 1, ISBN 90-247-2713-8.
G. Bennett Humphrey and Gerald B. Grindey, eds., Pancreatic Tumors in Children. ISBN 90-247-2702-2.
John J. Costanzi, ed., Malignant Melanoma 1. ISBN 90 247-2706-5.
C.T. Griffiths and A.F. Fuller, eds., Gynecologic Oncology. ISBN 0-89838-555-5.
Greco F. Anthony, ed., Biology and Management of Lung Cancer. ISBN 0-89838-554-7.
Walker, Michael D., ed., Oncology of the Nervous System. ISBN 0-89838-567-9.

Supportive Care
in Cancer Therapy

edited by

DONALD J. HIGBY

Department of Medical Oncology
Roswell Park Memorial Institute
Buffalo, New York, USA

1983 **MARTINUS NIJHOFF PUBLISHERS**
a member of the KLUWER ACADEMIC PUBLISHERS GROUP
BOSTON / THE HAGUE / DORDRECHT / LANCASTER

Distributors

for the United States and Canada: Kluwer Boston, Inc., 190 Old Derby Street, Hingham, MA 02043, USA
for all other countries: Kluwer Academic Publishers Group, Distribution Center, P.O. Box 322, 3300 AH Dordrecht, The Netherlands

Library of Congress Cataloging in Publication Data   CIP

Main entry under title:

Supportive care in cancer therapy.

    (Cancer treatment and research ; v. 13)
    Includes index.
    1. Cancer--Treatment--Addresses, essays, lectures.
I. Higby, Donald J. II. Series. [DNLM: 1. Neoplasms--
Therapy. W1 CA693 v. 13 / QZ 266 S959]
RC270.8.S9 1983   616.99'406   83-148
ISBN 0-89838-569-5

ISBN 0-89838-569-5

Copyright

PRINTED IN THE NETHERLANDS

DEDICATED TO MY WIFE, JOAN
WHO MAKES LIFE WORTH LIVING

Contents

Cancer Treatment and Research

Foreword

Where do you begin to look for a recent, authoritative article on the diagnosis or management of a particular malignancy? The few general oncology textbooks are generally out of date. Single papers in specialized journals are informative but seldom comprehensive; these are more often preliminary reports on a very limited number of patients. Certain general journals frequently publish good indepth reviews of cancer topics, and published symposium lectures are often the best overviews available. Unfortunately, these reviews and supplements appear sporadically, and the reader can never be sure when a topic of special interest will be covered.

Cancer Treatment and Research is a series of authoritative volumes which aim to meet this need. It is an attempt to establish a critical mass of oncology literature covering virtually all oncology topics, revised frequently to keep the coverage up to date, easily available on a single library shelf or by a single personal subscription.

We have approached the problem in the following fashion. First, by dividing the oncology literature into specific subdivisions such as lung cancer, genitourinary cancer, pediatric oncology, etc. Second, by asking eminent authorities in each of these areas to edit a volume on the specific topic on an annual or biannual basis. Each topic and tumor type is covered in a volume appearing frequently and predictably, discussing current diagnosis, staging, markers, all forms of treatment modalities, basic biology, and more.

In Cancer Treatment and Research, we have an outstanding group of editors, each having made a major commitment to bring to this new series the very best literature in his or her field. Martinus Nijhoff Publishers has made an equally major commitment to the rapid publication of high quality books, and world-wide distribution.

Where can you go to find quickly a recent authoritative article on any major oncology problem? We hope that Cancer Treatment and Research provides an answer.

WILLIAM L. McGUIRE
Series Editor

Preface

This book is meant as a ready reference for the physician whose specialty involves the care of the cancer patient. The topics were selected in an attempt to review and rationalize information which is not communicated in a formal way to those of us who have trained in cancer-related disciplines. Not unexpectedly, most cancer specialists use their learning time to update themselves on the direct treatment of the malignancy and rely on habit, innate communication skills, and occasionally other professionals for the delivery of supportive care to their patients. For instance, it is rare to find a cancer specialist who uses more than one or two anti-emetics in his practice or is familiar with pain control beyond the prescription of a favorite narcotic. It is unusual to discover a clinician who is familiar with the adjustments patients with breast cancer or patients who have enterostomies must face. Yet, a sizeable proportion of patients in a practice face these problems.

'Supportive Care' does not denote a discipline and my selection of topics would differ, I am sure, from those of other individuals. Therefore, the chapters in this book cover areas which I personally feel will be of use to the physician in practice, either now or in the near future. As cancer therapy becomes more aggressive, the practicing oncologist will be confronted more often with problems which heretofore have not been that common.

Some chapters will be of immediate practical benefit to the cancer physician; others may appear more arcane. Finally, some are included primarily to acquaint the physician with areas of great concern to the patient, but perhaps not within the physician's own purview. The theme running through the book is to compile in one volume state-of-the-art information concerning those areas of cancer patient management which involve optimization of life (acutely or chronically), but do not involve a direct attack on the tumor itself.

I personally have learned a great deal from all but one of the chapters in this book; whether this reflects my own state of ignorance or a more general situation in the physician community, I leave to the reader to determine.

Since all but two of the chapters are authored by others, I can express my delight at the thoughtful and comprehensive treatment they have given to their topics.

Hopefully, this book will have subsequent editions. I invite readers to comment on it and otherwise contribute towards an even more useful future edition.

I express my deepest appreciation to Ms Corrine Cesari for her dedicated efforts in the preparation of this book.

Donald J. HIGBY, M.D.

List of Contributors

ABRAMS, Ross A., M.D., Assistant Professor of Medicine, Medical College of Wisconsin, Dept. of Medicine, Section of Hematology/Oncology, Milwaukee County Medical Complex, 8700 West Wisconsin Avenue, Milwaukee, WI 53226, USA. Title: Hematopoietic Dysfunction Resulting from Antineoplastic Therapy: Current Concepts and Potential for Management

BANGERT, Jacqueline B., R.N., M.S., E.T., Enterostomal Therapy Consultant, The Illinois Cancer Council, 36 South Wabash Avenue, Chicago, IL 60603, USA. Title: Enterostomal Therapy: Supportive Care for the Cancer Patient

BRASS, Corstiaan, M.D., Assistant Professor of Medicine, Division of Infectious Disease, Dept. of Medicine, Buffalo General Hospital, 100 High Street, Buffalo, NY 14203, USA. Title: Fungal Infections in the Immunocompromised Host

CARL, William, D.D.S., Senior Cancer Dental Surgeon, Department of Dentistry & Maxillofacial Prosthetics, Roswell Park Memorial Institute, 666 Elm Street, Buffalo, NY 14263, USA; and Associate Clinical Professor of Fixed Prosthetics, State University of New York at Buffalo, Buffalo, NY. Title: Oral Complications of Cancer Patients Undergoing Chemotherapy and Radiation Therapy

CATALANO, Robert B., Pharm. D., Coordinator of Clinical Studies, Dept. of Medical Oncology, American Oncologic Hospital/Fox Chase Cancer Center, Central & Shelmire Avenues, Philadelphia, PA 19111, USA. Title: Medical Management of Chronic Pain Caused by Cancer

CERRA, Frank B., M.D., Associate Professor of Surgery, Dept. of Surgery, University of Minnesota Medical School, Phillips Wangensteen Building, 516 Delaware Street S.E., Minneapolis, MN 55455, USA. Title: Nutritional/Metabolic Support: Parenteral and Enteral

DE JONGH, Carlos A., M.D., Assistant Professor of Medicine, University of Maryland Cancer Center, University of Maryland School of Medicine & Hospital, 22 South Greene Street, Baltimore, MD 21201, USA.

Title: Bacterial infections in Neutropenic Patients

DOUGLASS, Harold O., Jr., M.D., F.A.C.S., Associate Chief, Dept. of Surgical Oncology, Roswell Park Memorial Institute, 666 Elm Street, Buffalo, NY 14263, USA; and Associate Professor of Research Surgery, State University of New York at Buffalo, Buffalo, NY. Title: Problems in Surgical Oncology: The Surgical Approach to Recurrent and Metastatic Cancer

DRAPKIN, Robert L., M.D., F.A.C.P., Clinical Assistant Professor of Medicine, University of South Florida at Tampa, Tampa, Florida; and Medical Oncologist, Radiation Therapy Oncology Center, 725 Virginia Street, Dunedin, Fl. 33528, USA. Title: Nausea and Vomiting Caused by Chemotherapy

GELBER, Sandra Shiller, M.S.W., Oncology Social Work Consultant, The Illinois Cancer Council, 36 South Wabash Avenue, Chicago, IL 60603, USA. Title: Enterostomal Therapy: Supportive Care for the Cancer Patient

GOODMAN, Robert L., M.D., Professor & Chairman, Departments of Radiation Therapy, University of Pennsylvania School of Medicine/Fox Chase Cancer Center, Hospital of the University of Pennsylvania, 3400 Spruce Street, Philadelphia, PA 19104, USA., Title: Psychological Adjustment in the Mastectomy Patient

HIGBY, Donald J., M.D., Head, Section of Supportive Care/Transplantation, and Associate Chief, Dept. of Medical Oncology, Roswell Park Memorial Institute, 666 Elm Street, Buffalo, New York 14263, USA; and Research Associate Professor of Medicine, State University of New York at Buffalo, School of Medicine, Roswell Park Division, Buffalo, New York. Titles: 1) Granulocyte Transfusion Therapy; 2) The Care of the Terminal Patient

LOGEMANN, Jerilyn A., Ph.D., Director of Cancer Control, The Illinois Cancer Council, 36 South Wabash Avenue, Chicago, IL 60603, USA. Title: Enterostomal Therapy: Supportive Care for the Cancer Patient

LYSNE, Jolynn, Pharm. D., Nutritional Support Service, University of Minnesota Hospitals and Clinics, University of Minnesota Medical School, Phillips Wangensteen Building, 516 Delaware Street, S.E. Minneapolis, MN 55455, USA. Title: Nutritional/Metabolic Support: Parenteral and Enteral

MARGOLIS, Gerald J., M.D., Clinical Associate Professor of Psychiatry, University of Pennsylvania School of Medicine/Fox Chase Cancer Center, Hospital of the University of Pennsylvania, 3400 Spruce Street, Philadelphia, PA 19104, USA. Title: Psychological Adjustment in the Mastectomy Patient

NUWER, Nancy, R.N., M.S., Nurse Clinician, Nutritional Support Service, University of Minnesota Hospitals and Clinics, University of Minnesota

Medical School, Phillips Wangensteen Building, 516 Delaware Street, S.E., Minneapolis, MM 55455, USA. Title: Nutritional/Metabolic Support: Parenteral and Enteral

POWERS, Mary, R.N., E.T., Director of Ostomy Services, Ingalls Memorial Hospital, Harvey, IL 60426, USA. Title: Enterostomal Therapy: Supportive Care for the Cancer Patient

SCHIFFER, Charles A., M.D., Head, Division of Hematologic Malignancies, University of Maryland Cancer Center; and Associate Professor of Medicine, University of Maryland School of Medicine, University of Maryland, 22 S. Greene Street, Baltimore, MD 21201, USA. Title: Platelet Transfusion Therapy for Patients with Cancer

SCHIMPFF, Stephen C., M.D., Director, University of Maryland Cancer Center; and Professor of Medicine, University of Maryland School of Medicine, University of Maryland Cancer Center, University of Maryland School of Medicine and Hospital, 22 S. Greene Street, Baltimore, MD 21201, USA. Title: Bacterial Infections in Neutropenic Patients

SHRONTS, Eva P., R.D., Dietician, Nutritional Support Service, University of Minnesota Hospitals and Clinics, University of Minnesota Medical School, Phillips Wangensteen Building, 516 Delaware Street, S.E., Minneapolis, MN 55455, USA. Title: Nutritional/Metabolic Support: Parenteral and Enteral

TEASLEY, Kathy M., M.S., R.Ph., TPN Pharmacist, Nutritional Support Service, University of Minnesota Hospitals and Clinics, University of Minnesota Medical School, Phillips Wangensteen Building, 516 Delaware Street, S.E., Minneapolis, MN 55455, USA. Title: Nutritional/Metabolic Support: Parenteral and Enteral

TEBBI, Cameron K., M.D., Director, Adolescent Unit. Roswell Park Memorial Institute, 666 Elm Street, Buffalo, NY 14263, USA. Title: Care for Adolescent Oncology Patients

WILLIS, Marilyn A., R.N., M.S., Assistant Director for Rehabilitation, The Illinois Cancer Council, 36 South Wabash Avenue, Chicago, IL 60603, USA. Title: Enterostomal Therapy: Supportive Care for the Cancer Patient

YATES, Jerome W., M.D., Associate Director, Centers and Community Oncology Program, Division of Resources, Centers, and Community Activities, National Cancer Institute, Blair Building, Room 732, Bethesda, MD 20205, USA. Title: Religion as Supportive Care

1. Bacterial Infections in Neutropenic Patients

CARLOS A. DE JONGH, and STEPHEN C. SCHIMPFF

INTRODUCTION

Granulocytopenia occurs in a variety of situations but most commonly in patients with illnesses characterized by bone marrow failure (e.g., acute leukemia). Patients with fewer than 1,000 granulocytes/μl are at a high risk of infection [1], the incidence and severity of the infectious episodes increasing at granulocyte counts of less than 500/μl, a steeper rise evidenced when the granulocyte count drops to less than 100/μl [2].

The duration of the granulocytopenic period constitutes also an important factor, severe infections and bacteremias occurring more frequently among patients with prolonged (more than 10 days), severe (<100/μl) granulocytopenia. This is of considerable importance today since current cancer chemotherapy regimens are designed in such a way that patients with acute leukemia, advanced lymphomas and selected solid tumors are rendered granulocytopenic for prolonged periods. Neutropenia is also the rule following bone marrow transplantation, usually persisting for the three to four weeks required for the graft to begin to function.

In association with granulocytopenia, other factors predispose to infection: combination chemotherapy generally produces a moderate to severe degree of damage to the mucosal membranes of the alimentary canal, thus allowing for invasion by colonizing organisms. Also, disruption is caused in the mucociliary mechanisms of the tracheobronchial tree, the subsequent accumulation of secretions allowing the development of infection. Damage to the integuments by venipunctures, bone marrow aspirates or biopsies or other invasive procedures break the natural barrier against a wide variety of potential pathogens.

Neutropenic patients undergo dynamic changes of their endogenous flora due to different circumstances: their primary illness, prolonged hospitalization, and therapy with antibiotics. They are likely to come in contact with

Higby, DJ (ed), Supportive Care in Cancer Therapy. ISBN 0-89838-569-5.
© *1983, Martinus Nijhoff Publishers, Boston. Printed in The Netherlands.*

different potential pathogens, usually becoming colonized by the organisms that reach their alimentary canal or skin. This factor becomes relevant once it is known that more than half of the infections occurring in patients with profound granulocytopenia are caused by organisms acquired in the hospital [3]. The responsible pathogens are few: aerobic gram-negative bacilli such as *Escherichia coli, Pseudomonas aeruginosa* and *Klebsiella pneumoniae* accounting for 60% of initial infectious episodes in large series [4], *Staphylococcus aureus* and, lately, *Staphylococcus epidermidis* are the most common gram-positive organisms isolated in these patients [4, 5].

Some major sources of acquired organisms are food, water, air and hands, Salads, particularly leafy vegetables, are frequently contaminated with gram-negative bacilli, poultry has been found to be contaminated with *Salmonella* species and some processed fruit juices have been found to have *Candida* species [6]. Water supplies are usually low in bacterial counts if processes such as chlorination and filtration have been followed. Air is the source of particles carrying bacteria such as *Staphylococcus aureus* and *Mycobacterium tuberculosis,* spores of fungi or respiratory viruses. Hands are a common source of *S. aureus* and gram-negative bacilli, medical and paramedical personnel not infrequently forgetting to wash their hands before and after patient contact unless there is gross contamination [7].

THE FEBRILE, NEUTROPENIC PATIENT

The presence of granulocytopenia is responsible for muted and often absent signs of infection except for fever which is almost invariably present [2]. If one reviews large series of febrile, neutropenic patients, it will be found that about 20% of the febrile episodes are due to bacteremias, 20% to nonbacteremic, microbiologically documented infections, another 20% to clinically documented infections while 40% will have equivocal or doubtful infections [4]. Therefore, fever represents documented infection in approximately 60% of all febrile episodes in this patient population.

Careful, meticulous evaluation is necessary in order to establish the site of infection. Although they can occur at any site, infections usually affect only five or six common areas: the alimentary canal, particularly at its beginning, e.g., oral cavity, pharynx and distal esophagus and at its end, e.g., lower colon, rectum and perianum; the lungs, the skin, paranasal sinuses and the urinary tract.

DIAGNOSIS

The initial step in the evaluation of the neutropenic patient with suspected infection should be a careful history and physical examination. The history should be meticulous enough to detect even minor symptoms such as pain on defecation or substernal pain which may be the first manifestation of perianal cellulitis or esophagitis, respectively. As mentioned above, the classic signs of infection are diminished, for example: even though most patients with pharyngitis will have fever and sore throat, less than a third will have exudate or submandibular nodes. Patients with pneumonia may present initially with no symptoms other than fever and even have a clear chest X-ray; subsequent examination however usually will detect shortness of breath, chest pain and some evidence of consolidation while the chest X-rays will eventually demonstrate a pulmonary infiltrate.

The examination should be *thorough* and must include a search for predisposing factors such as intravenous catheters or butterfly needles in place for more than 48 hours, urinary catheters, and areas of local trauma to the skin. A urinalysis performed by the physician, cultures taken from any clinically suspicious area plus at least two separate sets of blood cultures from different venipunctures, urine culture and a chest X-ray should complete the initial evaluation.

Other procedures may be of substantial help: surveillance cultures from gingiva and rectum taken before the administration of antibiotics will reveal the baseline microbial flora of the patient and alert to the possibility of infection due to an unusually resistant organism [8]. Needle aspiration of areas of cellulitis, transtracheal aspirates and/or fiberoptic bronchoscopy in a patient with pulmonary infiltrates or esophagoscopy in cases of suspected esophagitis may yield prompt etiologic diagnosis. Meningitis is only rarely responsible for febrile episodes in patients with neutropenia, therefore a spinal tap and spinal fluid examination and culture should only be done in cases where specific signs and symptoms point toward its presence.

Perhaps more important is to emphasize that periodically repeated evaluations are necessary whether the initial diagnostic workup is negative or positive. In cases of fever of unknown origin, history and physical examination should be complemented with repeated chest X-rays, as many as one every other day, and other studies directed to a specific source if any symptomatology is suggested. It is not infrequent for a critically ill patient not to show a definitive source of infection for two, three and even four days despite meticulous repeated evaluations.

THERAPY

Since a majority of febrile neutropenic patients will prove to have a documented infection, which may rapidly progress and become life threatening unless appropriate measures are taken, diverse therapeutic appoaches have been developed. One of them, the concept of empiric, broad spectrum antibiotic administration, was first reported in 1971 [9] and now constitutes accepted practice. The appropriate choice of antimicrobials to use in a given regimen has been based on the following factors: the antibiotic spectrum should be broad and include gram-positive as well as gram-negative organisms since it is difficult to differentiate on clinical grounds alone between infections caused by each of these two groups of pathogens; the drugs should be bactericidal even in the presence of severe granulocytopenia and if antibiotic combinations are used, synergistic activity against most common pathogens should be sought; the antibiotics should be administered intravenously and in appropriate doses, in order to have an assurance that adequate serum levels are always present; finally, toxicities should be minimal since 20 to 40% of the patients to be treated will not have a documented infection.

Of significant importance, the choice for an antibiotic regimen should be made taking into consideration the potential problem pathogen(s) in a certain institution, i.e., if *P. aeruginosa* is responsible for a majority of the gram-negative infections, the empiric regimen to use must have excellent activity against that particular pathogen (e.g., ticarcillin plus an aminoglycoside) while if the problem pathogen is *K. pneumoniae,* the same combination plus a cephalosporin or a cephalosporin plus an aminoglycoside would be appropriate choices.

PROGNOSTIC FACTORS

Response of a documented infection in granulocytopenic patients to a given antibiotic regimen is related to the increment in the granulocyte count in the peripheral blood and to susceptibility of the pathogen to the antimicrobials given. Even minimal increments in the circulating granulocytes result in improved response rates (Table 1). In patients with persistent, profound granulocytopenia susceptibility of the infecting organism to two antibiotics in a combination has been associated with higher improvement rates

Table 1. Recovery of granulocyte count and response among UMCC patients with gram-negative bacteremia and initial granulocyte count <100/μl, treated with empiric broad spectrum antibiotic combinations (January 1979 – September 1981).

Subsequent granulocyte count	Improved/total	(%)
Persisted <100/μl	9/36	(25) [a]
Increased to >100/μl	27/31	(87) [a]
Total	36/67	(54)

[a] $p = 0.000001$.

than if the pathogen is sensitive to only one or none of the antibiotics used.

ANTIBIOTIC REGIMENS

Inadequate overall response and rapid emergence of resistance among potential pathogens have been reported in the few trials that have attempted initial empiric therapy with single drugs.

Semisynthetic penicillins such as carbenicillin [10] ticarcillin [11] and mezlocillin [12] as well as aminoglycosides, such as gentamicin [9, 13, 14] and tobramycin [15] have yielded poor response rates when used alone. In a trial using mezlocillin as a single drug, Wade et al. [12] obtained a response rate of 52% despite excluding all patients known to be colonized with mezlocillin-resistant organisms; also, the investigators observed an increase in the minimum inhibitory concentration of mezlocillin against most gram-negative bacilli collected after the completion of the trial.

These reasons, plus the advantages of using combinations of antibiotics, to be explained below, make us reluctant to recommend the use of single agents, even those with very broad spectrum, despite the theoretical advantages of decreased toxicity and cost.

Broadening of the antibacterial spectrum from a qualitative point of view is not the only advantage of using combination therapy. It has been noted that patients with gram-negative bacteremia and profound ($<100/\mu l$) persistent granulocytopenia respond best if the infecting organism is susceptible to two drugs in an antibiotic combination as opposed to when the pathogen is susceptible to only one antibiotic [16]. Moreover, the use of antibiotic combinations provides the potential for synergism against specific pathogens, making the combination more effective than any of the drugs used alone; several studies have been reported in the literature associating the use of synergistic combinations with better clinical response rates than that of nonsynergistic ones [17–19]. Also, the bactericidal activity of sera from patients receiving antibiotic combinations has been correlated to clinical effectiveness and found to be higher among patients who received synergistic antibiotics [17–20].

Numerous combinations of antibiotics have been evaluated in the febrile, granulocytopenic patient; from a microbiological point of view, these combinations have in common spectrum against a wide range of pathogens and clinically have various degrees of efficacy.

A semisynthetic penicillin such as carbenicillin or ticarcillin plus an aminoglycoside has been used extensively in different institutions around the world yielding adequate clinical results with minimal toxicity [4, 14, 21].

Ticarcillin can be given in a lower dosage than carbenicillin, hence less sodium is administered to the patient with resultant decreased hypokalemia. The difference in efficacy among aminoglycosides appears to be a result of resistant patterns of gram-negative bacilli in different institutions, since when used against susceptible bacteria different aminoglycosides have provided identical response rates [21–23]. These combinations provide broad overall coverage and, generally, synergism against *P. aeruginosa* and *E. coli.* Poor responses against *K. pneumoniae* constitute what may be the major deficiency of the regimen. Although poor coverage against *S. aureus* is a potential defect, published data show that this type of combination is appropriate as initial therapy [4, 24].

New semisynthetic penicillins, such as mezlocillin, azlocillin and piperacillin, have added *K. pneumoniae* and *S. marcescens* to their spectrum while maintaining or even improving their anti-Pseudomonas activity. The combination of one of these agents plus an aminglycoside would seem to be an excellent regimen for the neutropenic patient; however, the results of recently reported clinical trials have failed to demonstrate increased efficacy over regimens such as ticarcillin plus an aminoglycoside [25].

A combination of a cephalosporin such as cephalothin or cefazolin plus an aminoglycoside has also been widely used in patients with suspected sepsis with good overall results. Synergism against *Klebsiella* sp. has been documented but only the aminoglycoside is active against *P. aeruginosa* and poor response rates can be expected when treating such pathogens [13, 14]. New cephalosporin-like compounds with anti-Pseudomonas activity have undergone extensive clinical trials and have been or are about to be released for use by the medical community. Some of these drugs have increased activity against Enterobacteriaceae and include *S. marcescens* and anaerobes in their spectrum. The combination of one of these drugs plus an aminoglycoside would be expected to produce significant improvement over the results that can be obtained with standard regimens, however, prospective, randomized clinical trials have so far failed to demonstrate increased efficacy [26].

Carbenicillin or ticarcillin plus cephalothin or cefazolin is also a commonly used combination with broad spectrum and proven therapeutic efficacy [4, 27]. Its main disadvantages are single coverage against two major pathogens: *P. aeruginosa* and *K. pneumoniae* and the occasional occurrence of gram-negative bacilli resistant to both antibiotics. Its main advantage is the lack of an aminoglycoside hence having less potential for nephrotoxicity.

The combination of one of the new 'third generation' cephalosporins (moxalactam, cefotaxime, cefoperazone) and one of the new acylampicillins (piperacillin, mezlocillin, azlocillin) would seem to be an excellent regimen, since it would provide double coverage against most pathogens and synergism has been reported against gram-negative bacteria. The lack of an aminoglycoside would substantially reduce the possibilities of nephrotoxicity and ototoxicity. There is, however, suggestion of antagonism in vitro against some pathogens [28] because of that reason extreme caution should be recommended if one attempts to use such combinations until the results of more laboratory evaluations as well as pertinent clinical trials are available.

Other drug combinations have been evaluated as potentially effective regimens in febrile, neutropenic patients including clindamycin plus gentamicin, carbenicillin plus polymixin and gentamicin plus chloramphenicol. No extensive experience however exists with any of these combinations, in addition, from a microbiological point of view they are less effective than most of the commonly used regimens mentioned above.

At least two studies have been reported in the literature reporting the use of carbenicillin or ticarcillin plus trimethoprim/sulfamethoxazole [29, 30], response rates have been equivalent to those obtained with carboxypenicillin–aminoglycoside combinations, suggesting a role for this antibiotic regimen. The recent popular acceptance of oral trimethoprim/sulfamethoxazole as prophylaxis of infection in granulocytopenic patients and the likelihood of some infections being caused in such patients by trimethoprim/sulfamethoxazole-resistant organisms, plus the possibility of a patient being infected with an organism resistant to both carbenicillin (or ticarcillin) and trimethoprim/sulfamethoxazole make us introduce a note of caution on the use of this combination as an empiric antibiotic regimen.

One frequently asked question involves the combination of three or more antibiotics in the hope of widening the antimicrobial spectrum and increase the possibility of employing a synergistic combination. Carbenicillin/ticarcillin plus an aminoglycoside and a cephalosporin has been a widely utilized regimen, however, despite the theoretical advantages, large trials have failed to demonstrate a benefit of these drug combinations over the standard two-drug regimens [31]. Similarly, the advisability of including a specific anti-staphylococcal agent to combinations such as antipseudomonal penicillin plus an aminoglycoside has been extensively discussed; it is the experience of many centers, including ours, that the use of this last regimen provides good initial coverage in cases of severe staphylococcal infections and that the appropriate modification can be made once the results of cultures and susceptibility tests are known without detriment to the possibilities of obtaining a good antibiotic response [4, 19, 24, 32].

DURATION OF THERAPY AND ADDITION OF OTHER ANTIBIOTICS

Considerable controversy still exists concerning the optimal duration of antibiotic therapy. Superinfection and/or subsequent infections have been found in zero to 25% of patients treated with empiric broad spectrum regimens [4, 26, 33, 34]. Persistent granulocytopenia and prolonged therapy with antibiotics have been implicated as significant predisposing factors. On the other hand, side effects of the drugs such as the hypokalemia induced by penicillins and nephrotoxicity and ototoxicity induced by the aminoglycosides may become a substantial problem in patients that are to be treated for prolonged periods. It seems to be essential then to discontinue the antibiotic administration as soon as a documented infection is appropriately treated. The compromised host should be treated for as long as the same type of infection in the normal host and occasionally longer. Below are guidelines used successfully at our institution at this time; we should emphasize however that every patient should be individualized and the decision making based on the clinical conditions of the patient and the status of the primary disease.

In general, we suggest 14 days of therapy for those patients with gram-negative or gram-positive bacteremia providing that they have had a favorable evolution on a particular regimen and the source of infection has healed or considerably improved. Serious, nonbacteremic infections, either clinically or microbiologically documented are also treated for the same period of time. Less severe infections are treated for a week to 10 days but, in all cases, the treatment is continued for at least 5 days after clinical resolution.

Patients with equivocal (possible) infections who have an apparent clinical response to antibiotic administration are treated until they have remained afebrile for four to five days, usually a total of about seven days of therapy. Patients who have a doubtful infection have their antibiotics discontinued as soon as repeated clinical assessment and results of complementary tests (X-rays, cultures) are available and negative, usually within four days.

Perhaps the most difficult dilemma involves the group of patients who, while still granulocytopenic, continue to be febrile and in whom no infection has been documented. Should antibiotics be discontinued and the patient reevaluated or the regimen modified or intensified? Diverse approaches have been reported in the literature and there is no consensus about what approach should be taken. The approach that we follow in our institution is based on the belief that most patients, even though severely granulocytopenic, will show specific symptoms or signs of infection in addition to fever after 72 to 96 hours providing that a careful clinical evaluation is repeated on a daily basis from the moment of the original febrile episode; this evaluation should include appropriate cultures and the obtainment of repeated chest X-rays, at least every other day. After approximately four days of empiric antibiotic therapy, if the patient's condition is unchanged and culture results and appropriate radiographs are unhelpful, the antibiotics are discontinued, the patient closely followed, recultured and restarted on antibacterials if necessary. This decision, however, should be individualized: if the patient appears toxic or there is conflicting evidence of infection, the antibiotic regimen is maintained, other drugs added if there is suspicion of the presence of a resistant organism, or empiric antifungal therapy initiated on the basis of a possible fungal infection. Epidemiological data plays an important role in the making of such decisions, thus a patient who shows an unusual or resistant organism in surveillance cultures may benefit from the inclusion of a drug active against that presumptive pathogen in the empiric antibiotic combination; on the other hand, a patient who shows a positive nose culture for *Aspergillus* species or who has been severely granulocytopenic for a prolonged period during which he has received several courses of broad spectrum antimicrobials, is a candidate for empiric therapy with amphotericin B.

Other approaches suggest a complete change in the therapy [35] or the addition of antifungal therapy in every patient with fever of unknown origin who has not responded to seven days of broad spectrum antibacterial antibiotics [36]. Without doubt, a large number of patients have fever with no documented infection but response rates to empiric antibiotic therapy have been generally high and, in fact, the proportion of patients in whom such decisions have to be made is relatively small as can be seen in the results of two large studies addressing that issue [36, 37] and summarized in Table 2 together with data from our cancer center (unpublished data). We believe that in making decisions on an individual basis in these patients who do not respond to the initial regimen, most infections and pathogens will be identified and side effects of antimicrobial therapy minimized.

Alteration of the therapy in patients with documented infections who have shown favorable response is seldom justified. We prefer to continue the patient on an antibiotic combination even after a specific pathogen is identified, particularly if the patient is still granulocytopenic, since the use of synergistic associations may have a favorable impact on the outcome of the episode. In cases of resistance to one of the antibiotics used or when a better alternative is available (i.e., a penicillinase-resistant penicillin in patients with *S. aureus* infections treated initially with carbenicillin or ticarcillin plus an aminoglycoside) therapy can be justifiably altered according to results of in vitro susceptibility tests and the clinical judgement of the physician.

Table 2. Patients without obvious source of infection (FUO), persistently granulocytopenic and febrile after at least four days of empiric therapy with broad spectrum antibiotics.

Initial study population (No. of episodes)	FUO; persistently granulocytopenic and febrile	(%)	Ref.
652	50	(7.7)	36
335	36	(10.7)	37
429	22	(5.1)	+ [b]
1,416 [a]	108 [a]	(7.6)	

[a] Total.
[b] UMCC unpublished data.

ANTIBIOTIC SIDE EFFECTS

The use of combination antibiotics as empiric therapy provides extended spectrum but carries with it a higher risk of drug-related toxicity than the use of single drug regimens. Since a significant proportion of the patients treated will not have a documented infection, the use of combinations of proven efficacy and at the same time minimal toxicity is of great importance. All antibiotic combinations have some side effects: the use of carbenicillin or ticarcillin as well as the newly developed acylampicillins includes the possibility of penicillin allergy and the development of some degree of hypokalemia which usually requires potassium supplementation, occasionally in the form of large intravenous dosages. Platelet function can be affected by these semisynthetic penicillins, however, the clinical significance of this phenomenon does not appear to be important: despite frequent use in patients with less than 20,000 platelets/μl we have rarely seen excessive bleeding and only in patients who, because of decreased renal function, inadvertently achieve very high serum levels of the antibiotics. Cephalosporins may also produce allergic reactions and although they are given to many patients with a history of penicillin allergy, precautions should be taken in patients with a history of immediate reactions to penicillin since some immunological studies have demonstrated crossreactivity in as many as 20% of such patients. Some degree of hypokalemia has been described in trials in which cephalosporin-containing combinations have been used [26]. The true mechanism of antibiotic-related hypokalemia is still unclear although it is obvious that granulocytopenic cancer patients experience potassium losses from several sources: vomiting or diarrhea secondary to chemotherapy, the use of other antibiotics or the primary disease. This suggests that many patients will be already potassium depleted at the moment that they initiate the antibiotic therapy and are more susceptible to any potassium loss.

Aminoglycosides are well known for their nephrotoxic potential and conflicting data exist concerning differences of the most commonly used of these drugs in their potential for producing renal damage [38, 39]. The combination of an aminoglycoside plus a semisynthethic penicillin, however, has been proven to have minimal toxicity [21, 25] even when the doses of the aminoglycoside have been increased to double the usually recommended doscs in ordcr to achieve therapeutic blood levels throughout the interval between doses. The use of cephalothin combined with an aminoglycoside, on the other hand, has been shown to have an incidence of nephrotoxicity above 15% and among individuals more than 50 years old, incidences as high as 30% have been reported [40]. This has not been the case when other cephalosporins have been used in combination with aminoglycosides. Large antibiotic trials involving patients receiving carbenicillin, amikacin and cefazolin [4] and moxalactam plus amikacin [26] did not show an increase in nephrotoxicity when the patients were compared with the control arms: carbenicillin plus amikacin or cefazolin and ticarcillin plus amikacin, respectively. Furthermore, at our institution we recently reviewed the clinical courses of 57 patients with fever and granulocytopenia treated empirically with cefazolin plus aminoglycosides and found a 3.5% incidence of nephrotoxicity. We are therefore hesitant to use a cephalothin–aminoglycoside combination and when the need exists for a cephalosporin plus an aminoglycoside, we currently recommend the use of cefazolin or the new agent, moxalactam.

Ototoxicity, although it has received less attention, is by no means less important, particularly in a patient population that tends to have repeated episodes of granulocytopenia and the resulting infectious complications, hence requiring multiple courses of therapy with aminoglycoside-containing combinations. In studies cited in the literature, the frequency of ototoxicity associated with aminoglycosides has ranged from 3 to 25%, the variation explained by differences in ototoxicity criteria employed. At the University of Maryland Cancer Center, a group of 89 patients had audiograms performed during and after aminoglycoside therapy, an overall 19% incidence of ototoxicity was found [41, 42], this incidence was higher than 30% when patients with repeated courses of therapy spanned over several months were considered. The hearing loss of high frequency sounds is particularly discouraging for the patient who, to some degree, loses a major route of interaction with those around him. Other antibiotics, used less frequently, have the potential for toxic effects: vancomycin can be nephrotoxic and ototoxic, trimethoprim/sulfamethoxazole can produce allergic reactions and there is controversy concerning its myelosuppressive effect.

12

SUMMARY

Patients with prolonged periods of granulocytopenia are likely to develop infection with colonizing gram-negative bacilli such as *P. aeruginosa, K. pneumoniae* and *E. coli*; and gram-positive cocci such as *S. aureus* and *S. epidermidis*. Fever is a reliable sign of infection in this patient population with impaired inflammatory response; approximately 60% of febrile episodes represent documented infections. The prompt use of empiric therapy with broad spectrum antibiotics, preferentially synergistic, has resulted in reasonable degrees of efficacy with minimal toxicity. A combination of a semisynthetic penicillin such as ticarcillin and an aminoglycoside such as amikacin provides broad antibacterial coverage but other combinations such as ticarcillin plus a cephalosporin or cefazolin plus an aminoglycoside may be adequate in individual institutions.

One of the acylampicillins or the anti-Pseudomonas cephalosporins plus an aminoglycoside have been shown to be appropriate empiric therapy, and a combination of one agent of each of these two groups of beta-lactams may prove to be as efficacious yet less toxic than the currently used regimens. Recovery of the granulocyte count and susceptibility of the pathogen to the antimicrobials used appear to be important prognostic factors. Patients with bacteremia or other severe infections are usually treated for 10 to 14 days; patients with less serious episodes usually require less therapy, but in all circumstances antibiotics should be continued until all evidence of infection has resolved and the patient has remained afebrile for four to five days. No concensus exists for the management of patients with persistent fever and granulocytopenia and no obvious source of infection. Prolonged courses of antibiotics may result in superinfection with resistant bacteria or fungus as well as make evident antibiotic side effects such as hypokalemia, nephrotoxicity and ototoxicity.

REFERENCES

1. Bodey GP, Buckley M, Sathe YS, Freireich EJ: Quantitative relationship between circulating leukocytes and infection in patients with acute leukemia. Ann Intern Med 63:328–40, 1966.
2. Schimpff SC: Therapy of infection in patients with granulocytopenia. Med Clin No Amer 61:1101–1118, 1977.
3. Schimpff SC, Young VM, Greene WH, Vermeullen D, Moody MR, Wiernik PH: Origin of infection in acute nonlymphocytic leukemia: Significance of hospital acquisition of potential pathogens. Ann Intern Med 77:707–714, 1972.
4. EORTC International Antimicrobial Therapy Project Group: Three antibiotic regimens in the treatment of infection in febrile granulocytopenic patients with cancer. J Inf Dis 137: 14–29, 1978.

5. Wade JC, Schimpff SC, Newman KA, Wiernik PH: *Staphylococcus epidermidis*: an increasing cause of infection in granulocytopenic patients. Ann Intern Med (in press).
6. Remington JS, Schimpff SC: Please don't eat the salads. N Engl J Med 304:433–35, 1981.
7. Albert RK, Condie F: Handwashing patterns in medical intensive care units. N Engl J Med 304:1465–66, 1981.
8. Newman KA, Schimpff SC, Young VM, Wiernik PH: Lessons learned from surveillance cultures in patients with acute nonlymphocytic leukemia: usefulness for epidemiologic, preventive and therapeutic research. Am J Med 70:423–31, 1981.
9. Schimpff SC, Satterlee W, Young VM, Serpick AA: Empiric therapy with carbenicillin and gentamicin for febrile patients with cancer and granulocytopenia. N Engl J Med 284:1061–65, 1971.
10. Klastersky J, Cappel R, Daneau D: Therapy with carbenicillin and gentamicin for patients with cancer and severe infection caused by gram-negative rods. Cancer 31:331–6, 1973.
11. Rodriguez V, Bodey GP, Horikoshi N, Inagaki J, McCredie KB: Ticarcillin therapy of infections. *Antimicrob Ag Chemother* 4:427–31, 1973.
12. Wade JC, Schimpff SC, Newman KA, Fortner CL, Moody MR, Young VM, Wiernik PH: Potential of mezlocillin as empiric single agent therapy in febrile granulocytopenic cancer patients. Antimicrob Ag Chemother 18:299–306, 1980.
13. Bodey GP, Middleman E, Umsawadi T, Rodriguez V: Infections in cancer patients: results with gentamicin sulfate therapy. Cancer 29:1697–1701, 1972.
14. Young LS: Gentamicin: clinical use with carbenicillin and in vitro studies with recent isolates of *Pseudomonas aeruginosa*. J Inf Dis 124(Suppl.):202–206, 1971.
15. Valdivieso M, Horikoshi N, Rodriguez V, Bodey GP: Therapeutic trials with tobramycin. Am J Med Sci 63:548–555, 1977.
16. Love LJ, Schimpff SC, Schiffer CA, Wiernik PH: Improved prognosis for granulocytopenic patients with gram-negative bacteremia. Am J Med 68:643–648, 1980.
17. Klastersky J, Cappel R, Daneau D: Clinical significance of in vitro synergism between antibiotics in gram-negative infections. Antimicrob Ag Chemother 2:470–475, 1972.
18. Anderson ET, Young LS, Hewitt WL: Antimicrobial synergism in the therapy of gram-negative rod bacteremia. Chemotherapy 24:45–54, 1978.
19. Lau WK, Young LS, Black RE, Winston DJ, Linne SR, Weinstein, RJ, Hewitt WL: Comparative efficacy and toxicity of amikacin-carbenicillin versus gentamicin-carbenicillin in leukopenic patients. A randomized prospective trial. Am J Med 62:959–966, 1977.
20. Klastersky J, Cappel R, Swings CT, Vanderborre L: Bacteriological and clinical activity of the ampicillin-gentamicin and cephalothin-gentamicin combinations. Am J Med Sci 262:283–90, 1971.
21. Love LJ, Schimpff SC, Hahn DM, Young VM, Standiford HC, Bender JF, Fortner CL, Wiernik PH: Randomized trial of empiric antibiotic therapy with ticarcillin in combination with gentamicin, amikacin or netilmicin in febrile patients with granulocytopenia and cancer. Am J Med 66:603–610, 1979.
22. Feld R, Valdivieso M, Bodey GP, Rodriguez V: Comparison of amikacin and tobramycin in the treatment of infections in patients with cancer. J Inf Dis 135:61–66, 1977.
23. Parry MF, Neu HC: A comparative study of ticarcillin plus tobramycin versus carbenicillin plus gentamicin for the treatment of serious infections due to gram-negative bacilli. Am J Med 64:961–966, 1978.
24. Sotman SB, Schimpff SC, Young VM: *Staphylococcus aureus* bacteremia in patients with acute leukemia. Am J Med 69:814–8188, 1980.
25. Wade JC, Schimpff SC, Newman KA, Fortner CL, Standiford HC, Wiernik PH: Piperacillin or ticarcillin plus amikacin: a double blind prospective comparison of empiric antibiotic

14

therapy for febrile granulocytopenic cancer patients. Am J Med 71:983–990, 1981.

26. De Jongh CA, Wade JC, Schimpff SC, Newman KA, Finley RS, Salvatore PC, Moody MR, Standiford HC, Fortner CL, Wiernik PH: Empiric antibiotic therapy for suspected infection in granulocytopenic cancer patients: a comparison between the combination of moxalactam plus amikacin and ticarcillin plus amikacin. Am J Med 73:89-96, 1982.

27. Klastersky J, Henri A, Hensgens C, Daneau D: Gram-negative infection in cancer: study of empiric therapy comparing carbenicillin-cephalothin with and without gentamicin. JAMA 227:45-48, 1974.

28. Kuch NA, Testa RT, Forbes M: In vitro and in vivo antibacterial effects of combinations of beta-lactam antibiotics. Antimicrob Ag Chemother 19:634–638, 1981.

29. Stuart RK, Braine HG, Saral R, Leitman PS, Feiller DJ: Carbenicillin-trimethoprim/sulfamethoxazole versus carbenicillin-gentamicin as empiric therapy of infection in granulocytopenic patients: a perspective, randomized, double blind study. Am J Med 68:876–885, 1980.

30. Keating MJ, Lawson R, Grose W, Bodey GP: Combination therapy with ticarcillin and sulfamethoxazole-trimethoprim for infections in patients with cancer. Arch Intern Med 141:926–932, 1981.

31. EORTC International Antimicrobial Therapy Project Group: Empiric antibiotic therapy in febrile granulocytopenic patients. In: Topics in Paediatrics I. Hematology and Oncology, Morris-Jones PH (ed). Pitman Medical, Kent, England, 1979, pp 113–124.

32. Schimpff SC, Aisner J: Empiric antibiotic therapy. Cancer Treat Rep 62:673–680, 1978.

33. Greene WH, Schimpff SC, Young VM: Empiric carbenicillin, gentamicin and cephalothin therapy for presumed infection in patients with granulocytopenia and cancer. Ann Intern Med 78:825, 1973.

34. Klastersky J, Hensgens C, Debusscher L: Empiric therapy for cancer patients: comparative study of ticarcillin-tobramycin, ticarcillin-cephalothin and cephalothin-tobramycin. Antimicrob Ag Chemother 7:640–645, 1975.

35. Rodriguez V, Burgess M, Bodey GP: Management of fever of unknown origin in patients with neoplasia and neutropenia. Cancer 32:1007–1012, 1973.

36. Pizzo PA, Robichaud KJ, Gill FA, Whitebsky FG: Empiric antibiotic and antifungal therapy for cancer patients with prolonged fever and granulocytopenia. Am J Med 72:101–111, 1982.

37. Klastersky J, Schimpff SC, Gaya H, Glauser M, Tattersall MHN, Zinner S, Weerts D, Buyse M, Masesa G, Hoffnen G, Porcellini A, and the EORTC Antimicrobial Therapy Project Group: A cooperative investigation of a rational management of granulocytopenic febrile cancer patients. Abstract C-259 in Proceedings of the 18th Annual Meeting of the American Society of Clinical Oncology, St. Louis, Missouri, 1982.

38. Smith CR, Baughman KL, Edwards CQ, Rogers JF, Lietman PS: Controlled comparison of amikacin and gentamicin. N Engl J Med 296:349–353, 1977.

39. Smith CR, Lipsky JJ, Laskin OL, Hellman DB, Mellitis ED, Longstreth J, Leitman PS: Double blind comparison of the nephrotoxicity and auditory toxicity of gentamicin and tobramycin. N Engl J Med 302:1106-1109, 1980.

40. Wade JC, Schimpff SC, Wiernik PH: Aminoglycoside-cephalosporin associated nephrotoxicity. Arch Intern Med 141:1789–1796, 1982.

41. Danhauer FJ, Fortner CL, Schimpff SC, De Jongh CA, Wesley MN, Wiernik PH: Ototoxicity in granulocytopenic cancer patients associated with pharmacokinetically dosed amikacin. (Submitted).

42. De Jongh C, Joshi J, Newman K, Danhauer F, Finley R, Moody M, Wiernik P, Schimpff S: Moxalactam plus piperacillin or amikacin: empiric antibiotic therapy for febrile granulocytopenic cancer patients. (Submitted).

2. Fungal Infections in the Immunocompromised Host

CORSTIAAN BRASS

INTRODUCTION

The awareness of fungal infections and their impact on the morbidity and mortality of patients with neoplastic disease dates back to studies in the late 1940s and 1950s [1–3]. Prior to 1945, the reports of fungal infections were rare [1]. The advent of chemotherapeutic drugs and the use of combination radiotherapy/chemotherapy for neoplastic diseases (especially the hematologic malignancies) resulted in an increase in the incidence of a variety of infections [5–7], but with the development of newer antibiotics and the use of empiric antibiotic therapy, mortality as a result of bacterial infections has been substantially reduced [8–10]. However, with more intensive chemotherapy for diseases such as leukemia, the protracted period of post therapy host-defense failure has been associated with an increase in secondary infections, of which the fungal infections are the most notable.

THE EPIDEMIOLOGY OF FUNGAL INFECTIONS

In 1947, Farber did not describe fungal infections in his retrospective review of untreated leukemic patients [4]. Since then, an incremental increase of fungal infections has been described [11–13]. Stefanini and Allegra [13] demonstrated an increase of fungal infection from the period of 1943–47 (9%) to 1948-1949 (14%) and a further increase to 22% was seen from 1954 to 1956. This was confirmed by Hutter and Collins [14] and also documented at the NCI, where the incidence of invasive fungal disease was 11% in the period from 1954–58 and 31% during the period 1959–64 [15]. The incidence of fungal infections has also been demonstrated by a number

Higby, DJ (ed), Supportive Care in Cancer Therapy. ISBN 0-89838-569-5.
© *1983, Martinus Nijhoff Publishers, Boston. Printed in The Netherlands.*

of studies based on post-mortem examination. The rates of fungal infections in these series range from 13% to 69% [16–20].

From ante-mortem studies, the incidence of fungal infection appears to be lower (0–25 of patients) [21–23]. A review of the experience at Roswell Park (1977–1980) with one leukemia protocol demonstrated fungal infections occurring in 25 of 78 patients (41%). Most of these patients were undergoing their first remission induction attempt. In 8 of these patients, the diagnosis was made only at post-mortem. Singer et al. demonstrated a similar experience in that 52% of the patients with documented bacteremia who were autopsied had fungal infections but only 45% of these were diagnosed ante-mortem [24]. The subpopulation of patients who have demonstrated the highest incidence of fungal infections have been the patients with hematologic malignancies, however there is evidence that an increase in frequency of fungal infections in the patients with solid tumors is also occurring [25]. Unfortunately, most of the above studies used patients at different stages of their disease, with varying (if not imprecise) definitions of fungal infection and patients with different neoplastic disorders. In addition, the studies in the literature tended to use either clinical diagnosis of mycosis or post-mortem diagnosis to estimate the incidence of fungal disease.

The most common fungus isolated is Candida species, of which *C. albicans* is the most frequent isolate. Aspergillus and Mucor are seen in 16–32% of patients with documented fungal infection and most commonly in patients with leukemia. Cryptococcal disease, especially meningitis, is also seen. Unusual causes of fungal infection include *Pseudopetrillidium boydii*, Blastomycosis, and, more recently, Trichosporon species.

ANTIFUNGAL AGENTS

Amphotericin B (AmB)

Amphotericin B is a polyene macrolide antibiotic produced by *Streptomyces nodosis* [26]. Analysis of the structure/activity relationships of amphotericin B have demonstrated the importance of the polyene structure and its antifungal activity [27]. It has also been shown that while the major impact of amphotericin B is the alteration of the membrane structure by direct binding [28, 29], irreversible inhibition of chitin synthetase occurs [30] which may augment the membrane effect of amphotericin B.

The in vitro activity of this drug has been demonstrated for a wide variety of fungi with the notable exception of *Pseudopetrillidium boydii*. The M.I.C. range from 0.1 to 15 µg/ml [31, 32]. At present, the relationship of M.I.C. to clinical outcome is unknown. It has been demonstrated that the M.I.C. determinations for amphotericin B are not inoculum-dependent, nor are they time-dependent (in contrast to the imidazole compounds) [33, 34]. The M.I.C.s, however, are temperature-dependent.

The pharmacology of amphotericin B is not completely understood. Oral absorption is poor, but intravenous infusion of doses of 0.65 mg/kg result in peak concentrations of 1.5–2.0 µg/ml [35]. The terminal half-life $(t_{\frac{1}{2}})$ is 14 days, but the initial $t_{\frac{1}{2}}$ is 24–48 hours [36]. It is 90% bound to serum proteins [37] and the volume of distribution is 4 l/kg. Less than 10% of the drug is excreted via the kidney. Amphotericin B does not require protection from light, as inactivation by light is of little consequence [38]. From the pharmacokinetic data available, it is evident that the peak concentrations achieved using 0.6 mg/kg are not significantly different from the concentrations demonstrated for 1 mg/kg, whereas the incidence of nephrotoxicity is substantially increased. Thus, the daily dose of amphotericin seldom need exceed 0.7 mg/kg. The use of alternate day therapy provides some increased patient comfort, but does not appreciably change the pharmacokinetics of the drug nor the peak concentrations. Rapid escalation to 0.3 mg/kg can be undertaken in the presence of life-threatening illness.

The major toxic side effects seen with amphotericin include chills, fever, phlebitis, headache, anemia [39], anorexia, and abnormal renal function. This may manifest as potassium-wasting nephropathy [40], distal tubular acidosis [41], and decreased glomerular filtration [42–44]. Amphotericin B has been demonstrated to result in vacuole formation in arteriolar walls and it has been demonstrated to have vascular constrictive properties [45]. Tubular damage has been associated with focal calcification [46]. Recently, the use of dopamine and saralasin has reversed the acute vasoconstrictive phenomena seen in dogs after amphotericin therapy [47]. The role of vasoconstriction in the pathogenesis of renal damage secondary to amphotericin in man and its reversibility remains to be determined.

Attempts to reduce the incidence and severity of renal damage in man have included the administration of mannitol or bicarbonate [41, 45]. The administration of mannitol resulted in a more uniform decrease in renal function, but in no way protected the patient from the onset of renal damage; nor did it diminish the extent of damage. The use of bicarbonate has not been extensively evaluated, but its utility appears doubtful.

For a large number of fungal infections amphotericin B remains the drug of choice; however, there is only limited clinical data to document the dosages required in patients with compromised host defenses.

Miconazole

Miconazole is a synthetic imidazole which was developed in the early 1970s. It was demonstrated to inhibit d-methylation at the C-14 position of ergosterol precursors [48–50]. This secondarily results in permeability changes due to the inhibition of incorporation of the required steroids into the cell wall. There is also evidence that miconazole may also bind to sterol groups resulting in altered permeability characteristics [51].

The in vitro spectrum of activity includes most yeasts, the dimorphic fungi, and dermatophyte species [52]. However, members of the Rhizopus, Mucor, and Aspergillus species demonstrate resistance in vitro. *Pseudope-trillidium boydii* is sensitive to miconazole [53]. Miconazole is poorly absorbed from the gastrointestinal tract [52] (less than 20% of administered dose) and is primarily given as an intravenous preparation. It requires a camphor base for solution. Protein binding of this drug is on the order of 90% and peak concentrations of the drug after a 500 mg dose range from 2–9 μg/ml [52]. Miconazole can penetrate into infected joints, peritoneal fluid, vitreous humor, and to a lesser extent, cerebrospinal fluid [54, 55]. Terminal half-life is about 20–25 hours [56]. However, miconazole can be given every eight hours (at doses of 10 mg/kg) without evidence of significant accumulation. There is no change in the distribution or elimination half-life in the presence of renal failure.

A wide variety of side effects have been reported including phlebitis (28%), pruritis (21%), nausea (18%), fever and chills (11%), rashes, diarrhea, drowsiness, hyperlipidemia, thrombocytosis, leukopenia, hyponatremia, and rarely, anaphylactoid reactions [52]. The incidence of hyponatremia was especially high in the series reported by Stevens [57]. This was tentatively linked to inappropriate antidiuretic hormone (ADH) secretion, as well as the administration of large quantities of free water used for infusion of miconazole.

Hypertriglyceridemia, anemia [58], thrombocytosis, and rouleau formation in the peripheral blood smears are common occurrences. Miconazole has also been demonstrated to enhance the activity of warfarin [55]. Acute psychotic reactions and, in rare instances, seizures have been noted with this drug. There is no evidence of hepatic or renal damage with this drug.

Therapeutic efficacy. Unfortunately, all the clinical data obtained for the use of miconazole has been in the form of ancedotal reports or open-ended noncomparative trials. Many of the patients entered had failed amphotericin B therapy. The quality of reporting varies considerably in the definition of patient population, diagnosis of disease, and criteria for response. Patient follow-up is also not consistent. For these reasons, comments as to the utility of this drug and its place relative to amphotericin B in the therapeutic arsenal must remain tentative.

Ketoconazole
Ketoconazole is also an imidazole derivative with a substitution (pipera-

zine moiety) which resulted in solubility of the compound in an acid aqueous solution allowing for oral absorption.

The mechanism of action and spectrum of activity is similar to miconazole, but *Pseudopetrillidium boydii* does not appear to be sensitive in vitro [59, 60].

The pharmacokinetics of this drug have not been well defined, but preliminary data [61] suggests that oral absorption requires the presence of gastric acid production. Absorption is substantially reduced in the presence of cimetidine. Administration with meals does not impair absorption substantially [61]. There is an apparent first pass effect which is seen at the lower doses of ketoconazole (200 mg or less) [61]. The protein binding of ketoconazole is 90% and the drug has been demonstrated in infected soft tissue, joint fluid, saliva, and cerebrospinal fluid (CSF) [61]. There is no change in distribution or elimination half-life in the presence of renal failure [61]. The presence of hepatic dysfunction may appreciably alter the elimination of ketoconazole. Only 15% of the active drug is excreted in the urine.

Side effects include nausea and vomiting (3%), pruritis, somnolence, dizziness, SGOT abnormalities, hepatitis, and headache (less than 1%) [62]. Gynecomastia has also been reported [63]. Severe hepatic toxicity has been occasionally seen [64]. There is no interaction with warfarin [61]. The use of cytochrome P450 enzyme inducers (e.g., rifampicin) may alter the disposition of ketoconazole [61].

FUNGAL DISEASE IN MAN

Candidiasis

I. Epidemiology. Candida albicans is an obligate commensal of humans and animals and not an environmental contaminant [66]. It is commonly isolated from the gastro-intestinal tract, mouth, and vagina [67, 68]. It is rarely isolated from the skin of individuals under 60 or from the blood, urine, or bronchial secretions of normal individuals [68]. Colonization of the skin is greater in incidence in older individuals and the hospitalized patient [69, 70]. Colonization of the bladder or other body sites is often facilitated by the presence of indwelling appliances. Other species of Candida (specifically *C. tropicalis* and *C. parapsilosis*) can live in water as well as soil [71]. Unlike *C. albicans* infection, acquisition of these fungi may thus be from exogenous sources as well. Person to person transmission has yet to be demonstrated except in the case of Candida balanitis.

II. Clinical manifestations. Invasive candidiasis can manifest as a local infection of one of the mucosal surfaces, invasion into the bloodstream, or dissemination into one or more organs. Oral thrush is usually a superfical infection [72], however, it has the capacity for invasion of tissue and blood vessels [72, 73]. Thus, these lesions may be a source of further dissemination.

The involvement of the gastrointestinal tract is 100% in patients with leukemia who have evidence of disseminated candidiasis at autopsy [74], but only 27% of patients who had autopsy evidence of gastrointestinal invasive disease demonstrated disseminated disease at autopsy [75]. Gastrointestinal involvement may involve any part of the gastointestinal tract, but one of the more common sites is the esophagus [76–79]. The most common symptom is dysphagia, often associated with retrosternal pain or burning and a feeling of fullness in the neck. Occasional patients are asymptomatic. Barium swallow is useful at best in only 50% of cases [80]. The findings can be confused with herpetic esophagitis [81]. In one series, barium swallow did not identify any esophagitis [82]. Furthermore, since 30% of esophagitis seen in this patient population is a result of herpetic infection [83] and cannot be distinguished on barium swallow from candidal infection, esophagoscopy is the diagnostic procedure of choice. Invasion of the stomach and small intestine is not uncommon and may present as an ulcerating lesion or pseudo-membrane formation [84]. Penetrating ulcers and perforation have also been demonstrated.

Pulmonary candidiasis is most often a result of hematogenous spread rather than from a primary inoculation of lung tissue [85, 86]. The latter situation has been documented only rarely [87]. One study attempted to distinguish aspiration from hematogenous spread [85]; however, the criteria were imprecise and the study was done retrospectively, so that there was no standardization for estimation of involvement of the lung nor regarding sampling methodology. In addition, many of the patients had other complicating pulmonary pathology, such that it was determined that only 3 of 30 patients had significant involvement of the lung by candida. Pulmonary involvement is therefore unusual in the compromised host. When it occurs, the radiologic manifestations are indistinguishable from other etiologic agents [88]. Fine nodular infiltrates are occasionally seen [85].

Urinary tract candidiasis is most often seen in diabetics but can be seen in the compromised host [89]. The species most frequently associated with infections arising from the urinary tract is *C. tropicalis* [90]. *C. albicans* can be isolated from the urine if hematogenous spread of the infection involves the kidney parenchyma [91]. Retrograde spread of infection occurs but is uncommon. Cystitis due to Candida may occur after prolonged Foley catheter use [92].

Catheter-related candidemia (*C. albicans* and *C. glabrata*) occurs in up to 20% of patients who are on hyperalimentation for long periods of time [93–95].

Disseminated candidiasis (involvement of more than one organ) can be demonstrated in up to 87% of infected patients who are autopsied [96, 97]. The frequency with which disseminated infection is demonstrated depends on the ability of the pathologist to define the extent of disease as well as the characteristics of the patient population and geographic locale in which the survey is carried out. Detection of disseminated candidiasis ante-mortem ranges from 15–40% [99, 100]. The most common sites for dissemination include the kidney, brain, myocardium, and the eye. Endo-opthalmitis can be seen in up to 9.9% of patients who are on hyperalimentation for more than 3 weeks [101, 102]. The characteristic finding on examination is the presence of a focal, white lesion that demonstrates invasion onto the retinal surface and into the vitreous. This lesion may be covered with a pre-retinal haze [103]. Involvement of liver and spleen with no other overt involvement has been demonstrated in up to 67% of patients and the physical signs and laboratory parameter abnormalities may be very subtle [107, 108]. Involvement of the meninges is quite variable ranging from 5–75% of autopsied cases [103–106]. There are no distinguishing characteristics of the CSF, except for the positivity of the CSF for candidal organisms in approximately 40% of cases [95]. Nodular erythematous lesions of the skin are seen almost exclusively in leukemic patients and are of significance since biopsy will allow the diagnosis to be made within 24 hours of obtaining the specimen instead of waiting for growth of the organism on the culture plate [109–110].

III. Diagnosis. The diagnosis of candidal infection hinges on the demonstration of tissue invasion by the organism on histology or isolation from a site that is highly unlikely to be contaminated.

Ante-mortem blood cultures in patients with disseminated candidiasis have been negative in 62–100% of cases reviewed [15, 18, 74, 111]. Cultures from the urine are only of significance if obtained from a non-catheterized patient [112]. There is no way to distinguish colonization from invasion unless the blood cultures are positive for the identical fungus. Sputum and bronchial washing cultures are useless in the diagnosis of pulmonary candidiasis [112, 113]. There is no way to distinguish colonization from invasion unless the blood cultures are positive for the identical fungus. Sputum and bronchial washing cultures are useless in the diagnosis of pulmonary candidiasis [112, 113]. The only acceptable diagnostic test for pulmonary candidiasis is open lung biopsy and demonstration of tissue invasion. The utility of surveillance cultures has been demonstrated [114]. Sandford et al. [114] demonstrated that surveillance cultures from stool or urine that were positive on two consecutive occasions had a predictive value of 83%, whereas negative cultures from all sites had a predictive value of 100% in ruling out candidal disease.

The isolation of Candida from the blood must be considered to be indicative of possible candidal infection but it should be noted that in one series reviewing positive blood cultures in patients with hematologic malignancies, 23% of 48 patients had transient benign candidemia, of which 72% were catheter-related infections [111].

It is clear that the demonstration of Candida by culture will not identify a substantial proportion of patients with invasive or disseminated disease. Several serologic tests have been investigated in an effort to improve the detection ante-mortem [115–125]. There are several problems in the evaluation of these results. These include: 1) differing composition of the antigen preparation; 2) differing source of antigen and antigen preparation; 3) observer variability; 4) definition of endpoint (especially with the agglutinating antibody); and 5) criteria for endpoint determination. These tests are further complicated by the fact that different populations of patients were studied at either unspecified time intervals or were not critically evaluated for contributing demographic characteristics. Furthermore, the definition of invasive candidiasis differs not only from paper to paper but also within certain studies. The major serologic markers that have been utilized include the agglutinating titer, precipitin titer, complement fixation titer, and immunofluorescent antibody test. There have been a number of recent reports using variations of the precipitin and agglutinin titer-counter-immunoelectrophoresis and double diffusion [126, 127]. A critique of the entire literature is beyond the scope of this chapter, but can be summarized. The complement fixation test, the immunofluorescent antibody test, and the agglutinin titer are all associated with a high rate of false positivity. Using a rise in agglutinin titer, there is still a rate of false positivity that is twice that of the precipitin test. Although some authors [115, 116] claim that the agglutinin test is more reliable, a calculation of the predictive value of the precipitin test and the agglutinin test from these papers (using the documented incidence of fungal disease in the study of 9%) demonstrates that the precipitin test is more sensitive than the agglutinin (predictive value of agglutinin test in the population at risk = 0.43; predictive value of precipitin test in population at risk = 0.55). Review of the experience with agglutinin and precipitin titers in the leukemia population demonstrates quite a variable predictive value, with the highest value being 60% [115, 116, 128, 129]. Newer variations of the antibody detection methods have demonstrated similar positivity rates, but none of these has been tested on significant number of patients to demonstrate their overall utility. Of the antibody tests available, the only one that demonstrates an acceptable rate of false positivity is the precipitin test. It is useful as an adjunct in the diagnosis of invasive candidiasis in surgical patients and those patients without hematologic malignancies (predictive value = 90%) [130]. There is no data that defines the use of this test in the therapeutic decision-making process regarding patients who are known to be at high risk for candidal infection.

The continued failure of serologic and mycologic methods to adequately identify the patient population with disease (especially in the hematologic malignancies) resulted in the search for antigens present in body fluids that might allow for earlier detection of invasive candidal disease. These methods have included detection and quantitation of mannan antigenemia by radioimmune assays [132] and the enzyme-linked immuno-absorbant assay [131, 133, 134]; detection of lipid and other components by gas-liquid chromatography [138–141]; and the detection and quantitation of arabinotol using high pressure liquid chromatography [135–137]. To date only selected populations have been studied using these methods, and although these methods appear promising, larger series of patients are required before the utility of these tests can be defined.

IV. Therapy. There are two major decisions that confront the clinician dealing with the possibility of candidal infection in the immunocompromized host: 1) indications for therapy, and 2) choice of therapy.

The indications for therapy can be stratified into two categories: indications for the neutropenic patient and indications for non-neutropenic patients. Indications for therapy in the neutropenic host include persistent fever in the face of seven to ten days of broad spectrum antibacterial chemotherapy, positive blood cultures regardless of site, candidal retinitis, isolation of Candida from any sterile site, greater than 100 colonies of Candida from a mid-stream urine in the absence of a urinary catheter, and the demonstration of esophageal candidal involvement. Those individuals with extensive oropharyngeal involvement are also treated. It is recognized that a portion of patients have transient candidemia which may be catheter-related, but since no reliable criteria are evident to discern those who will resolve spontaneously from those who will disseminate, treatment is recommended for all. It should be noted that in individuals who have recently completed courses of antibiotic therapy (within 14 days of initiation of the next round of chemotherapy) and who are then exposed to further chemotherapy (either as further antileukemic therapy or for conditioning for bone marrow transplantation), the time to onset of overt fungal disease may be much shorter [142, 143]. The empiric use of amphotericin may be considered in such patients if the clinical condition deteriorates after 72 hours of appropriate empiric, broad spectrum antibacterial chemotherapy.

The indications for therapy in non-neutropenic individuals is similar to that for neutropenic hosts. However, the need to treat empirically in the absence of an isolate or site of infection is unusual. In addition, candidemia need not be treated unless any or more of the following criteria are met: 1) continued positive cultures 48 hours after extraction of an indwelling intravenous catheter; 2) clinical deterioration; 3) evidence of visceral dissemination; 4) no indwelling venous catheter at the time of fungemia; and 5) precipitin titer of greater than 1/16.

The therapy of choice for candidal infection had been amphotericin B. This was based primarily on the experience with this drug in the treatment of candidiasis in other settings and ancedotal reports of its efficacy in patients with malignancies [144-151]. The literature, however, contains scant data to address this issue in the neutropenic host, and what data is available suggests that recovery of marrow function is the major determinant of adequate response in the leukemia patient. One recent report is illustrative [152]; of 21 patients with candidemia and neutropenia, one responded to amphotericin B. The experience of Roswell is not dissimilar; 3 of 7 patients with documented candidal disease responded (2 of which had only oral infection). This may be a result of a number of factors: 1) late intervention with anti-fungal therapy; 2) initiation of therapy in patients whose probability surviving an adequate course of amphotericin B are remote; and 3) failure of normal bone marrow to recover.

The use of adjunctive therapy, such as rifampicin or 5-flucytosine (5-FC), has been advocated [95, 157], but there is no clinical data that suggests that it is superior to amphotericin B alone. The data supporting these combinations arise from animal experiments and in vitro data [153-157]. There is no need to use 5-FC or rifampicin while waiting for amphotericin to be escalated, since amphotericin B can be escalated to therapeutic doses within 48 hours of the test dose.

The duration of therapy is a matter of considerable debate. Suggestions for low dose therapy, arbitrary limits of 1-2 gm of amphotericin B, and tailoring therapy to either AmB serum levels or clinical and/or mycologic cure have been made by various authors [148, 158-162]. None of these suggestions has been shown to be of utility in any substantial number of patients, and no data exists as to the optimal daily dose, duration of therapy, or total dose required to ensure success. The following general guidelines are offered.

1. For individuals that have evidence of disseminated disease or sustained candidemia in the absence of venous catheters, amphotericin B should be given to a total dose of 1.5-2.0 gm or until resolution of all observable clinical abnormalities and laboratory values for 14 days. For those indi-

viduals with concomitant neutropenia at the onset of therapy, duration of therapy should be continued until the PMN count remains over 1000/mm^3 for 7 days.

2. For individuals with esophagitis and oropharyngeal involvement, therapy should be continued until the lesions are completely healed and the PMN count is greater than 1000/mm^3 for 5 days.

3. For individuals with suspected but not proven disease, duration of therapy should be maintained until resolution of fever and/or the PMN count is greater than 1000/mm^3 for 5 days. Those individuals still febrile after the PMN count is greater than 1000/mm^3 should be thoroughly re-evaluated for an occult focus of infection.

Alternative anti-mycotic agents have been developed and their utility has been the subject of case reports and one significant open study [163–171]. The article by Heel et al. [172], describes results with miconazole in 58 patients with various manifestations of fungal infection who had leukemia or lymphoma. Some of these patients are not easily identifiable as to the nature or extent of response to antimycotic therapy. The reported responses range from 59–71%. In the one series by Jordan et al. [173], a response rate of 41% was demonstrated. It should be noted that the majority of responses were in patients with blood culture positivity alone. The experience at Roswell is similar to that in the published literature, in that the majority of responses were seen in individuals who had oral or esophageal disease (6/12 patients). The response in disseminated disease was disappointing (1/4 patients).

The newest anti-mycotic to reach the marketplace is ketoconazole. This compound has been tried on a very limited basis in leukemic and lymphoma patients. In our experience, ketoconazole has produced response in esophageal disease, candidemia with and without dissemination, and oropharyngeal infection. A number of these individuals had progressed after receiving AmB. or miconazole. We are currently conducting a randomized trial of AmB versus ketoconazole in the therapy of documented candidiasis in neutropenic leukemia and bone marrow transplant patients. We hope this will provide a response rate for both AmB and ketoconazole in a similar patient population and allow for comparison of the relative efficacy and toxicity of each.

Aspergillosis

I. Epidemiology. Aspergillus is a ubiquitous organism that is found in the air of most hospitals and can be demonstrated in certain building materials, pasta products, and the feces of pigeons [174–176]. The most common portal of entry is the respiratory tract, although the gastrointestinal tract may also be the site of invasion in a proportion of patients [177]. The nasopharynx is another site for infection and invasion. A few studies have demonstrated the contamination of hospital air by Aspergillus and have shown that the use of a high efficiency air filtration system can reduce or eliminate aspergillosis in patients so protected [23, 178].

II. Clinical manifestations. The lung is the most common site of infection; 90% of documented cases have lung lesions [177, 179–181]. Clinical manifestation may range from acute progressive dyspnea and cough to hemoptysis. Pulmonary infarction is not uncommon, but nodular formation and cavitation are usually seen only in the presence of a recovering peripheral white count [182]. Radiologic examination can give variable results ranging from within normal limits to an interstitial process or a mass-like density that crosses fissure lines [183, 196]. Histologically, Aspergillus is a septate hyphal form with acute branching. Vascular invasion is common. On some series, aspergillus may accompany other pulmonary infections frequently (74%). Dissemination occurs in 20–50% of cases [18, 177, 195], of which the commonest site is the brain (60–70%) [18, 184, 193]. Gastrointestinal involvement and invasion of the liver, myocardium, and kidney are also seen [177, 184, 185, 186, 193]. In one series the incidence of gastrointestinal involvement was substantial [177]. Incidence of aspergillosis ranges from 0–5% to 35% of fungal disease identified at autopsy [11, 17, 18]. Combined infections with Candida and Aspergillus are not uncommon [177].

III. Diagnosis. Cultures of body fluids or secretions are of limited value in the diagnosis of aspergillosis and thus, a negative culture does not rule out the disease. Culture positivity from any site ante-mortem ranges from 0–34% [15, 18, 177, 194]. Post-mortem cultures may also be negative in 30–58% of cases [180, 187, 193]. Because of the rarity of aspergillus isolation, any isolate from sputum, urine, throat or skin should be considered presumptive evidence for Aspergillus. Isolation from blood has on occasion been associated with false positivity [187], but in the face of clinical signs, should be considered presumptive evidence of infection.

Serologic testing has been used in an effort to increase the identification of patients with aspergillosis. Studies using precipitin tests have reached variable conclusions [188–191]. In one series the detection rate was 6 of 14 [190] and in the other, the rate of detection was 13/55 [91]. In the latter study the diagnosis allowed for some overlap between invasive aspergillosis and non-invasive disease.

Aspergillus antigen detection has been demonstrated in animal models. The rate of detection is similar to that seen for antibodies in human infections [192].

IV. Therapy. This organism shows variable sensitivity in vitro to amphotericin B [197, 198]. It appears resistant in vitro to ketoconazole and miconazole [2, 8]. The therapeutic efficacy of AmB alone [15, 177] or with the addition of 5-FC has not been very encouraging [199, 200]. If involvement of the brain is demonstrated, AmB will be useful only in conjunction with surgical removal of the lesion in the brain. At best, AmB alone will only halt the progression of the lesions, but containment in the neutropenic host requires the recovery of the bone marrow [194–195]. Since only 10% of normal patients [200] demonstrate spontaneous lysis of fungus balls, residual lesions in immunocompromised hosts should be excised if they can be demonstrated to be in one localized area or if only a single lesion exists. When aggressive chemotherapy and surgical excision are attempted, cure can occasionally be demonstrated. One encouraging development is the demonstration of the efficacy of amphotericin B and rifampicin in three ancedotal cases [202–204]. This synergy is also demonstrated by in vitro experiments as well as limited animal studies [207, 208].

Duration of therapy is arbitrary, but has been as long as one year [112]. The most reliable endpoint for therapy is the resolution of all clinical and biochemical evidence of disease. The excision of remaining lesions may be advantageous, either because of slowly progressive increase of lesions or failure to resolve the radiologic abnormality. Since most cancer patients require aggressive chemotherapy to maintain remission, the presence of residual lesions and the resulting possibility of reactivation is a real problem. In those individuals in which it is possible, we have found that excision of lesions in conjunction with 2–3 gm of amphotericin B and rifampicin 600–900 mg per day can reduce the incidence of recurrence as evidenced by clinical and radiologic parameters as well as failure to demonstrate residual disease at autopsy [205.].

Miconazole and ketoconazole have been used in a few cases of aspergillosis [172, 206] with reports of some success. In view of demonstrated in vitro resistance, however, these antifungals should be used only when there is progression of unresectable invasive disease that has been treated with at least 1–2 gm total dose of AmB and rifampicin.

Mucormyocosis

I. Epidemiology. Mucor represents 4–29% of all fungal infections in patients with neoplastic disease [209–211]. In our institution, we see 2–3 cases of mucor per year. The incidence in one series of leukemia patients was 4%. The mode of entry is thought to be by inhalation, since the spores of this organism are demonstrable in ambient air [212, 213]. Another mode of entry may be the gastrointestinal tract [214]. This is becoming a more frequent site for invasion in the patients with lymphoma and leuke-mia [209].

II. Clinical manifestations. The usual site (50–80% of cases) for infection in the patient with malignancy is the lung [214, 216, 218, 219]. The next most frequent site for infection is the brain (30–35% of cases) [221]. Rhinocere-bral involvement in those patients occured but was unusual. Meyer et al. demonstrated rhinocerebral presentation in 4/9 cases with cerebral involve-ment [209]. All the patients had leukemia.

Clinical manifestations included peri-orbital cellulitis, sinus tenderness, palatal ulceration and gangrene. Respiratory distress, cough, hemoptysis and clinical signs of pneumonia are common. Pulmonary infarction may be seen. Chest X-rays are variable in appearance and do not have pathogno-monic features. Cavitating lesions may be larger than those seen in Asper-gillus and progression may be more rapid [215]. Gastrointestinal involve-ment may be manifest by abdominal pain or evidence of localized bleeding. Hepatitic involvement is demonstrated only by hepatic enzyme abnormali-ties; histologic evidence usually demonstrates infarction.

III. Diagnosis. Diagnosis is by demonstration of non-septate hyphae on clinical material or isolation of the organism from a clinically suspicious area. Unfortunately, identification of the organism is usually diffi-cult [214].

IV. Therapy. The diagnosis of mucormycosis in cancer ante-mortem is rare and reports of treatment are few. Successful treatment has been reported with amphotericin B in individual cases of pulmonary infection [219, 220]. The importance of control of acidosis, weaning of steroid doses, and ade-quate debridement of necrotic tissue in rhinocerebral disease cannot be overly stressed [220, 221]. The aggressive removal of solitary lesions in the lung that do not resolve completely may be advised to prevent recurrence, since most of these patients will require extensive immunosuppressive ther-apy to maintain a remission of the underlying disease. The utility of these interventions including AmB are ancedotal, and as such, is very much in doubt.

Cryptococcosis

I. Epidemiology. Cryptococcus can be isolated from the soil, most reproduc-ibly from soil around chicken coops and pigeon roosts [222, 223]. It has also been isolated from fruit juice and non-pasteurized milk from cows with cryptococcal mastitis [224]. Serotype A is the most common type associated with infection [232]. Cryptococcus can be isolated from the gastrointestinal tract [226] and from the respiratory tract of normal man [113]. Cryptococcal disease is most frequently associated with the presence of lymphoma, particularly Hodgkin's disease [98, 100, 227].

II. Clinical manifestations. Pulmonary and CNS cryptococcosis are the most frequent manifestations of disease in the cancer patient. Cryptococcal infection varies in extent and severity of disease over time. It produces only a mild to moderate inflammatory response in the normal host and even less in the immunocompromised host [229]. Spontaneous recoveries and exacerbations can be seen in the immunocompromised host [112].

The manifestations of pulmonary cryptococcosis include pulmonary nodules or a localized infiltrate. On occasion, only hilar lymphadenopathy is noted [112]. The natural history of this disease in the immunocompromised host is not known. In the non-compromised host, 6 % of patients with pulmonary cryptococcosis will proceed to involvement of the meninges [228].

Cryptoccocal meningitis can be insidious in onset. The most common symptom is headache and fever, both occurring in 97 % of patients [229–233]. Mental aberrations are not uncommon, as well as decreased level of consciousness. Cranial nerve palsies as well as other mass effects have also been described [223]. Endophthalmitis can also be seen [231]. Seventy-seven percent of patients die by 6 months and 100 % are dead by one year if left untreated [231]. Other manifestations, including renal infection, have been seen [234–236].

III. Diagnosis. Demonstration of the organism in spinal fluid by india ink preparation is seen in up to 40 % of cases of cryptococcal meningitis [183]. Demonstration of the organism in sputum smears is considered non-diagnostic and requires confirmation by lung biopsy. The organism can be isolated from the spinal fluid in most individuals with meningitis but may require repeated sampling to provide a positive culture [231, 237] as only 77 % of patients are positive on the first tap. The organism can also be demonstrated in urine in 40 % of patients with cryptococcal disease [238]. Isolation from blood culture is unusual and usually correlates with a poor prognosis [239].

The detection of cryptococcal capsular antigen by later agglutination in blood or spinal fluid has been a very reliable indicator of the presence of cryptococcal disease [237–243]. False positives are seen only in the presence of rheumatoid disease [224], but with the incorporation of a rheumatoid control, and modification of the test, it has been possible to reduce the incidence of false positives to a very low level. The complement fixation test, which does not have false positives, can help confirm false positivity, but, unfortunately, the C.F. test has a sensitivity of only 63% [238]. The latex agglutination test is positive in the spinal fluid of most patients with meningeal disease, although repeated taps may be required for detection of the antigen [240]. The sensitivity of this test is 92% if sampling of the serum and CSF are performed simultaneously [241]. The L.A. test is much less sensitive for extra-neural disease [224]. The detection of antibodies to cryptococcal antigen are of little value [239].

Characteristics of the spinal fluid include 40–400 cells/mm^3, predominantly lymphocytes, with an elevated protein and low sugar. Poor prognostic factors include low protein, low glucose, high white count, and L.A. titer of greater than 32 [238]. Persistent positive India ink preparations throughout the course of therapy correlates with an increased incidence of relapse [230].

IV. Therapy. The therapy of choice for cryptococcal meningitis is the combination of AmB (0.3 mg/kg/day) and 5-flucytosine (150 mg/kg/day in four divided doses) [248, 249]. This has been associated with a lower relapse rate than seen with single drug therapy [245–247], and there appears to be a trend for more frequent response in the combination group. This therapy is continued for 6 weeks. Trials are now underway to determine whether 4 weeks of therapy are as effective as 6 weeks.

Therapy of pulmonary crytococcosis should be undertaken in the patients with neoplasia, as the incidence of dissemination is unknown and the containment of this disease by the host is not assured. The duration of therapy is open to question, but should be tailored to the clinical and radiologic response of the lesion. If resolution of the lesion does not occur after the administration of 1–2 gm of AmB, consideration for removal of solitary lesions under AmB coverage may be initiated. Follow-up for both extraneural and meningeal disease should be maintained for at least two years, by which time most of the relapses to therapy should be evident [238].

MISCELLANEOUS FUNGI

Pseudopetrillidium boydii

This saprophytic fungus is found in soil, decaying matter, and other natural sources [250]. Infection results usually from inhalation of spores or by accidental inoculation. It can present as a pulmonary infiltrate or sinus involvement in the leukemic host [251, 252]. The actual incidence is unknown, but invasive pulmonary involvement is almost exclusively seen in immunocompromised hosts [253]. Identification by culture is the only definitive way of making the diagnosis, although the presence of acute septated hyphae in the lung without evidence of vascular invasion should alert one to this possibility [253]. The differentiation of this species from Aspergillus (with which it is often confused) is important in that amphotericin B is of no value in this infection [254], and the drug of choice is miconazole [254, 255].

Trichosporon species

This fungus is a cause of white piedra, a common problem in dermatologic practice [256]. It has recently been demonstrated to cause systemic disease in immunocompromised hosts [257–262]. Most patients have demonstrated multiple organ involvement and the organism has been isolated from the blood, urine, and skin. The M.D. Anderson group reported a substantial number of isolations per year from urine and other body sites. In review of our mycologic data, we have demonstrated that isolation of Trichosporon from urine, feces, and throat occur 12–18 times per year. In the last year (1981), we have had two deaths with disseminated Trichosporon sepsis, one of which began with diffuse gastrointestinal invasion, suggesting that this may have been the site of entry for that patient.

Success with antifungal therapy has been infrequent, with the only response being a patient who was treated with amphotericin B. One patient treated with miconazole died, and three died within 96 hours of institution of amphotericin B.

Coccidioidomycosis

The occurrence of this disease in the immunocompromised host is seen primarily in patients with prior history of disease or who have recently travelled through an endemic region [263]. Diagnosis rests on demonstrating either the spherule on biopsies or demonstration of C.F. titer to coccidiodin of greater than 32 for disseminated disease, or precipitin positivity and C.F. titer positivity for newly acquired pulmonary disease [264, 265]. The therapy of choice at present is amphotericin B [266], but the use of ketoconazole appears to be of great benefit at least for the cutaneous manifestations [267, 268]. Ketoconazole has also been useful in the therapy of bone and joint involvement and chronic pulmonary infection [267, 269]. The utility of ketoconazole in the treatment of coccidioidal disease in the immunocompromised host remains to be determined.

Histoplasmosis

The occurrence of histoplamosis in the immunocompromised host is seen in situations similar to those seen in patients with coccidioidal disease. Diag-

32

nosis rests entirely on the isolation of the fungus or detection by histology [270, 271]. The presence of histoplasmosis in tissue can be confirmed by detection of organism-associated antigens in fixed tissue using immunofluorescence techniques [272]. The treatment of choice is amphotericin B [272–274]. The utility of other agents is at present undetermined for the immunocompromised host, but ketoconazole in disseminated disease appears to be effective [275, 276]. However, more patients need to be treated and followed for substantial lengths of time before the efficacy of this drug and the relapse rate can be determined.

SUMMARY

As can be witnessed by the above discussion of the opportunistic fungi, there remains much to be delineated as to the natural history, host–pathogen interrelationships, and therapy. It will require a concerted effort by all the disciplines of medicine and basic science to come to an understanding of the infections that represent one of the major threats to the short-term survival of many of the patients with neoplastic disease. It is also imperative that the data base be generated to allow for a reasoned approach to the diagnosis and therapeutic intervention in the leukopenic host.

REFERENCES

1. Keye JD, Magee WE: Fungal disease in a general hospital. Amer J Clin Pathol 26:1235, 1956.
2. Craig JM, Farber S: The development of disseminated visceral mycosis during therapy for acute leukemia. Amer J Pathol 29:601, 1953.
3. Gruhn JG, Sanson J: Mycotic infection in leukemic patients at autopsy. Cancer 16:61, 1963.
4. Farber S: Quoted as a personal communication by Zimmerman LE: Candida and aspergillus endocarditis. Arch Pathol 50:591, 1950.
5. Ketchel SJ, Rodriquez V: Acute infections in cancer patients. Sem in Oncol 5:167, 1978.
6. Levine AS, Deisseroth AB: Recent developments in the supportive therapy of acute myelogenous leukemia. Cancer 42(Suppl):883, 1978.
7. Schimpff SC: Therapy of infection in patients with granulocytopenia. Med Clinics of N Amer 61:1101, 1977.
8. Pennington JE: Fever, neutropenia, and malignancy: a clinical syndrome in evolution. Cancer 39:1345, 1977.
9. The EORTC International Antimicrobial Therapy Project Group: Three antibiotic regimens in the treatment of infection in febrile granulocytopenic patients with cancer. J Infect Dis 137:14, 1978.
10. Love LJ, Schimpff SC, Schiffer CA, Wiernik PH: Improved prognosis for granulocytopenic patients with gram-negative bacteremia. Amer J Med 68:643, 1980.

11. Baker RD: Leukopenia and therapy in leukemia as factors predisposing to fatal mycoses. Amer J Clin Pathol 37:358, 1962.
12. Schumacher HR, Ginns DA, Warren WJ: Fungus infection complicating leukemia. Amer J Med Sci 247:313, 1964.
13. Stefanini M, Allegra S: Pulmonary mucormycosis in acute histiocytic leukemia. New Engl J Med 163:1026, 1957.
14. Hutter RVP, Collins HS: The occurrence of opportunistic fungus infections in a cancer hospital. Lab Invest 11:1035, 1962.
15. Bodey GP: Fungal infections complicating acute leukemia. J Chronic Dis 19:667, 1966.
16. Burgess MA, deGruchy GC: Septicemia in acute leukemia. Med J Austral 1:1113, 1969.
17. Hughes WT: Fatal infections in childhood leukemia. Amer J Dis Child 122:283, 1971.
18a. Mirsky HS, Cuttner J: Fungal infections in acute leukemia. Cancer 30:348, 1972.
18b. Rosen PR: Opportunistic fungal infections in patients with neoplastic diseases. Pathol Ann 11:255, 1976.
19. Sickles EA, Young VM, Greene WH, Wiernik PH: Pneumonia in acute leukemia. Ann Intern Med 79:528, 1973.
20. Meunier-Carpentier F, Kiehn TE, Armstrong DA: Fungemia in the immunocompromised host. Amer J Med 71:363, 1981.
21. Rodriquez V, Gutterman JU, McMullan GK, Heckman AA, Jr: The spectrum of infections in patients with acute leukemia and malignant lymphoma in a military hospital. Milt Med 137:199, 1972.
22. Hughes WT, Smith DR: Infection during induction of remission in acute lymphocytic leukemia. Cancer 31:1008, 1973.
23. Levine AS, Siegel SE, Schreiber AD et al.: Protected environments and prophylactic antibiotics. New Engl J Med 288:477, 1973.
24. Singer C, Kaplan MH, Armstrong D: Bacteremia and fungemia complicating neoplastic disease. Amer J Med 62:731, 1977.
25. Cho SY, Choi HY: Opportunistic fungal infection among cancer patients. Amer J Clin Pathol 72:617, 1979.
26. Ganes P, Avotabile G, Mechlinski et al.: Polyene macrolide antibiotic, amphotericin B. Crystal structure of the N-acetyl derivative. J Amer Chem Soc 93:4560, 1971.
27. Kotler-Brajtburg J, Medoff G, Kobayashi GS et al.: Classification of polyene antibiotics according to chemical structure and biological effects. Antimicrob Agents & Chemo (AAC) 15:716, 1979.
28. Hoogevest P et al.: Effects of amphotericin B on cholesterol containing liposomes of egg phosphatyldyl-choline and didoeosesylphosphoatydlcholine. Biochim Biophys Acta 511(3):397, 1978.
29. Hamilton-Miller JMT: Chemistry and biology of the polyene macrolide antibiotics. Bacteriol Rev 37:166, 1973.
30. Rast DA, Bartnichi-Garcia S: Effects of amphotericin B, nystatin, and other polyene antibiotics on chitin synthetase. Proc Natl Acad Sci (USA) 78:1233, 1981.
31. Shadomy S, Shadomy HJ, McKay J, Utz J: In vitro susceptibility of cryptococcus to amphotericin B, namycin, and 5-flucytosine. Antimicrob Agents & Chemo 8:452, 1968.
32. Gold W, Stout HA, Jagans JF, Dorovick R: Antifungal antibiotics produced by a streptomyces. I. In vitro studies. Antibiotic Annals 579, Medical Encyclopedia, Inc. New York, NY, pp 1955–56.
33. Brass C, Shainhouse JZ, Stevens DA: Variability of agar dilution-replicator method of yeast susceptibility testing. AAC 15:763, 1979.
34. Galgiani JN, Stevens DA: Antimicrobial susceptibility testing of yeasts: A turbidometric technique independent of inoculum size. AAC 10:721, 1978.

35. Bindschadler DD, Bennett JE: A pharmacologic guide to the clinical use of amphotericin B. J Infect Dis 120:427, 1969.
36. Atkinson AJ, Bennett JE: Amphotericin pharmacokinetics in humans. AAC 13:271, 1978.
37. Block ER, Bennett JE, Livoti W et al.: Flucytosine and amphotericin B: Hemodialysis effects on the plasma concentrations and clearance. Ann Intern Med 80:613, 1974.
38. Block ER, Bennett JE: Stability of amphotericin B in infusion bottles. AAC 4:648, 1973.
39. MacGregor RR, Bennett JE, Erslew AJ: Erythropoietin concentration in amphotericin B-induced anemia. AAC 14:270, 1978.
40. Butler WT, Bennett JE, Alleng DW et al.: Nephrotoxicity of amphotericin B. Ann Intern Med 61:175, 1964.
41. McCurdy DK, Frederic M, Elkinton JR: Renal tubular acidosis due to amphotericin B. New Engl J Med 278:124, 1968.
42. Douglas JB, Healy JK: Nephrotoxic effects of amphotericin B including renal tubular acidosis. Amer J Med 46:154, 1969.
43. Bhathena DB, Bullock WE, Nuttal CE et al.: The effects of amphotericin B therapy on the intra-renal vasculature and renal tubules in man. Clin Nephro 9:103, 1978.
44. Beard HW, Rohert JH, Taylor RA: The treatment of deep mycotic infections with amphotericin B with particular emphasis on drug toxicity. Amer Rev Resp Dis 81:43, 1960.
45. Bullock WE, Luke RG, Nuttal CE, Bhathena DB: Can mannitol reduce amphotericin B nephrotoxicity? AAC 10:555, 1976.
46. Wertlake PT, Buller WT, Hill GJ, Utz JP: Nephrotoxic tubular damage and calcium deposition following amphotericin B therapy. Amer J Pathol 43:449, 1963.
47. Reiner NE, Thompson WL: Dopamine and saralasin antagonism of renal vasoconstriction and oliguria caused by amphotericin B. J Infect Dis 140:564, 1979.
48. DeNollin S, Van Belle H, Goossens F et al.: Cytochemical and biochemical studies of yeasts after in vitro exposure to miconazole. AAC 11:500, 1977.
49. deNollin S, Borgers M: The effects of miconazole on the ultrastructure of Candida albicans. Proc Royal Soc Med 70(Suppl):9, 1977.
50. Van den Bossche H, Willemsens G, Cools W et al.: Biochemical effects of miconazole of fungi. II. Inhibition of ergosterol biosynthesis in Candida albicans. Chemico-Biol Interactions 21:50, 1978.
51. Yamaguchi H: Antagonistic action of lipid components of membranes from Candida albicans and various other lipids on two imidazoles, antimycotics, clotrimazole and miconazole. AAC 12:16, 1977.
52. Heel RC, Brodgin RN, Pokes GF, Speight TM et al.: Miconazole: a preliminary review of its therapeutic efficacy in systemic fungal infections. Drugs 19:7, 1980.
53. Lutwick WI, Galgiani JN, Johnson RH et al.: Visceral fungal infections due to petrillidium boydii. Amer J Med 61:632, 1976.
54. Deresinski SC, Galgiani JN, Stevens DA: Miconazole treatment in human coccidioidomycosis: status report. In: Coccidioidomycosis: Current Clinical and Diagnostic Studies, Ajello J (ed). Symposia Specialists, Miami, Florida, 1977, p 207.
55. Deresinski SC, Lilly RB, Levine HB et al.: Treatment of fungal meningitis with miconazole. Amer Rev Resp Dis 113:71, 1976.
56. Stevens DA, Levine HB, Deresinski SC: Miconazole in coccidioidomycosis. II. Therapeutic and pharmacologic studies in man. Amer J Med 60:191, 1976.
57. Stevens DA: Miconazole in the treatment of systemic fungal infections. Amer Rev Resp Dis 116:801, 1977.
58. Marmion LC, Desse KB, Lilly RB, Stevens DA: Reversible thrombocytosis and anemia

due to miconazole therapy. AAC 10:447, 1976.

59. Van den Boosche H, Willemsens G, Corts W et al.: In vitro and in vivo effects of the antimycotic drug ketoconazole on sterol synthesis. AAC 17:922, 1980.

60. Dixon D, Shadomy S, Shadomy HJ, Espinel- Ingroff A: Comparison of the in vitro anti-fungal activities of miconazole and a new imidazole R41400. J Infect Dis 138:245, 1978.

61. Brass C, Galgiani JN, Blaschke T et al.: Disposition of ketoconazole, an oral antifungal in humans. AAC 21:151, 1982.

62. Symoens J, Moens M, Dom D et al.: An evaluation of two years of clinical experience with ketoconazole. Rev Infect Dis 2:674, 1980.

63. DeFelice R, Johnson DG, Galgiani JN: Gynecomastia with ketoconazole. AAC 19:1073, 1981.

64. Petersen EA, Alling DW, Kirkpatrick CH: Treatment of chronic mucocutaneous candid-iasis with ketoconazole. A controlled trial. Ann Intern Med 93:791, 1980.

65. Brass C, Galgiani JN, Campbell SC et al.: Therapy of coccidioidomycosis with oral keto-conazole. In: Current Chemotherapy and Infectious Disease. Proc of the 11th Internatl Congress in Chemotherapy, Vol 2, Amer Soc for Microbiol, Washington, DC, 1980, p 965.

66. Hurley R: Pathogenicity of the genus Candida. In: Symposium on Candida Infections, Winner JI and Hurley R (eds). Edinburgh, E & S Livingstone, 1966, pp 13-14.

67. Cohen R, Roth FJ, Delgado E et al.: Fungal flora of the normal human small and large intestine. New Engl J Med 280:638, 1969.

68. Taschdjian CL, Seelig MD, Kozinn PJ: Serologic diagnosis of candidal infections. CRC Critical Reviews in Clin Lab Sci 4:13, 1973.

69. Kahanpaa A: Yeast fungus flora in patients in a geriatric hospital. Acta Pathol et Microbiol Scand 82:81, 1974.

70. Somerville DA: Yeasts in a hospital for patients with skin diseases. J Hygiene 70:667, 1972.

71. Ahearn DG: Identification and ecology of yeasts of medical importance. In: Opportunistic Pathogens, Prier JE and Friedman H (eds). Baltimore: University Park Press, 1974, pp 129–146.

72. Lehner T: Systemic candidiasis and renal involvement. Lancet 1:1414, 1964.

73. Symmers W, St. C: Septicemic candidosis. In: Symposium on Candida Infections, Winner HE and Hurley R (eds). Edinburgh, E & S Livingstone, 1966, pp 196–212.

74. Myerowitz RL, Allen CM, Pazin GJ: Disseminated candidiasis. Changes in incidence, underlying diseases, and pathology. Amer J Clin Pathol 68:29, 1977.

75. Eras P, Goldstein MJ, Sherlock P: Candida infection of the gastrointestinal tract. Medicine 51:367, 1972.

76. Goldberg HI, Dodds WJ: Cobblestone esophagus due to monilial infection. Amer J of Roent Rad, Thera and Nucl Med 104:608, 1968.

77. Sheft DJ, Shrago G: Esophageal moniliasis. The spectrum of the disease. JAMA 213:1859, 1970.

78. Seaman WB: The case of the painful swallow. Hospital Practice 9:131, 1974.

79. Gonzalez-Crussi F, Lung OS: Esophageal moniliasis as a cause of death. Amer J Surg 109:634, 1964.

80. Jensen KB, Stenderup A, Thomsen JB, Bichel J: Esophageal moniliasis in malignant neo-plastic disease. Acta Med Scand 175:455, 1964.

81. Nash G, Ross JS: Herpetic esophagitis – a common cause of esophagitis – a common cause of esophageal ulceration. Human Pathol 5:339, 1974.

82. Kodsi BE, Wickremesinghe PC, Kozinn PJ et al.: Candida esophagitis. Gastro 71:715,

1976.

83. Muller SA, Hermann EC, Jr, Winkelmann RK: Herpes simplex infections in hematologic malignancies. Amer J Med 52:102, 1972.

84. Edwards JE, Jr: Candida species. In: Principles and Practice of Infectious Diseases, Mandell GL, Douglass RG, Jr and Bennett JE (eds). New York, John Wiley & Sons, 1979, pp 1981-2001.

85. Masur J, Rosen PP, Armstrong D: Pulmonary disease caused by candida species. Amer J Med 63:914, 1977.

86. Rosenbaum RB, Barber JV, Stevens DA: Candida albicans pneumonia. Amer Rev Resp Dis 109:373, 1974.

87. Ramirez G, Schuster M, Kozub W, Pribor JC: Fatal acute candida albicans bronchopneumonia. Report of a case. JAMA 199:340, 1967.

88. Rose JD, Sheth NK: Pulmonary candidiasis. Arch Intern Med 138: 964, 1978.

89. Goldman HJ, Littman ML, Oppenheimer GD et al.: Monilial cystitis-effective treatment with instillations of amphotericin B. JAMA 174:359, 1960.

90. Wise GJ, Goldberg P, Kozinn PJ: Genitourinary candidiasis: diagnosis and treatment. J Urol 116:778, 1976.

91. Kozinn PJ, Taschdjian CL, Goldberg PK et al.: Advances in the diagnosis of renal candidiasis. J Urol 119:184, 1978.

92. Janosko EO, McRoberts JW: Evaluation and treatment of urinary candidiasis. South Med J 72:1578, 1979.

93. Henderson DK, Edwards JE, Jr, Montgomerie JZ: Hematogenous candida endophthalmitis in patients receiving parenteral hyperalimentation fluids. J Infect Dis 143:655, 1981.

94. Aisner J, Schimpff SC, Sutherland JC et al.: Torulopsis glabrata infections in patients with cancer. Amer J Med 61:23, 1976.

95. Edwards JE. Jr (moderator): Disseminated candidiasis: trends, manifestations, and diagnosis. In: UCLA Conference, Severe Candida Infections. Clinical Perspectives, Immune Defense Mechanisms, and Current Concepts of Therapy. Ann Intern Med 89:91, 1978.

96. Louria DB, Stiff DP, Bennett B: Disseminated moniliasis in the adult. Medicine 41:307, 1962.

97. Valdivieso M, Luna M, Bodey GP et al.: Fungemia due to Torulopsis glabrata in the compromised host. Cancer 38:1750, 1976.

98. Casazza AR, Duvall CP, Carbone PP: Infection in lymphoma. Histology, treatment and duration in relation to incidence and survival. JAMA 197:710, 1966.

99. Hart PD, Russell E, Jr, Remington JS: The compromised host and infection. II. Deep fungal infection. J Infect Dis 120:169, 1969.

100. Feld R, Bodey GP, Rodriguez V, Luna M: Causes of death in patients with lymphoma. Amer J Med Sci 268:97, 1974.

101. Montgomerie JZ, Edwards JE, Jr: Association of infection due to Candida albicans with intravenous hyperalimentation. J Infect Dis 137:197, 1978.

102. Fishman LS, Griffin JR, Sapico FL, Hecht R: Hematogenous candida endophthalmitis – a complication of candidemia. New Engl J Med 286:675, 1972.

103. Edwards JE, Jr, Foos RY, Montgomerie JZ et al.: Ocular manifestations of Candida septicemia: review of 76 cases of hematogenous candida endophtalmitis. Medicine 53:47, 1974.

104. Bernhardt HE, Orlando JC, Benfield JR, Hirose FM, Foos RY: Disseminated candidiasis in surgical patients. Surg Gynecol Obstet 134:819, 1972.

105. Taschdjian CL, Kozinn PJ, Toni EF: Opportunistic yeast infections with special reference to candidiasis. Ann NY Acad Sci 174:606, 1970.

106. Parker JC, Jr, McCloskey JJ, Lee RS: The emergence of candidosis – the dominant post-

mortem cerebral mycosis. Amer J Clin Pathol 70:31, 1978.

107. Wald BR, Ortega JA, Ross L et al.: Candidal splenic abscesses complicating acute leukemia of childhood treated by splenectomy. Pediatrics 67:296, 1981.

108. Page CP, Coltman CA, Robertson HD, Nelson EA: Candidal abscess of the spleen in patients with acute leukemia. Surg Gynecol Obstet 151:604, 1980.

109. Kressel B, Szewczyk C, Tuazon CU: Early clinical recognition of disseminated candidiasis by muscle and skin biopsy. Arch Intern Med 138:429, 1978.

110. Jacobs MI, Magid MS, Jarowski CI: Disseminated candidiasis – newer approaches to early recognition and treatment. Arch Dermatol 116:1277, 1980.

111. Young RC, Bennett JE, Geelhoed GW, Levine AS: Fungemia with compromised host resistance. A study of 70 cases. Ann Intern Med 80:605, 1974.

112. Krick JA, Remington JS: Opportunistic invasive fungal infections in patients with leukemia and lymphoma. Clin Haematol 5(2):249, 1976.

113. Kahanpaa A: Bronchopulmonary occurrence of fungi in adults especially according to cultivation material. Acta Pathol en Microbiol Scand 82 (Suppl):81, 1972.

114. Sandford GR, Merz WG, Wingard JR, Charache P, Saral R: The value of fungal surveillance cultures as predictors of systemic fungal infections. J Infect Dis 142:503, 1980.

115. Preisler HD, Hansenclever HF, Henderson ES: Anti-candida antibodies in patients with acute leukemia. Amer J Med 51:352, 1971.

116. Preisler HD, Hansenclever HF, Levitan AA, Henderson ES: Serologic diagnosis of disseminated candidiasis in patients with acute leukemia. Ann Intern Med 70:19, 1969.

117. Taschdjian CL, Seelig MS, Kozinn PJ: Serological diagnosis of candidal infections. CRC Critical Reviews of Laboratory Sciences 4:19, 1973.

118. Harding SA, Sandford GR, Merz WG: Three serologic tests for candidiasis. Amer J Clin Pathol 65:1001, 1976.

119. Merz WG, Eveans GL, Shadomy S et al.: Laboratory evaluation of serological tests for systemic candidiasis: A cooperative study. J Clin Micro 5:596, 1977.

120. Meckstroth KL, Reisse E, Keller JW, Kaufman L: Detection of antibodies and antigenemia in leukemic patients with candidiasis by enzyme linked immunosorbent assay. J Infect Dis 144:24, 1981.

121. Myerowitz RL, Layman H, Petursson S, Yee RB: Diagnostic value of candida precipitins determined by counterimmunoelectrophoresis in patients with acute leukemia. Amer J Clin Pathol 72:963, 1979.

122. Filice G, Yu B, Armstrong D: Immunodiffusion and agglutination tests for candida in patients with neoplastic disease: inconsistent correlation of results with invasive infections. J Infect Dis 135:349, 1977.

123. Laforce FM, Mills DM, Iverson K et al.: Inhibition of leukocyte candidacidal activity by serum from patients with disseminated candidiasis. J Lab & Clin Med 86:657, 1975.

124. Gaines JD, Remington JS: Diagnosis of deep infection with candida. A study of candida precipitins. Arch Intern Med 132:699, 1973.

125. Hellwege HH, Fisher K, Blaker F: Diagnostic value of candida precipitins (Letter to the Editor). Lancet 2:386, 1972.

126. Glew RH, Buckley HR, Rosen HM et al.: Serologic tests in the diagnosis of systemic candidiasis. Amer J Med 64:586, 1978.

127. Oches FC, Evan EGV, Holland KT: Detection of candida precipitin. A comparison of double diffusion and counterimmunoelectophoresis. J Immunol Methods 7:211, 1975.

128. Rosner G, Gabriel FD, Taschdjian CL et al.: Serological diagnosis of candidiasis in patients with acute leukemia. Amer J Med 51:54, 1971.

129. Taschdjian CL, Kozinn PJ, Cuesta MB, Toni EF: Serodiagnosis of candidal infection. Amer J Clin Pathol 57:195, 1972.

38

130. Remington JS, Gaines JD, Gilmer MA: Demonstration of candida precipitins in human sera by counterimmunoelectrophoresis. Lancet 1:413, 1972.

131. Warren RC, Richardson MD, White LO: Enzyme-linked immunosorbent assay of antigens from *Candida albicans* circulating in infected mice and rabbits: the role of mannan. Mycopathologia 66:179, 1978.

132. Weiner MH, Coats-Stephen M: Immunodiagnosis of systemic candidasis: mannan antigenemia detected by radioimmunoassay in experimental and human infections. J Infect Dis 140:989, 1979.

133. Segal E, Berg RA, Pizzo PA, Bennett JE: Detection of candida antigen in sera of patients with candidiasis by E.L.I.S.A. inhibition technique. J Clin Micro 10:116, 1979.

134. Kerkering TM, Espinel-Ingroff A, Shadomy S: Detection of candida antigenemia by counterimmunoelectrophoresis in patients with invasive candidiasis. J Infect Dis 140:659, 1979.

135. Kiehn TE, Bernard EM, Gold JWM, Armstrong D: Candidiasis: detection by gas-liquid chromatography of d-arabinitol, a fungal metabolite in human serum. Science 205:577, 1979.

136. Eng RHK, Chmel H, Buse M: Serum levels of arabinitol in the detection of invasive candidiasis in animals and humans. J Infect Dis 143:677, 1981.

137. Roboz J, Suzuki R, Holland JF: Quantification of arabinitol in serum by selected ion monitoring as a diagnostic technique in invasive candidiasis. J Clin Micro 12:594, 1980.

138. Gangopadhyay PK, Thadepalli H, Roy I, Ansari A: Identification of species of candida, Cryptococcus, and torulopsis by gas-liquid chromatography. J Infect Dis 140:952, 1979.

139. Miller GG, Witwer MW, Braude AI, Davis CE: Rapid identification of *Candida albicans* septicemia in man by gas-liquid chromatography. J Clin Invest 54:1235, 1974.

140. Monson TP, Wilkinson KP: Mannose in body fluids as an indicator of invasive candidiasis. J Clin Mivro 14:557, 1981.

141. Weiner MH, Yount WJ: Mannan antigenemia in the diagnosis of invasive candida infections. J Clin Invest 58:1045, 1976.

142. Winston DJ, Gale RP, Meyer DV, Young LS: Infectious complications of human bone marrow transplantation. Medicine 58:1, 1979.

143. Neiman PE, Thomas ED, Reeves WC et al.: Opportunistic infection and interstitial pneumonia following marrow transplantation for aplastic anemia and hematologic malignancy. Transplantation Proc 8:663, 1976.

144. Seabury JH, Dascomb HE: Results of the treatment of systemic mycosis. JAMA 188:509, 1964.

145. Utz JP, Andriole VT: Analysis of amphotericin treatment failures in systemic fungal disease. Ann NY Acad Sci 89:277, 1960.

146. Seabury JH, Dascomb HE: Experience with amphotericin B. Ann NY Acad Sci 89:202, 1960.

147. Medoff G, Dismukes WE, Meade RH, III, Moses JM: A new therapeutic approach to candida infections. Arch Intern Med 130:241, 1972.

148. Gauto A, Law EJ, Holder IA, MacMillan BG: Experience with amphotericin B in the treatment of systemic candidiasis in burn patients. Amer J Surg 133:174, 1977.

149. Medoff G, Dismukes WE, Meade RH, III, Moses J: Therapeutic program for candida infection. AAC 10:286, 1970.

150. Emmons C: Antimycotics (Editorial). AAC 11:609, 1961.

151. Meunier-Carpentier F, Kiehn TE, Armstrong D: Fungemia in the immunocompromised host. Amer J Med 71:363, 1981.

152. Block ER, Bennett JE: The combined effect of 5-fluorocytosine and amphotericin B in the

therapy of murine cryptococcosis. Proc Soc Exp Biol Med 142:476, 1973.

153. Medoff G, Comfor M, Kobayashi GS: Synergistic action of amphotericin B and 5-fluoro-cytosine against yeast-like organisms. Proc Soc Exp Biol Med 138:571, 1971.

154. Rabinovich S, Shaw BD, Bryant T, Donata ST: Effect of 5-fluorocytosine and ampho-tericin B on *Candida albicans* infection in mice. J Infect Dis 130:28, 1974.

155. Montgomerie JZ, Edwards JE, Jr, Guze L: Synergism of amphotericin B and 5-fluoro-cytosine for Candida species. J infect Dis 132:82, 1975.

156. Beggs WH, Sarosi GA, Andrews FA: Synergistic action of amphotericin B and rifampin on *Candida albicans*. Amer Rev Resp Dis 110:671, 1974.

157. Krick JA, Remington JS: Treatment of fungal infections (Editorial). Arch Intern Med 135:344, 1975.

158. Drutz DJ, Spickar A, Rogers DE, Koenig MG: Treatment of disseminated mycotic infec-tions – a new approach to amphotericin B therapy. Amer J Med 45:405, 1968.

159. Sutliff WB: Therapeutic trial of curative drugs for systemic fungus disease, AAC 1:359, 1961.

160. Procknow JJ: Treatment of opportunistic fungus infection. Lab Invest 11:1218, 1962.

161. Rose HD, Varkey B: Deep mycotic infection in the hospitalized adult: a study of 123 patients. Medicine 54:499, 1975.

162. Hermans PE: Antifungal agents used for deep-seated mycotic infections. Mayo Clinic Proc 52:687, 1977.

163. Wust HJ, Lennartz H: Successful treatment of yeast sepsis with miconazole. Deutsch Med Wschr 99:2515, 1974.

164. Tytgat GN, Surachno S, de Groot WP, Schellekens PT: A case of chronic oropharynoe-sophageal candidiasis with immunological deficiency: Successful therapy with miconazole. Gastro 72:563, 1977.

165. Rutgeerts L, Verhaegen H: Intravenous miconazole in the treatment of chronic esophageal candidiasis. Gastro 72:316, 1977.

166. Wade TR, Jones HE, Chanda JJ: Intravenous miconazole therapy of mycotic infections. Arch Intern Med 139:784, 1979.

167. Verhaegen H: Miconazole treatment in candidal esophagitis. Proc Royal Soc Med 70 (Suppl 1):48, 1977.

168. Iwand A, Deppermann D: Miconazole in systemic mycosis. Proc Royal Soc Med 70 (Suppl 1) *et al.*43, 1977.

169. Sung JP, Rajani K, Chopra DR et al.: Miconazole therapy for systemic candidiasis in a conjoined (siamese) twin and a premature newborn. Amer J Surg 138:688, 1979.

170. Evers KG, Knoop UF: Miconazole treatment of candida sepsis in an aminophenazone-induced agranulocytosis. Acta Paediatr Belg 31:151, 1978.

171. Katz ME, Cassileth PA: Disseminated candidiasis in a patient with an acute leukemia – successful therapy with miconazole. JAMA 237:1124, 1977.

172. Heel RC, Brogden RN, Pakes GE, Speight TM, Avery GS: Miconazole: a preliminary review of its therapeutic efficacy in systemic fungal infections. Drugs 19:7, 1980.

173. Jordan WM, Bodey GP, Rodriguez V et al.: Miconazole therapy for treatment of fungal infections in cancer patients. AAC 16:792, 1979.

174. Aisner J, Schimpff SC, Bennett JE, Sutherland JC, Young VM, Wiernik PH: Aspergillus infections in cancer patients: an association with fire-proofing materials. JAMA 235:411, 1976.

175. Burton JR, Zachery JB, Bessin R et al.: Aspergillosis in four renal transplant patients. Diagnosis and effective treatment with amphotericin B. Ann Intern Med 77:383, 1972.

176. Christensen CM, Kennedy BW: Filamentous fungi and bacteria in macroni and spaghetti products. Appli Micro 21:144, 1971.

177. Young RC, Bennett JE, Vogel CL et al.: Aspergillosis – the spectrum of disease in 98 patients. Medicine 49:147, 1970.
178. Rosen PP, Sternber SS: Decreased frequency of aspergillosis and mucormycosis. New Engl J Med 295:1319, 1976.
179. Aisner J, Schimpff SC, Wiernik PH: Treatment of invasive aspergillosis: relation of early diagnosis and treatment to response. Ann Intern Med 86:539, 1977.
180. Meyer BR, Young LS, Armstrong D, Yu B: Aspergillosis complicating neoplastic disease. Amer J Med 54:6, 1973.
181. Gurwith MJ, Stenson EB, Remington JS: Aspergillus infection complicating cardiac transplantation. Arch Intern Med 128:541, 1971.
182. Gerrcovich FG, Richman SP, Rodriguez V et al.: Successful control of systemic aspergillus niger infections in two patients with acute leukemia. Cancer 36:2771, 1976.
183. Levine AS, Schimpff SC, Graw RG, Jr, Young RC: Hematologic malignancies and other marrow failure states: progress in the management of complicating infections. Seminars Hematol 11:141, 1974.
184. Fetter BF, Klintworth GK, Hendry WS: Mycoses of the central nervous system. Baltimore, Williams & Wilkins, 1967, p. 214.
185. Walsh TJ, Bulkley BH: Aspergillus pericarditis: clinical and pathologic features in the immunocompromised patient. Cancer 49:48, 1982.
186. Cooper JAD, Weinbaum DL, Aldrich TK, Mandell GL: Invasive aspergillus of the lung and pericardium in a non-immunocompromised 33-year old man. Amer J Med 71:903, 1981.
187. Young RC, Bennett JE, Vogel CL et al.: Fungemia with compromised host resistance. A study of 70 cases. Ann Intern Med 80:605, 1974.
188. Baradana EJ, Jr: Measurement of humoral antibodies to aspergilli. Ann NY Acad Sci 221:64, 1974.
189. Young RC, Bennett JE: Invasive aspergillosis: absence of detectable antibody response. Amer Rev Resp Dis 104:710, 1971.
190. Schaefer JC, Yu B, Armstrong D: An aspergillus immunodiffusion test in the early diagnosis of aspergillosis in adult leukemia patients. Amer Rev Resp Dis 113:325, 1976.
191. Gold JWM, Fisher B, Yu B, Chein N, Armstrong D: Diagnosis of invasive aspergillosis by passive hemagglutinin assay of antibody. J Infect Dis 142:87, 1980.
192. Shaffer PJ, Medoff G, Kobayashi GS: Demonstration of antigenemia by radioimmunoassay in rabbits experimentally infected with aspergillus. J Infect Dis 139:313, 1979.
193. Fisher BD, Armstrong D, Yu B, Gold JW: Invasive aspergillosis: Progress in early diagnosis and treatment. Amer J Med 71:571, 1981.
194. Aisner J, Murilo J, Schimpff SC, Steere AC: Invasive aspergillosis in acute leukemia: Correlation with nose cultures and antibiotic use. Ann Intern Med 90:4, 1979.
195. Sinclair AJ, Rossof AH, Coltman CA: Recognition and successful management in pulmonary aspergillosis in leukemia. Cancer 42:2019, 1978.
196. Orr DP, Myerowitz RL, Dubois PJ: Pathoradiologic correlation of invasive pulmonary aspergillosis in the compromised host. Cancer 41:2028, 1978.
197. Brandsberg JW, French ME: In vitro susceptibility of isolates of aspergillus and sprorthrix schenkii to amphotericin B. AAC 2:402, 1972.
198. Sawyer PR, Brogden RM, Pinder RM, Speight TM, Avery GS: Miconazole: a review of its antifungal activity and therapeutic efficacy. Drugs 9:406, 1977.
199. Fields BT, Jr, Meredith WR, Galbraith JE, Hardin HF: Studies with amphotericin B and 5-fluorocytosine in aspergillosis. Clin Res 22:32A, 1974.
200. Atkinson K, Isreal HL: 5-fluorocytosine treatment of meningeal and pulmonary aspergillosis. Amer J Med 55:496, 1973.

201. Hammerman KJ, Christianson CS, Huntington I et al.: Spontaneous lysis of aspergilloma-ta. Chest 64:697, 1973.
202. Adelman BA, Bentman BA, Rosenthal A: Treatment of aspergillosis in leukemia. Ann Intern Med 91:323, 1979.
203. Beyt BE, Cannon RO, Tuteur PG: Successful treatment of invasive pulmonary aspergillosis in the immunocompromised host. South J Med 71:1164, 1978.
204. Ribner B, Keusch GT, Hanna BA, Perlopff M: Combination amphotericin B/rifampin therapy for pulmonary aspergillosis in a leukemia patient. Chest 70:681, 1976.
205. Brass C: Unpublished observations.
206. Symoens J, Moens M, Dom J et al.: An evaluation of two years of clinical experience with ketoconazole. Rev Infect Dis 2:674, 1980.
207. Ketahara M, Seth VK, Medoff G et al.: Activity of amphotericin B, 5-fluorocytosine and rifampin against six clinical isolates of aspergillus. AAC 9:915, 1976.
208. Arroyo J, Medoff G, Kabayashi G: Therapy of murine aspergillosis with amphotericin B in combination with rifampin or 5-fluorocytosine. AAC 11:21, 1977.
209. Meyer RD, Rosen P, Armstrong D: Phycomycosis complicating leukemia. Ann Intern Med 77:871, 1972.
210. Meyer RD, Armstrong D: Mucormycosis-changing status. CRC Critical Rev Clin Lab Sci 4:421, 1973.
211. Symmers WSC: Histopathologic aspects of the pathogenesis of some opportunistic fungal infections as exemplified in the pathology of aspergillosis and the phycomycetoses. Lab Invest 11:1073, 1962.
212. Sayer WJ, Shean DB, Ghosseiri J: Estimation of airborne fungal flora by the Andersen sampler versus the gravity settling culture plate. J Allergy 44:214, 1969.
213. Noble WC, Clayton YM: Fungi in the air of hospital wards. J Gen Micro 32:397, 1963.
214. Lehrer RI (Moderator): Mucormycosis. Ann Intern Med 93:93, 1980.
215. Bragg DG, Janis B: The radiographic presentation of pulmonary opportunistic inflammatory disease. Rad Clin of North Amer 11:357, 1973.
216. Pagani JJ, Libshitz HI: Opportunistic fungal pneumonias in cancer patients. Amer J Rad 137:1033, 1981.
217. Murray JW: Pulmonary mucormycosis with massive fatal hemoptysis. Chest 68:65, 1975.
218. Medoff G, Kobayashi GS: Pulmonary mucormycosis. New Engl J Med 286: 86, 1972.
219. Murray JF, Haegelin GF, Gewitt WL et al.: Opportunistic pulmonary infections. Ann Intern Med 65:655, 1966.
220. Battock DJ, Grausz H, Bobrowsky M, Littman Ml: Alternate-day amphotericin B therapy in the treatment of rhinocerebral phycomycosis. Ann Intern Med 68:122, 1968.
221. Landau JW, Newcomer VD: Acute cerebral phycomycosis. J Pediatr 61:363, 1962.
222. Powell KE, Dahl BA, Weeks RJ et al.: Airborne *Cryptococcus neoformans*: particles from pigeon excreta compatible with alveolar deposition. J Infect Dis 125:412, 1972.
223. Buechner HA, Furcolow ML, Farness OJ et al.: Epidemiology of the pulmonary mycoses. Chest 58:68, 1970.
224. Diamond RD: *Cryptococcus neoformans*. In: Principles and Practices of Infectious Diseases, Mandell GL, Douglas RG, Jr, Bennett JE (eds). John Wiley & Sons, 1979, p 2023.
225. Bennett JE, Kwon-Chung KJ, Howard DH: Epidemiologic differences among serotypes of *Cryptococcus neoformans*. Amer J Epidemiol 10:582, 1977.
226. Littman ML, Zimmerman LE: Cryptococcosis. Torulosis or European blastomycosis. New York, Grune & Stratton, 1956, p 205.

42

227. Kaplan MH, Rosen PP, Armstrong D: Cryptococcosis in a cancer hospital. Cancer 39:2265, 1977.
228. Hammerman KJ, Powell KE, Christianson CS et al.: Pulmonary cryptococcosis: clinical forms and treatment. Amer Rev Resp Dis 108:1116, 1973.
229. Littman ML, Walter JE: Cryptococcosis: current status. Amer J Med 45:922, 1968.
230. Sarosi GA, Parker JD, Doto IL, Tosh FE: Amphotericin B in cryptococcal meningitis. Long-term results of therapy. Ann Intern Med 71: 1079, 1969.
231. Mosberg WH, Jr, Arnold JG, Jr: Torulosis of the central nervous system: review of the literature and report of 5 cases. Ann Intern Med 32:1153, 1950.
232. Spickard A: Diagnosis and treatment of cryptococcal disease. South Med J 66:26, 1973.
233. Pontifex AH, Richards AG: Cryptococcal meningitis. Canadian Med Assoc J 98:772, 1968.
234. Heenan PJ, Dawkins RL: Cryptococcosis and multiple squamous cell tumors associated with a T cell defect. Cancer 47:291, 1981.
235. Hinchey WW, Someren A: Cryptococcal prostatitis. Amer J Clin Pathol 75:257, 1981.
236. Hellman RN, Hinrichs J, Sicard G et al.: Cryptococcal pyelonephritis and disseminated cryptococcosis in a renal transplant recipient. Arch Intern Med 141:128, 1981.
237. Berger MP, Paz J: Diagnosis of cryptococcal meningitis. JAMA 236:2157, 1976.
238. Diamond RD, Bennett JE: Prognostic factors in cryptococcal meningitis. Ann Intern Med 80:176, 1974.
239. Bindschadler DD, Bennett JE: Serology of human cryptococcosis. Ann Intern Med 69:45, 1968.
240. Snow RM, Dismukes WE: Cryptococcal meningitis. Arch Intern Med 135:1155, 1975.
241. Prevost E, Newell R: Commercial cryptococcal latex kit: clinical evaluation in a medical center hospital. J Clin Micro 8:529, 1978.
242. Kauffman CA, Bergman AG, Severance PJ, McClatchey KD: Detection of cryptococcal antigen. Amer J Clin Pathol 75:106, 1981.
243. Bloomfield N, Gordon MA, Elmendorf DF, Jr: Detection of *Cryptococcus neoformans* antigen in body fluids by latex particle agglutination. Proc Soc Exper Biol Med 114:64, 1963.
244. Bennett JE, Bailey JW: Control for rheumatoid factor in the latex test for cryptococcosis. J Clin Pathol 56:360, 1971.
245. Bardana EJ, Jr, Kaufman L, Benner EJ: Amphotericin B and cryptococcal infection. Arch Intern Med 122:517, 1968.
246. Pickard A, Butler WT, Andriole V, Utz JP: The improved prognosis of cryptococcal meningitis with amphotericin B therapy. Ann Intern Med 58:66, 1963.
247. Sarosi GA, Parker JD, Doto IL, Tosh FF: Amphotericin B in cryptococcal meningitis. Ann Intern Med 71:1079, 1969.
248. Utz JP, Garriques Il, Sandi MA et al.: Therapy of cryptococcosis with a combination of flucytosine and amphotericin B. J Infect Dis 132:368, 1975.
249. Bennett JE, Dismukes WE, Duma, RJ et al.: Comparison of amphotericin B alone with amphotericin B plus 5-flucytosine in cryptococcal meningitis. New Engl J Med 301:126, 1979.
250. Ajello L: The isolation of *Allescheria boydii* shear, an etiologic agent of mycetomas from soil. Amer J Trop Med Hyg 1:227, 1952.
251. Gluckman SJ, Ries K, Abrutyn E: *Allescheria (petrillidium) boydii* sinusitis in a compromised host. J Clin Microbiol 5:481, 1977.
252. Winston DJ, Jordan MC, Rhodes J: *Allescheria boydii* Infections in the immunocompromised host. Amer J Med 63:830, 1977.
253. Bennett JE: Miscellaneous fungi. In: Principles and Practices of Infectious Disease, Man-

dell GL, Douglas RG, Jr, Bennett JE (eds). Wiley & Sons, New York, 1979, p 2080.

254. Lutwick LI, Galgiani JN, Johnson RH et al.: Visceral fungal infections due to *Petrillidium boydii (Allescheria boydii).* Amer J Med 61:632, 1976.

255. Lutwick LI, Rytel MW, Yaniz JP, Galgiani JN, Stevens DA: Deep infections from *Petrillidium boydii* treated with miconazole. JAMA 241:272, 1979.

256. Rippon JW: Piedra. In: Medical Mycology: The Pathogenic Fungi and the Pathogenic Actinomycetes, W.B. Saunders, Philadelphia, 1974, p 91.

257. Yung CW, Hanauer SB, Fretzin D, Rippon JW et al.: Disseminated *Trichosporon beigelii* (cutaneum). Cancer 48:2107, 1981.

258. Gold JWM, Poston W, Mertelsmamm R et al.: Systemic infection with *Trichosporon cutanium* in a patient with acute leukemia. Cancer 48:2163, 1981.

259. Evans HL, Kletzel M, Lawson RD, Frankel LS, Hopfer RL: Systemic mycosis due to *Trichosporon cutanium.* Cancer 45:367, 1980.

260. Winston DJ, Baisley GE, Rhodes J, Linne SR: Disseminated *Trichosporon capitatum* Infection in an immunosuppressed host. Arch Intern Med 137:1192, 1977.

261. Rivera R, Cangir A: Trichosporon sepsis and leukemia. Cancer 36:1106, 1975.

262. Watson KC, Kalichurum S: Brain abscess due to *Trichosporon cutaneum.* J. Med Microbiol 3:191, 1970.

263. Deresinski SC, Stevens DA: Coccidioidomycosis in compromised hosts. Medicine 45:377, 1974.

264. Smith CE, Saito MT: Serologic reactions in coccidioidomycosis. J Chronic Dis 5:571, 1957.

265. Pappagianis K: Coccidioidomycosis. In: Immunological Disease (2nd edition), Samter M (ed). Boston, Little Brown & Company, 1975.

266. Stevens DA: *Coccioides immitis.* In: Principles and Practices of Infectious Disease, Mandell G, Douglas R, Bennett J (eds). New York, Wiley & Sons, 1979, p. 2053.

267. Brass C, Galgiani JN, Campbell SC, Stevens DA: Therapy of disseminated or pulmonary coccidioidomycosis with ketoconazole. Rev Infect Dis 2:656, 1980.

268. Stiller RL, Defelice R, Brass C et al.: Therapy of cutaneous coccidioidomycosis with imidazoles: comparison of results with miconazole and ketoconazole. Fifth Internatl Conference on the Mycoses (PAHO) 396:375, 1980.

269. Graybill JR, Lungberg D, Donovan W et al: Treatment of coccidioidomycosis with ketoconazole. Clinical and laboratory studies in 18 patients. Rev Infect Dis 2:661, 1980.

270. Goodwin Ra, Jr, DesPrez RM: Histoplasmosis. Amer Rev Resp Dis 117:929, 1978.

271. Vanek J, Schwarz J: The gamut of histoplasmosis. Amer J Med 50:89, 1971.

272. Kaplan W: Application of the fluorescent antibody technique to the diagnosis and study of histoplasmosis. In: Histoplasmosis, Proceedings of the Second National Conference. Ajello L, Chick EW (eds). Springville, Illinois, Charles C. Thomas, Chapter 41, 1971.

273. Sarosi GA, Voth DW, Dahl BA et al.: Disseminated histoplasmosis: results of long-term follow-up. Ann Intern Med 75:511, 1971.

274. Furcolow ML: Comparison of treated and untreated severe histoplasmosis. JAMA 183:121, 1963.

275. Negroni R, Robles AM, Arechavala A, Tuculet MA, Galimberti R: Ketoconazole in the treatment of paracoccidioidomycosis and histoplasmosis. Rev Infect Dis 2:643, 1980.

276. Reomarz JZ, Mader JT, Masek JL: Ketoconazole therapy for disseminated histoplasmosis. Presented at the 20th Interscience Conference on Antimicrobial Agents and Chemotherapy, New Orleans, Louisiana, Septembre 22–24, 1980.

3. Platelet Transfusion Therapy for Patients with Cancer

CHARLES A. SCHIFFER

INTRODUCTION

A number of important advances have occurred in the area of platelet transfusion therapy in recent years. As recently as 10 years ago, the greatest problem in many centers was simply obtaining sufficient numbers of units of platelets for the increasing population of patients with cancer and leukemia being treated more intensively and successfully with newer chemotherapeutic agents. Improvements in bag design and plastics, an increased understanding of the many factors which influence platelets during storage, the development of sophisticated and well organized hospital and regional blood centers and the proliferation of apheresis equipment in these centers, have all helped to make platelets readily available in almost all medical centers. Different problems have arisen however which still limit the effectiveness of platelet transfusions in many patients. In particular, the provision of histocompatible platelets for alloimmunized patients remains a difficult and expensive challenge, and this issue and others will be discussed in this review.

PLATELET COLLECTION AND STORAGE

Most platelets for transfusion are prepared as a byproduct of whole blood donation. Platelets are the lightest formed elements in blood and can be effectively separated from red blood cells and most leukocytes by a slow centrifugation of whole blood which produces a supernatant layer termed platelet rich plasma (PRP). PRP is then centrifuged at a higher speed to produce cell free plasma and a platelet pellet which is resuspended in 50–60 ml of residual plasma to form a platelet concentrate (PC). A single PC or

Higby, DJ (ed), Supportive Care in Cancer Therapy. ISBN 0-89838-569-5.
© 1983, Martinus Nijhoff Publishers, Boston. Printed in The Netherlands.

platelet 'unit' should contain about $0.7–0.9 \times 10^{11}$ platelets or approximately 75–80% of the platelets contained in the original unit of blood [1].

A number of studies have demonstrated that PC can be stored prior to transfusion and that stored platelets can maintain near normal transfusion recovery, survival and hemostatic effectiveness [2–5]. Until recently, storage had been limited to 72 hours. Current regulations permit storage of PC for up to five days prior to transfusion. The development of thinner bags constructed of plastics with increased permeability to oxygen permitted this extension of shelf life which should in turn increase platelet availability [6]. Platelets undergo continuous metabolic activity during storage and strict attention must be paid to a number of procedural details to allow adequate platelet preservation even after short periods of storage [2–5]. In general, all of these factors interact to minimize platelet activation and aggregation and allow continued aerobic platelet metabolism. Gentle to and fro agitation, physical separation of the bags, and avoidance of excessively high concentrations of platelets by using adequate plasma volumes when preparing PC, all serve to help guarantee adequate oxygen delivery to the platelets [4]. Decreases in plasma pO_2 with resultant anaerobic metabolism is associated with accumulation of lactate, fall in pH and loss of viability and clinical effectiveness [2]. It is unclear at this time whether it is the fall in pH to levels of 6.1–6.2 per se which is harmful to the platelets or whether the damage is secondary to the depletion of metabolites and the switch to anaerobic metabolism which occurs under certain conditions. This issue is important because buffering systems are available which can maintain pH at near normal levels despite ongoing platelet metabolism [7].

Although published guidelines appear relatively simple, the quality of platelet preparation and storage varies considerably amongst blood centers. There are also possible additional deleterious effects which can occur during transport from blood centers to hospitals. Current mandated 'quality control' testing is minimal and probably inadequate to detect moderate degrees of damage which may occur during collection and storage due to practices in individual blood banks. It is therefore important that clinicians provide careful post transfusion follow-up so that any possible difficulties due to platelet storage can be detected and corrected [8]. This is particularly important as the use of the 'five day' platelet bags increases. It may well be that the major impact of these improved bags will be to better guarantee the quality of platelets stored 48–72 hours rather than to extend storage to five days. This could represent a considerable improvement in the stored products being supplied by many blood centers at this time.

Multiple units of platelets can also be obtained from single donors by repeated manual centrifugation techniques [9] or using a variety of cytopheresis machines. Equipment is available which can process large volumes of blood either in a continuous flow fashion [10, 11] or by an intermittent flow technique which 'batch processes' the blood in a uniquely designed centrifuge bowl [12, 13]. All the available techniques separate platelets by differential centrifugation according to cell density and can produce between 4-12 units of normally functional platelets from one donor in 90-180 minutes. The degree of RBC and lymphocyte contamination varies according to collection technique and some preparations require an additional centrifugation to remove RBC in the case of donor/recipient ABO incompatibility [13]. The collection procedures produce a fall in donor platelet count which generally recovers within 1-2 days, and donors can donate on multiple occasions if required [14]. All of the systems have excellent safety records although symptoms related to hypovolemia or transient hypocalcemia due to chelation by the citrate anticoagulant can occur in some donors. Of theoretic concern is the removal of substantial numbers of lymphocytes which can occur after repeated donations of platelets and granulocytes [15]. No untoward acute or long term immunologic changes have been described and it is unlikely that this is an important issue for most platelet donors particularly as machines are developed which minimize lymphocyte loss [11, 12].

INDICATIONS FOR PLATELET TRANSFUSIONS

The likelihood of hemorrhage in a given thrombocytopenic patient is related to the platelet count, the functional quality of the circulating platelets, the etiology of the thrombocytopenia and the presence of other clinical factors such as coagulation disorders, infection and potential bleeding sites. The decision to administer platelet transfusions depends on an assessment of all these factors. There are few prospective clinical trials to provide guidelines for platelet transfusions in individual patients. In addition, there is no reliable test of in vivo hemostasis which correlates with the onset of bleeding episodes in thrombocytopenic patients.

The template bleeding time is the only standardized test of in vivo platelet function [16, 17]. Small, replicate incisions are made in the forearm, the blood from these incisions is repeatedly absorbed with filter paper and the time to cessation of hemorrhage is recorded. With functionally normal platelets there is an inverse relationship between the bleeding time and the platelet count [17]. As the platelet count falls below 100,000 μl the bleeding time, normally 3-5 minutes, increases in a linear fashion such that at a count of 50,000/μl the bleeding time is approximately 15 minutes. At counts of 20,000 μl or less, the bleeding time is greater than 25-30 minutes and many patients do not stop bleeding from the small incisions. Nevertheless, despite marked prolongation of the bleeding time, many patients do not develop spontaneous hemorrhage at platelet counts of 10,000/µl or below. Conversely, minor hemorrhagic phenomena such as petechiae in dependent areas, occult blood in the stools or microscopic hematuria may develop in some patients at higher platelet counts although they do not necessarily presage the onset of more clinically significant bleeding. In addition, life-threatening hemorrhage can develop rapidly at higher platelet counts and shorter bleeding times during episodes of infection, fever, chemotherapy administration with tumor lysis, and disturbances of coagulation, particularly disseminated intravascular coagulation (DIC). Lastly, diagnostic and therapeutic procedures can be done safely in otherwise stable thrombocytopenic patients at platelet counts (40–50,000/µl) associated with 3–4 fold prolongation of bleeding times. Because of these discrepancies with clinical observations and the cumbersome nature of the test, the bleeding time is used infrequently as a guideline for platelet transfusion therapy.

Platelet transfusions can be administered both to prevent hemorrhage and to slow or stop already established bleeding. Strictly prophylactic platelet transfusions to otherwise stable recipients are usually administered to patients with leukemia and severe (less than 15–20,000/µl) thrombocytopenia who are expected to remain aplastic for weeks following therapy [18]. This general approach has been validated by a prospectively randomized study reported by Higby et al. [19]. Transfusions are administered at the 10–20,000/µl range because it is known that the platelet count is likely to fall further in these intensively treated patients and because it is at these levels that the incidence of serious hemorrhage increases significantly [20, 21]. In addition these patients are usually concurrently granulocytopenic and at risk for infection, have mucosal damage due to chemotherapy and frequently have protracted emesis with increased intracranial pressure and oral and ocular sites of hemorrhage. The impact of these factors on the onset of hemorrhage can be substantial. It is common to observe leukemia patients in relapse who remain hemorrhage free when clinically stable who promptly develop significant bleeding at the same platelet count during or shortly after courses of chemotherapy. Prophylactic transfusions are less often required in patients with solid tumors because of the shorter periods of marrow aplasia which accompany the treatment of these disorders [20, 22] and should not be utilized in stable patients with aplastic anemia because of the indefinite duration of transfusion support which may be required in such patients. These patients must be followed by experienced physicians with ready access to platelet transfusions.

Because many clinical factors influence the development of hemorrhage at any given count, it is often appropriate to administer platelets at higher counts to seriously ill patients with serious infection, DIC, chemotherapy related mucosal injury, and/or 'precarious' sites of tumor involvement (e.g., intracranial tumors). A recent study by Solomon et al. [23] confirmed other clinical observations that the liberal use of platelets, often at platelet counts greater than 20,000 to 30,000/µl in patients in high-risk groups, can effectively prevent hemorrhage in adult patients with acute nonlymphocytic leukemia. These investigators demonstrated that a rapid fall in platelet count from day to day is a helpful clinical clue suggesting a need for transfusion. Thus, for patients with other active clinical problems, it appears that a transfusion policy of this sort is superior to a rigid prophylactic approach based solely on platelet count. In addition, efforts should be made to treat these other medical problems promptly with appropriate antibiotics, antiemetics, heparin for DIC occurring with progranulocytic leukemia, etc. Menses should be also suppressed during periods of thrombocytopenia in younger women as it is usually easier to prevent uterine hemorrhage than to stop bleeding with platelet transfusions.

In seriously ill patients with these or other active medical problems, it is advisable to maintain the platelet count in at least the 20–30,000/µl range. Patients receiving heparin for DIC or patients with high blast counts undergoing treatment with resulting rapid cytolysis should probably have platelet counts of 40–50,000/µl during the first few days of active therapy when their risk of bleeding is highest. There is of course considerable individual variation in the levels at which patients experience bleeding with or without other medical problems. Should bleeding continue at platelet counts greater than 50–60,000/µl, however, one should be concerned that other, 'non-platelet' etiologies (coagulopathy, anatomic causes) are the major cause of the continued hemorrhage.

Although invasive procedures should be minimized in thrombocytopenic patients, many tests (e.g. bone marrow aspirates and biopsies, lumbar punctures) must be done either at diagnosis or during treatment. There are no data which provide guidelines as to the platelet count at which various procedures can be done safely. Some procedures, such as bone marrow aspirates and radial arterial punctures, in which it is possible to apply direct pressure to the puncture site, can clearly be done without undue hazard at counts less than 20,000/µl. If the patient is already scheduled to receive platelet transfusions the same day, however, it is best to perform the procedure after the transfusion if possible. Other procedures, such as bronchoscopy, are more problematic because even a small amount of bleeding can be catastrophic. It is sometimes possible to predict the likelihood of hemorrhage after more extensive procedures by the amount of bleeding which occurred during recent more limited 'trauma' such as the placement of arterial lines, cutdowns, dental work, etc. In general, it has been our experience that larger procedures, including major surgery, can be done safely with platelet counts in the 40–50,000/μl range in the absence of co-agulation abnormalities. Although higher counts may be preferable during and immediately after surgery, it is clearly not necessary to achieve post transfusion counts in the 'normal' range to perform even large-scale abdominal surgery with relative safety [24]. Major procedures should not be done unless an adequate supply of platelets is readily available and unless it has been demonstrated that platelet counts of this level can consistently be achieved and maintained.

The 'dose' of platelets required varies according to the size of the recipient and the desired elevation in platelet count. Because it is not required to raise the platelet count to the normal range to achieve hemostasis, an appropriate level for most patients is a platelet count of 50–70,000/μl one hour after transfusion. As a rough guide, this post-transfusion count can be achieved by transfusion of 1 unit of PC/10 kg of lean body weight. A transfusion to an average, uncomplicated adult should contain 6–8 units of PC and result in an increment of approximately 10,000/μl/unit shortly after transfusion. Approximately 60–70% of transfused platelets are recovered immediately post-transfusion with the remainder being sequestered in the spleen and liver [25]. Normal platelet survival is 8–9 days with a $t\frac{1}{2}$ of about 4 days. It is uncommon to have perfectly normal platelet survival, however, because of the presence of complicating clinical factors in the usual recipients of platelet transfusions. Because of variations in recipient size and the number of platelets in different bags of PC, it is often helpful to express increments using a formula [9] which corrects for these factors:

$$\text{corrected count increment (CCI)} = \frac{\text{Absolute increment} \times \text{body surface area (m}^2)}{\text{\# of platelets transfused } (\times 10^{11})}$$

Thus if a 2 m^2 patient received 3×10^{11} platelets and had an increase in platelet count from 10 to 40,000/μl, the CCI = (30,000/3) × 2 = 20,000. Clinically stable patients have CCI of approximately 20–22,000 one hour post transfusion.

A number of side effects can accompany platelet transfusion, the most common of which are listed in Table 1. The major problem however is the development of alloimmunization with refractoriness to platelets from random donors. Indeed, it is concern about the development of alloimunization which has prompted some investigators to caution against the overuse of prophylactic platelet transfusions. A recent study, however, has demonstrated that there is no relationship between the number of platelet transfusions administered and the development of alloimmunization [40]. For reasons which probably relate to immunosuppression from chemotherapy and the underlying disease, a substantial proportion of patients (40–60%) never

Table 1. Hazards of platelet transfusion.

Side effect	Mechanism	Frequency	Treatment
Transfusion reactions	Alloimmunization to platelets and WBC; IgA deficiency	See text 1/700 patients at risk	Histocompatible platelets; remove leucocytes prior to transfusion [26]; wash and resuspend in plasma-free media [27]
Circulatory congestion	Each transfusion has 300–500 ml of plasma	Particularly in elderly patients or pediatric population	Recentrifuge pooled PC and remove most of plasma; must then be transfused immediately
Post-transfusion hepatitis [28]	Cytomegalovirus, Type 'B', 'Non A, Non B'	Prob. >50% incidence of 'Non A-Non B' hepatitis in leukemia patients receiving multiple transfusions [29]	Improved donor screening with development of assay for 'Non A, Non B' vector
Graft-versus-host disease [30, 31]	Infusion of donor lymphocytes	Extremely rare except in bone marrow transplant recipients or severely immunocompromised hosts	Irradiate (1500 R) blood products; not necessary for adult patients with leukemia or solid tumors
Hemolysis of recipient RBC [32]	Infusion of incompatible plasma	Rare with pooled PC because of small amount of plasma from each donor	Donor antibody screens (not necessary for random donor transfusions)
Alloimmunization to RBC [33, 34]	Infusion of incompatible RBC	Unknown; uncommon to be a major clinical problem	Type-specific platelets (not necessary for routine transfusions); possibly Rh immune globulin for selected Rh negative female recipients
Bacteremia from contaminated platelets [35]	Probable contamination at time of collection with proliferation during storage	Very rare [36, 37] but probably underreported	Strict attention to sterile technique; possibly new sterile docking technology
Alloimmunization to histocompatibility antigens	Development of antibody to platelet/leucocyte antigens	Estimates vary but probably <50% in leukemia patients [34, 38–40] lower in solid tumor patients [41]	See text

become alloimmunized despite receiving large numbers of platelet transfusions over a period of many weeks to months [42]. Conversely, some patients become rapidly sensitized after only a few transfusions. It is not possible to distinguish prospectively between these groups of patients. However, because sensitization does not appear to be 'dose-related', platelet transfusions should not be withheld from severely thrombocytopenic patients expressly to prevent alloimmunization.

MANAGEMENT OF ALLOIMMUNIZATION

Diagnosis

Alloimmunization should be suspected in patients who fail to achieve adequate platelet count increments after transfusion. Although many clinical factors can modify post-transfusion kinetics, in most circumstances platelet survival is affected more profoundly than platelet recovery [43, 44]. Thus, even patients with severe infection or DIC can have relatively normal immediate post-transfusion recoveries accompanied by much shortened survivals. Massive splenomegaly, shock, or perhaps massive hemorrhage represent exceptions to this observation. Alloimmunized patients tend to have both markedly decreased platelet recoveries and survivals [44]. It is therefore usually possible to distinguish alloimmunization from other complicating medical factors by measurement of platelet count increments one hour after transfusion. If poor (CCI less than 5 to 7,000) increments are achieved at 24 hours after transfusion, all such patients should have 1-hour counts done following their next transfusion. One-hour transfusion of CCIs of less than 7,500 are highly suggestive of alloimmunization in the absence of splenomegaly, or overwhelming infection [44]. The 1-hour increment should be done after the transfusion of fresh platelets because it is possible, depending on the quality of storage conditions, that the poor increments observed could be the results of transfusion of partially damaged platelets.

Measurement of lymphocytotoxic antibody, which now can be done at many regional blood centers and hospitals, can help confirm the diagnosis. Antibody measurements are particularly helpful in seriously ill patients with splenomegaly in whom it can be difficult to determine by assessment of count increments alone whether apparent refractoriness is secondary to immune or clinical factors or both. A total of 210 transfusion sequences in 189 patients with acute leukemia treated by our group were analyzed recently [45]. Eighty-eight percent of patients with lymphocytotoxic antibody (cytotoxicity against greater than 20% of a lymphocyte panel) had poor platelet count increments at both 1 and 24 hours after transfusion with only

7 % of the antibody positive patients having good increments at both post-transfusion times. In contrast, only 7 % of patients with negative antibody had poor increments at both 1 and 24 hours. A number of patients had good increments at 1 hour but poor increments at 24 hours and subsequently developed antibody positivity. This suggests that low levels of antibody might have been present at the time of transfusion which was sufficient to affect platelet survival but not platelet recovery.

Donor selection

Platelets have HLA antigens which are shared with all other tissues and tested for most easily on lymphocytes, as well as platelet-specific antigens expressed on their surface [46]. Although antibodies against platelet-specific antigens account for refractoriness in a small percentage of patients [46, 47], most alloimmunized patients can be successfully supported with platelets matched at the HLA and B loci [47–52]. Most alloimmunized patients develop multi-specific antibody (i.e. directed against large numbers of HLA antigens) and because of this are less likely to respond successfully to platelets which are partially matched but also mis-matched for other HLA antigens. Thus, if HLA typing is not immediately available and one attempts to use family members as donors, it is best to utilize sibling donors first.

Because of the extreme polymorphism of the HLA system, the number of perfectly matched donors available per patient is often quite low [53, 54]. Many patients, however, will respond to platelets which are only partially matched and specifically mis-matched for antigens which may be serologically cross-reactive (i.e. antigenically similar) with the patient's antigens [55]. This strategy markedly increases the number of potential donors available per patient although the number of donors may still be limited, particularly when one considers donor non-availability due to illness, vacation, lack of desire to donate on repeated occasions, etc. It is difficult to distinguish serologically between patients who are more or less likely to respond to partially matched platelets. Generally, however, we have noted that patients with antibodies which are cytotoxic against greater than 90 % of the cells in a large panel are likely to respond only to very closely matched platelets. Conversely, patients with cytotoxicity against a smaller number of cells and possibly against a smaller number of antigens, may more often respond to platelets which are either partially matched or mis-matched for cross-reactive antigens.

There have been a number of attempts to analyze which antigens can more likely be successfully mis-matched. Duquesnoy et al. have demonstrated that mis-matches for certain common and probably 'strong' HLA antigens, (e.g. HLA-A2), are usually associated with poor results [59]. Additional patients may also be refractory because of antibodies against the dial-lelic system of W4/W6 [57] or because of an additive effect that ABO mis-matching may have when partially HLA-matched platelets are administered to some alloimmunized patients [58]. Another study did not confirm this latter observation, however [59]. Because HLA-C antigens are weakly ex-pressed on platelets, it is likely that matching for this locus is unimpor-tant [60, 61].

Analyses of large numbers of selectively mis-matched transfusions may provide further clues regarding the relative importance of other antigens. This is of particular importance with respect to antigens such as HLA-B12 which can have variable expression on platelets compared to lymphocytes from the same individual [62]. In many individuals, HLA-B12 is weakly expressed on platelets [62] and platelets mis-matched for HLA-B12 can have normal recoveries and survivals [18, 63] despite positive lymphocyto-toxic cross-matches. The HLA-B12 group [BW 44, 45] is found in approxi-mately 25% of the Caucasian population [64] and therefore it would repre-sent a considerable increase in potential donors if one could routinely mis-match for these or other antigens (e.g. HLA-B8) which may not be fully expressed on platelets [62]. Preliminary analysis of large numbers of trans-fusions performed at the University of Maryland Cancer Center, indicate that at least 50% of transfusions mis-matched for the HLA-B12 group were successful in alloimmunized patients.

PLATELET ANTIBODY TESTING

It is difficult to estimate the incidence of refractoriness due to antibody against platelet specific antigens. Because most investigators present data on transfusions from donor–recipient pairs, it is probable that 'difficult' pa-tients who receive large numbers of unsuccessful transfusions are over-represented in many of these publications. Thus, although a review of the literature suggests that the failure rate of perfectly matched platelet *transfu-sions* is between 15 and 30%, at our center only about 5% of clearly refrac-tory *patients* do not have lymphocytotoxic antibody present [45] and/or are refractory to perfectly HLA matched platelets [46]. In these patients, anti-body directed against the platelet itself could be detected in only about half of the patients [45]. Nonetheless, because of the expense of HLA typing, the failure rate of HLA-matched platelets and the logic that it is best to perform a cross-match with the cell which is actually being transfused, there has been considerable interest in the use of platelet antibody testing as a means of cross-matching for platelet transfusion. Dozens of antiplatelet antibody tests using a variety of different approaches and endpoints are available, this large number probably reflecting the insensitivity and lack of reproducibility of some of these assays [46, 65]. Recently, however, assays [66–69] have become available which are quite sensitive and can measure picogram amounts of platelet-associated IgG (PAIgG). There is preliminary evidence from a number of laboratories that some of these tests may be helpful in selecting donors for refractory patients although it is not clear that the over-all results are superior to selection by HLA typing [47, 70, 71]. None of these assays have been repeated on a large scale to verify their applicability. Further studies are thus necessary prior to utilizing platelet antibody testing for donor selection. In addition, it is mandatory that any platelet cross-matching test be done utilizing some sort of preserved platelets. It is impractical to expect donors to come to the blood center on multiple occasions for cross-matching to return on subsequent dates should the cross-match suggest compatibility.

PREVENTION OF ALLOIMMUNIZATION

There are a number of theoretical approaches by which one might choose to either prevent or modify the pattern of alloimmunization in multiply-transfused patients. Unfortunately, it has been impossible to either prospectively or retrospectively identify groups of patients who are more or less likely to become alloimmunized after receiving multiple blood products [42]. Therefore, any 'prevention strategy' must presently be directed at the entire group of multi-transfused patients and one may be utilizing complex or expensive technology for a large group of patients who would never require histocompatible platelets in any event.

There are experimental data in rodent models to indicate that platelets administered alone without contaminating lymphocytes are minimally if at all immunogenic [72–74]. Administration of a 'pure' population of platelets can provoke an anamnestic response in previously sensitized mice however-er [72, 74]. In canines, the administration of platelets alone infrequently sensitizes recipients of marrow grafts whereas leukocyte 'rich' platelets induce sensitization and subsequent graft rejection [75]. Early observations in humans produced parallel results. It was difficult to sensitize individuals to subsequent skin grafts by the intradermal injection of platelets alone, where-as most individuals became rapidly sensitized following intradermal administration of platelets plus leukocytes [76].

On the basis of these observations, Eernisse and Brand administered leukocyte-depleted platelets to a heterogeneous group of patients and compared the results retrospectively to a group of patients treated in the early 1970s [77]. A markedly decreased rate of alloimmunization was noted in the

56

patients receiving leukocyte-poor platelets, suggesting that this might be a useful approach on a more widespread basis. There are a number of questions to be raised about this most intriguing study, however. First, the retrospectively studied group of patients contained a disproportionate number of multiparous females who may have been previously sensitized. Second, these investigators were able to reduce the leukocyte contamination of standard platelet concentrates to less than 10^7 per unit. It has been difficult in our laboratory, even using the same centrifugation spins, to produce leukocyte depletion of this magnitude. Lastly, patients with different diseases were studied and a variety of types of chemotherapy was administered. Nonetheless, this is a provocative study and we are presently attempting to verify these results in a prospectively randomized study in patients with acute non-lymphocytic leukemia, all of whom are receiving identical cytotoxic therapy. It should also be pointed out that it is necessary to utilize leukocyte-poor blood if one is attempting to eliminate alloimmunization. Our patients all receive frozen blood in an attempt to isolate the antigenic exposure to the platelet transfusions alone. This represents a considerable increase in effort on the part of the blood bank and a marked increase in the expense of blood products for the patient. This factor should be borne in mind should consideration be given to using approaches such as this on a more widespread scale*.

Another approach which has been considered is the use of single donor platelet transfusions which are either closely or partially HLA matched in an effort to prevent alloimmunization. There are no comprehensive published data dealing with this strategy and one can only speculate about the results. One must have initial concern that if closely HLA-matched platelets are utilized, then one might select for the development of antibody against platelet-specific antigens which are extremely difficult to detect reliably at this time. Experiments in dogs by O'Donnell and Slichter [78] indicate that platelet transfusions from DLA-matched litter mates can result in a high incidence of refractoriness probably due to platelet-specific antigens. These same experiments demonstrated an equivalent rate of alloimmunization but a more rapid onset of sensitization when the use of non-matched single donor platelets was compared to a series of pooled PC from multiple random donors. Furthermore, the use of single donor platelets exclusively would strain the pheresis capabilities of most centers so that it would be more difficult to supply histocompatible platelets and granulocytes for patients who clearly need and could benefit from them. In addition, the number of HLA-typed donors available per patient is usually quite limited and the cost of single donor platelets is considerable. Certainly, further information regarding the utility and cost effectiveness is needed before single donor platelets are utilized as standard transfusion support. The current

* *Note added in proof.* Recent analysis of this trial with a total of 98 patients entered on study has failed to demonstrate a significant difference in alloimmunization rate between controls and patients receiving leukocyte-depleted platelets [82].

practice of administering random donor platelets to be followed by single donor platelets should alloimmunization develop, is justified by both economic and scientific reasoning at this time [79].

PLATELET CRYOPRESERVATION

Another approach to the management of alloimmunization is to utilize autologous frozen platelets. In our center, we have organized a program of platelet cryopreservation which has expanded markedly over the last 10 years. Patients with leukemia are platelet-pheresed during remission with the platelets frozen using dimethylsulfoxide (DMSO) for subsequent transfusion during later courses of chemotherapy [80, 81]. Approximately 200–250 autologous transfusions are administered to 30–40 different patients annually. The technology is relative simple and suitable for use in most blood bank settings. An emphasis is placed on obtaining platelets from alloimmunized patients and, in particular, attempts are made to platelet-pherese patients who develop a thrombocytosis upon entering remission, in an effort to harvest as many platelets as possible at a single donation. The

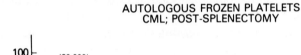

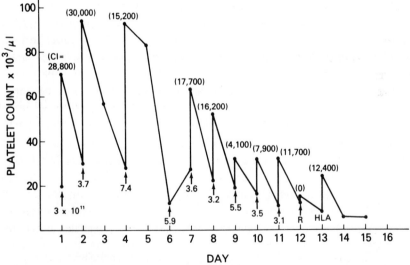

Figure 1. This alloimmunized patient with chronic myelogenous leukemia (CML) in blast crisis was supported with autologous frozen platelets obtained 1–2 years earlier while she was in chronic phase. Advanced pneumonia and bacteremia contributes to shortened platelet survival, although no hemorrhage occurred during a stormy clinical course. R = random donor platelet; CI = corrected increments.

58

patient described in Figure 1 had platelet-pheresis done at a time when her chronic myelogenous leukemia was associated with a high platelet count. The equivalent of ten platelet transfusions were obtained in only two donations. The results using this technology have been quite stable during the years with post-transfusion recovery averaging 60–65% of that expected using fresh platelets with approximately normal post-transfusion survival. For many patients, autologous frozen platelets have represented the only source of platelet transfusion, and without this technology, it would have been difficult to safely administer further maintenance therapy. This approach should also be suitable for the increasing number of patients with hematological malignancies or solid tumors who are receiving very intensive therapy followed by autologous bone marrow rescue.

SUMMARY

Substantial progress has been made in the twelve years since the first reports of HLA-matched platelet transfusion were published. Ongoing research should help to further refine donor selection for alloimmunized patients and reduce the number of unsuccessful transfusions. Randomized studies in progress should help define the role of leukocyte-depleted and single donor platelets as means of preventing or delaying alloimmunization. Whereas in the early 1970s it was unusual to find an unrelated donor compatible with an alloimmunized patient, we now are frustrated when we cannot find large numbers of such donors for our patients on short notice. In addition, improvement in short- and long-term platelet storage methods will likely continue, further increasing the availability of high quality platelets for transfusion. As a consequence of these advances, fewer patients are dying of hemorrhage and are therefore able to receive the potential benefits of more intensive chemotherapy, which has resulted in increased survival and cure in some patients with hematologic malignancies.

REFERENCES

1. Slichter SJ, Harker LA: Preparation and storage of platelet concentrates. Brit J Haemat 34:395–402, 1976.
2. Murphy S, Gardner FH: Platelet storage at 22 °C; metabolic, morphologic and functional studies. J Clin Invest 50:370–377, 1971.
3. Filip DJ, Aster RH: Relative hemostatic effectiveness of human platelets stored at 4 °C and 22 °C. J Lab Clin Med 91:618–624, 1978.
4. Holme S, Vaidja K, Murphy S: Platelet storage at 22 °C: effect of type of agitation on morphology, viability, and function in vitro. Blood 52:425–436, 1978.

5. Slichter SJ, Harker LA: Preparation and storage of platelet concentrates: II. Storage variables influencing platelet viability and function. Brit J Haemat 34:403–418, 1976.
6. Murphy S, Simon T: Characteristics of prolonged platelet storage in a new container. Transfusion 21:637, 1981.
7. Kotelba-Witkowska B, Harmening-Pittiglio DM, Schiffer CA: Storage of platelet concentrates using ion exchange resin charged with dibasic phosphate. Blood 58:537–543, 1981.
8. Schiffer CA: International Forum: What are the parameters to be controlled in platelet concentrates in order that they may be offered to the medical profession as a standardized product with specific properties? Vox Sang 40:122–124, 1981.
9. Daly PA, Schiffer CA, Aisner J, Wiernik PH: A comparison of platelets prepared by the Haemonetics Model 30 and multiunit bag plateletpheresis. Transfusion 19:778–781, 1979.
10. Hester JP, Kellogg RM, Mulzet AP et al.: Variable anticoagulant (AC) flow rates for plateletpheresis in the dual stage disposable channel. Blood 54(Suppl 1):124a, 1979.
11. Katz AJ, Genco PV, Blumberg N et al.: Platelet collection and transfusion using the Fenwal CS-3000 cell separator. Transfusion 21:560–563, 1981.
12. Slichter SJ: Efficacy of platelets collected by semi-continuous flow centrifugation (Haemonetics Model 30). Brit J Haemat 38:131–140, 1978.
13. Aisner J, Schiffer CA, Wolff JH et al.: A standardized technique for efficient platelet and leukocyte collection using the Model 30 Blood Processor. Transfusion 16:437–445, 1976.
14. Schiffer CA, Buchholz DH, Wiernik PH: Intensive multiunit plateletpheresis of normal donors. Transfusion 14:388–394, 1974.
15. Koepke JA, Parks WM, Goeken JA, Klee GG, Strauss RG: The safety of weekly plateletpheresis: effect on the donor's lymphocyte population. Transfusion 21:59–62, 1981.
16. Mielke CH, Kaneshiro MM, Maher IA et al.: The standardized normal Ivy bleeding time and its prolongation by aspirin. Blood 34:204–215, 1969.
17. Harker LA, Slichter SJ: The bleeding time as a screening test for evaluation of platelet function. N Engl J Med 287:155–159, 1972.
18. Schiffer CA, Aisner J, Wiernik PH: Platelet transfusion therapy for patients with leukemia. In: The Blood Platelet in Transfusion Therapy, Greenwalt TJ, Jamieson GA (eds). Alan R. Liss, Inc, New York, 1978, pp 267–279.
19. Higby DJ, Cohen E, Holland JF, Sinks L: The prophylactic treatment of thrombocytopenic leukemic patients with platelets: a double blind study. Transfusion 14:440–446, 1974.
20. Belt RJ, Leite C, Haas CD et al.: Incidence of hemorrhagic complications in patients with cancer. JAMA 239:2571–2574, 1978.
21. Roy AJ, Jaffe N, Djerassi I: Prophylactic platelet transfusions in children with acute leukemia: a dose response study. Transfusion 13:283–290, 1973.
22. Dutcher JP, Schiffer CA, Aisner J, O'Connell BA, Levy C, Kendall JA, Wiernik PH: Incidence of thrombocytopenia and bleeding among patients with solid tumors. Cancer. (In press).
23. Solomon J, Bofenkamp T, Fahey JL et al.: Platelet prophylaxis in acute non-lymphoblastic leukemia. Lancet 1:267, 1978.
24. Simpson MB: Platelet function and transfusion therapy in the surgical patient. In: Platelet Physiology and Transfusion, Schiffer CA (ed). Washington, DC, Amer Assoc Blood Banks, 1978, pp 51–67.
25. Aster RH, Jandl JB: Platelet sequestration in man. I. Methods. J Clin Invest 13:843–852, 1961.
26. Herzig RH, Herzig GP, Bull MI et al.: Correction of poor platelet transfusion responses with leukocyte poor HLA-matched platelet concentrates. Blood 46:743, 1975.
27. Silvergleid AJ, Hafleigh EB, Harabin MA et al.: Clinical value of washed-platelet concentrates in patients with non-hemolytic transfusion reactions. Transfusion 17:33, 1977.
28. Alter HJ, Holland PV, Purcell RH et al.: Post-transfusion hepatitis after exclusion of

60

commercial and hepatitis-B antigen-positive donors. Ann Intern Med 77:691, 1972.
29. Barton JC, Conrad ME: Beneficial effects of hepatitis in patients with acute myelogenous leukemia. Ann Intern Med 90:188, 1979.
30. Cohen D, Weinstein H, Mihm M et al.: Nonfatal graft-versus-host disease occurring after transfusion with leukocytes and platelets obtained from normal donors. Blood 53:1053–1057, 1979.
31. Ford JM, Cullen MH, Lucey JJ et al.: Fatal graft-versus-host disease following transfusion of granulocytes from normal donors. Lancet 2:1167–1172, 1976.
32. Zoes C, Dube VE, Miller HG et al.: Anti-A_1 in the plasma of platelet concentrates causing a hemolytic reaction. Transfusion 17:29, 1977.
33. Goldfinger D, McGinniss MH: Rh-incompatible platelet transfusions-risks and consequences of sensitizing immunosuppressed patients. N Engl J Med 284:942, 1971.
34. Schiffer CA, Lichtenfeld JL, Wiernik PH et al.: Antibody response in patients with acute non-lymphocytic leukemia. Cancer 37:2177–2182, 1976.
35. Buchholz DH, Young VM, Friedman NR et al.: Bacterial proliferation in platelet products stored at room temperature. N Engl J Med 285:429, 1971.
36. Silver H, Sonnenwirth AC, Beisser LD: Bacteriologic study of platelet concentrates prepared and stored without refrigeration. Transfusion 10:315, 1970.
37. Katz AJ, Tilton RC: Sterility of platelet concentrates stored at 25°C. Transfusion 10:329, 1970.
38. Green D, Tiro A, Basiliere J et al.: Cytotoxic antibody complicating platelet support in acute leukemia. JAMA 236:1044, 1976.
39. Howard JE, Perkins HA: The natural history of alloimmunization to platelets. Transfusion 18:496, 1978.
40. Dutcher JP, Schiffer CA, Aisner J et al.: Alloimmunization following platelet transfusion: the absence of a dose response relationship. Blood 57:395-398, 1980.
41. Holohan TV, Terasaki PI, Deisseroth AB: Suppression of transfusion-related alloimmunization in intensively treated cancer patients. Blood 58:122–128, 1981.
42. Dutcher JP, Schiffer CA, CA, Aisner J, Wiernik PH: Long-term follow-up of patients with leukemia receiving platelet transfusions: identification of a large group of patients who do not become alloimmunized. Blood 58:1007-1011, 1981.
43. Slichter SJ: Controversies in platelet transfusion therapy. Ann Rev Med 31:509-540, 1980.
44. Daly PA, Schiffer CA, Aisner J et al.: Platelet transfusion therapy — one hour post-transfusion increments are valuable in predicting the need for HLA-matched preparations. JAMA 243:435-438, 1980.
45. Hogge D, Dutcher J, Aisner J, Schiffer C: Lymphocytotoxic antibody is a predictor of response to random donor platelet transfusion. Am J Hematology. (in press).
46. Schiffer CA: Clinical importance of antiplatelet antibody testing for the blood bank. In: A Seminar on Antigens on Blood Cells and Body Fluids, Bell CA (ed). Washington, DC, Am Assoc Blood Banks, 1980, pp 189–208.
47. Brand A, van Leeuwen A, Eernisse JG et al.: Platelet transfusion therapy. Optimal donor selection with a combination of lymphocytotoxicity and platelet fluorescence tests. Blood 51:781–788, 1978.
48. Yankee RA, Grumet FC, Rogentine GN et al.: Platelet transfusion therapy. The selection of compatible platelet donors for refractory patients by lymphocyte HL-A typing. N Engl J Med 281:1208-1212, 1969.
49. Lohrmann HP, Bull MI, Decter JA et al.: Platelet transfusions from HL-A compatible unrelated donors to alloimunized patients. Ann Intern Med 80:9-14, 1974.
50. Duquesnoy RJ, Filip DJ, Rodey GE et al.: Successful transfusion of platelets 'mismatched'

for HLA antigens to alloimmunized thrombocytopenic patients. Am J Hemat 2:219–226, 1977.

51. Aster RH: Matching of blood platelets for transfusion. Am J Hemat 5:373–378, 1978.
52. Gmur J, von Felten A, Frick P: Platelet support in polysensitized patients: role of HLA specificities and crossmatch testing for donor selection. Blood 51:903–909, 1978.
53. Opelz G, Mickey MR, Terasaki PI: Unrelated donors for bone-marrow transplantation and transfusion support: pool sizes required. Transpl Proc 6:405–409, 1974.
54. Duquesnoy RJ, Vieira J, Aster RH: Donor availability for platelet transfusion support of alloimmunized thrombocytopenic patients. Transpl Proc 9:519–521, 1977.
55. Duquesnoy RJ, Filip DJ, Rodey GE et al.: Successful transfusion of platelets 'mismatched' for HLA antigens to alloimmunized thrombocytopenic patients. Am J Hemat 2:219–226, 1977.
56. Duquesnoy RJ, Filip DJ, Aster RH: Influence of HLA-A2 on the effectiveness of platelet transfusions in alloimmunized thrombocytopenic patients. Blood 50:407–412, 1977.
57. McElligott MC, Menitove JE, Duquesnoy RJ, Hunter JB, Aster RH: Effect of HLA Bw4/Bw6 compatibility on platelet transfusion responses of refractory thrombocytopenic patients. Blood 59:971–975, 1982.
58. Duquesnoy RJ, Anderson AF, Tomasulo PA, Aster RH: ABO compatibility and platelet transfusions to alloimmunized thrombocytopenic patients. Blood 54:595–599, 1979.
59. Tosato G, Applebaum FR, Deisseroth AB: HLA-matched platelet transfusion therapy of severe aplastic anemia. Blood 52:846–854, 1978.
60. Duquesnoy RJ, Filip DJ, Tomasulo PA, Aster RH: Role of HLA-C matching in histocompatible platelet transfusion therapy of alloimmunized thrombocytopenic patients. Transpl Proc 9:1827–1828, 1977.
61. Mueller-Eckhardt G, Hauck M, Kayer W, Mueller-Eckhardt C: HLA-C antigens on platelets. Tissue Antigens 16:91–94, 1980.
62. Aster RH, Szatkowski N, Liebert M, Duquesnoy RJ: Expression of HLA-B12, HLA-B8, w4, and w6 on platelets. Transpl Proc 9:1695–1696, 1977.
63. Thorsby E, Helgesen A, Gjemdal T: Repeated platelet transfusions from HL-A compatible unrelated and sibling donors. Tissue Antigens 2:397–404, 1972.
64. Daly PA, Simon R, Schiffer C et al.: A study of HLA antigens and haplotypes in a population of Caucasians with acute non-lymphocytic leukemia. Leuk Res 3:75–82, 1979.
65. Kahn RA, Harmon JA, Miller MV: Detection of platelet antibodies. In: A Seminar on Immune Mediated Cell Destruction, Bell CA (ed). Amer Assoc Blood Banks, Wash, DC, 1981, pp 151–198.
66. Dixon R, Rosse W, Ebbert L: Quantitative determination of antibody in idiopathic thrombocytopenic purpura. N Engl J Med 292:230–236, 1975.
67. Kr. von dem Borne AEG, Verheugt FWA, Oosterhof F et al.: A simple immunofluorescence test for the detection of platelet antibodies. Brit J Haemat 39:195–207, 1978.
68. Cines DB, Schreiber AD: Immune thrombocytopenia. Use of a Coombs antiglobulin test to detect IgG and C3 on platelets. N Engl J Med 300:106–111, 1979.
69. Gudino M, Miller WV: Application of the enzyme linked immunospecific assay (ELISA) for the detection of platelet antibodies. Blood 57:32–37, 1981.
70. Myers TJ, Kim BK, Steiner M, Baldini MG: Selection of donor platelets for alloimmunized patients using a platelet-associated IgG assay. Blood 58:444–450, 1981.
71. Slichter SJ: Selection of compatible platelet donors. In: Platelet Physiology & Transfusion, Schiffer CA (ed). Amer Assoc Blood Banks, Wash, DC, 1978, pp 83–92.
72. Batchelor JR, Welsh KI, Burgos H: Transplantation antigens per se are poor immunogens within a species. Nature 273-4-56, 1978.
73. Claas FHJ, Smeenk RJT, Schmidt R, van Steenbrugge GJ, Eernisse JG: Alloimmunization

62

against the MHC antigens after platelet transfusions is due to contaminating leukocytes in the platelet suspension. Exp Hematol 9:84–89, 1981.

74. Welsh KI, Burgos H, Batchelor JR: The immune response to allogeneic rat platelets; Ag-B antigens in matrix form lacking Ia. Eur J Immunol 7:263–267, 1977.
75. Storb R, Deeg HG, Weiden PL et al.: Marrow graft rejection in DLA-identical canine littermates: antigens involved are expressed on leukocytes and skin epithelial cells but probably not on platelets and red blood cells. Transpl Proc 9:504–506, 1979.
76. Dausset J, Rapaport FT: Transplantation antigen activity of human blood platelets. Transplantation 4:182–193, 1966.
77. Eernisse JG, Brand A: Prevention of platelet refractoriness due to HLA antibodies by administration of leukocyte-poor blood components. Exp Hematol 9:77–83, 1981.
78. O'Donnell MR, Slichter SJ: Platelet (PLT) alloimmunization – correlation with donor source. Clin Res 27:390, 1979.
79. Schiffer CA, Slichter SJ: Platelet transfusions from single donors. N Engl J Med 307:245–248, 1982.
80. Schiffer CA, Aisner J, Wiernik PH: Frozen autologous platelet transfusion for patient with leukemia. N Engl J Med 299:7–12, 1978.
81. Schiffer CA, Aisner J, Dutcher JR, Daly PA, Wiernik PH: A clinical program of platelet cryopreservation. In: Cytopheresis and Plasma Exchange: Clinical Indications, Vogler WR (ed). Alan R. Liss Inc, 1982, pp 165–180.
82. Schiffer CA, Dutcher J, Aisner J et al.: A randomized trial of leukocyte-depleted platelet transfusion to modify alloimmunization in patients with leukemia. Blood 60: 182a, 1982.

4. Granulocyte Transfusion Therapy

DONALD J. HIGBY

INTRODUCTION AND BACKGROUND

There is much controversy surrounding granulocyte transfusion therapy today. Questions about the clinical utility of granulocyte transfusions once thought to be settled are now rightly being raised again. A historical perspective is useful as a first step towards addressing this issue.

In the 1960s, the speciality of medical oncology began to develop in response to the discovery that in a few rare malignancies chemotherapy was occasionally curative and often palliative. For example, the attitude towards patients with leukemia changed from one of hopelessness to one of hope. The discovery that cytosine arabinoside was strikingly effective in remission induction of acute myeloid leukemia (compared to previous agents) led investigators to develop more intensive regimens in an attempt to improve remission rate and remission duration. It became possible to eradicate leukemia, and the consequences of pancytopenia became the major problem facing the clinician. The demonstration that platelet transfusions could control the consequences of thrombocytopenia left infection as the major cause of death during remission induction [1, 2]. However, the management of the neutropenic patient was hampered by the availability of effective antibiotics and there was inadequate understanding of why these patients became infected. A survey of the literature on the subject during this period reflects the state of the art; five-drug antibiotic combinations were advocated [3] and total gut sterilization was attempted [4]. A surge of interest in total protected isolation led to the construction of laminar flow units at great expense in several centers; even books, games, and writing materials were sterilized before they could be used by the patient. Nevertheless, results of such studies were disappointing [5–8].

In those days, remission induction for acute myelocytic leukemia often was followed by four to eight weeks of bone marrow aplasia. Seminal stud-

Higby, DJ (ed), Supportive Care in Cancer Therapy. ISBN 0-89838-569-5.
© *1983, Martinus Nijhoff Publishers, Boston. Printed in The Netherlands.*

ies by Bodey [9] showed that the rate of acquisition of infection rose as the duration of neutropenia increased. This was also the period in which Freireich and his colleagues began to use buffy coats from patients with chronic myelocytic leukemia to replace granulocytes in these patients [10, 11], and the impressive results of this therapy led to the development of in-line centrifugation equipment for extracting granulocytes from normal individuals for the same purpose [12]. Filtration leukapheresis, invented by Djerassi, came to the forefront as an alternate method for collection of large quantities of transfusable granulocytes [13]. For a while, granulocyte procurement technology proliferated and granulocyte transfusions became available to patients in most larger centers where leukemia was agressively treated.

Three developments followed. First, it was found that the combination of anthracycline antibiotics and cytosine arabinoside not only greatly increased remission rates for patients with acute myeloid leukemia, but in addition, the use of this combination was associated with a marked reduction in the duration of the post-induction pancytopenia. In our institution, the median time to remission prior to and following the institution of these newer regimens dropped from 42 days to 28 days. Second, the development of improved broad spectrum antibiotic agents (the cephalosporins, the aminoglycosides, and the synthetic antipseudomonal penicillins) greatly improved the ability to manage intercurrent infections. Third, as granulocyte collection became commonplace, attention to quality, quantity, storage conditions, and rational use of granulocyte concentrates became more lax. In sum, the great strides in management of the neutropenic leukemic patient coupled with the much broader definition of what constitutes a granulocyte transfusion, have led to current questions about the exact role of granulocytes in the management of the patient undergoing remission induction for acute leukemia.

Today, there are few who would advocate granulocyte transfusions for every patient (or even every seriously infected patient) with neutropenia. There are others who have come to believe that such transfusions have no value at all in the management of such patients. It is not unlikely that with further developments in infection prevention and treatment, and increasing specificity of cancer treatments, a day will come when granulocyte transfusion therapy will become a historical curiosity. However, the short-term, rational use of granulocyte concentrates will continue to salvage some patients who would otherwise expire.

PROCUREMENT

Granulocyte concentrates can be prepated in several ways. Simple bag apheresis and buffy coat concentration can be used to obtain functional

polymorphonuclear neutrophils from patients with untreated chronic myelocytic leukemia (CML); larger yields can be obtained using in-line centrifugation equipment. These granulocytes are functionally normal or near-nor-
mal and still constitute the only reasonable source of extremely large doses
of granulocytes. In addition to the problems having to do with alloimmunization (common to all blood products), untreated CML patients are rare.
Of theoretical concern is the possibility that the disease (CML) can be transmitted in this way, although the evidence for this is lacking.

More commonly, granulocyte concentrates are prepared by in-line centrifugation equipment (Figure 1). One system exists in which blood is with-
drawn, buffy coat is collected, and red cells and plasma recombined and
returned to the donor in a continuous operation. Other instruments withdraw aliquots of donor blood, remove the buffy coat, and return the red
cells and platelets to the donor in an intermittent fashion. With both the
continuous and intermittent systems, the conduit for blood is closed and
disposable and the devices are automated and require only moderate oper-
ator skill. The ability to obtain transfusable numbers of granulocytes from
normal donors obviates several problems existing when granulocytes are
obtained from donors with chronic leukemia: a much larger donor pool
exists; the theoretical objection to using 'malignant' cells is met; and per-

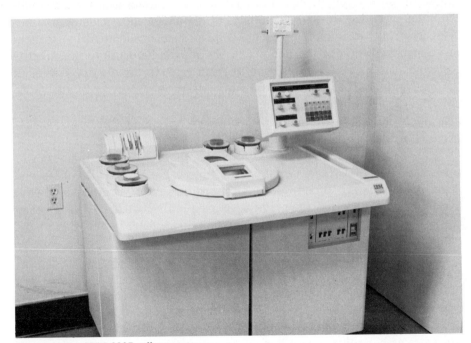

Figure 1. The IBM 2997 cell separator.

haps most importantly, donors can be selected so that alloimmunization problems can be overcome.

Hydroxyethyl starch is often used in conjunction with these instruments to cause roleux formation of red blood cells and more rapid sedimentation as a result [14], and many investigators administer glucocorticosteroids to donors prior to the procedure to provoke a neutrophilic leukocytosis and thus increase substantially the yield of granulocytes [15, 16. 17]. Both adjunctive pharmaceutical maneuvers are extremely safe.

'Filtration' leukapheresis is not widely used at present. This technique involves the passage of heparinized donor blood over nylon wool filters. Granulocytes adhere to the fibers while cells of other types pass through and are returned to the donor. After loading the filters, granulocytes can be eluted by rising with a calcium-chelating agent such as acid citrate dextrose (ACD) or EDTA [13, 18]. Although very large yields were possible, granulocytes prepared by this technique showed varying functional defects: they did not circulate well; chemotactic properties were diminished; and transfusion reactions were high [19]. Of greatest concern, however, was the demonstration of complement activation in the donor [20] and the incidence of donor reactions ranging from mild fever and chills to more serious disorders such as priapism requiring surgical correction [21] and cramping pelvic pain with occasional vaginal spotting in women [22].

Also, those working in this field have noted a variation in the quality of the filters provided, so that side effects in the donor and yields of granulocytes were not predictable. Although it is probable that attention to adequate heparinization of the donor and the concomitant use of glucocortiscosteroids can greatly diminish the reaction rates in the donors as well as the recipients and improve the function of the granulocytes in the product [23, 24], the wide availability of the more dependable centrifugation instruments and improvements in their design have made 'filtration' leukapheresis a rarely used procedure.

Djerassi has described a method for obtaining transfusable quantities of granulocytes from a single donor by multiple bag pheresis without special instrumentation [25]. Blood collected is sedimented after admixture with hydroxyethyl starch, and the granulocyte-rich buffy coat obtained can then be separated with standard blood bank equipment. After red cells and plasma are returned to the donor, second and subsequent procedures can be performed so that a single donor can provide in a few hours, a yield of granulocytes sufficient for a transfusion. Although this procedure is not widely used, it is extremely inexpensive and does not require technical skills other than those necessary in the operation of any blood procurement center. Blood product suppliers who rarely are required to obtain granulocyte concentrates have this method as an option.

Finally, granulocyte concentrates are prepared in some centers as a by-product of platelet-pheresis. In-line centrifugation equipment used for platelet collection can be adjusted so that buffy coats can also be collected. Pools of buffy coats, either from the same donor or from multiple donors having the same blood type, can so be obtained and issued as granylocyte concentrates.

GRANULOCYTE KINETICS

The granulocyte mass in man is primarily extravascular. In an uninfected individual, autologous labeled granulocytes are cleared from the circulation with a half-time of about 3–6 hours [26]. Granulocytes in the circulation are essentially in transit from the marrow to tissues and studies on animals and man with transiently induced aplasia indicate that with recovery, the marrow compartment, the marginated pool, and tissue areas with heightened chemotactic stimulus (infected areas, etc.) are repopulated with granulocytes before the circulating pool is filled [27]. The common observation that patients recovering from remission induction therapy for acute leukemia often show defervescence, clearing of infection, and improvement in their physical condition several days before the end of their neutropenic period, illustrates this phenomenon.

For these reasons, a given granulocyte transfusion to a neutropenic patient results in a markedly lower increment relative to total cells transfused than does a transfusion of red blood cells or platelets, both of which remain predominantly in the circulation as demonstrated by autologous transfusion experiments. Nevertheless, a granulocyte transfusion should contain sufficient cells so that a measurable circulating increment is seen at one hour following the transfusion. The increment is obviously dependent on fever, severity of infection, blood volume of the recipient, and alloimmunization of the recipient, but a detectable increment at least assures that the cells available for treatment of infection are at a workable threshold. Studies have indicated that doses of cells of at least 10^{10} should be used in a granulocyte transfusion [28, 29], and the larger the dose, the better. In many of the 'negative' clinical experiments, significantly smaller doses of granulocytes were given [30, 31], whereas in contrast, the most dramatic results associated with granulocyte transfusion therapy have been noted when very large doses of chronic myelocytic leukemia polymorphonuclear neutrophils were used [32, 11].

GRANULOCYTE CONCENTRATE STORAGE

Polymorphonuclear neutrophilic leukocytes are highly reactive endstage cells, which after activation rapidly undergo autolytic processes [19, 33, 34].

The cells are metabolically active–more so than platelets or red blood cells. Under ideal conditions, granulocytes may be preserved intact for 24–48 hours [35], although under the conditions available in most blood banks, the antibiotic efficacy of granulocytes deteriorates with time so that far less granulocytes are functional at 24 hours. Time in transit or on a hospital ward prior to transfusion, can further shorten their useful life. As such, it is best to arrange transfusion of granulocytes on the same day as procurement.

TRANSFUSION

Granulocytes obtained by centrifugation or sedimentation techniques can be transfused relatively easily. A granulocyte concentrate consisting of $1-5 \times 10^{10}$ freshly obtained neutrophilic leukocytes should be administered over a period of one hour. Other reasons than donor alloimmunization can cause mild transfusion reactions, and simple fevers and chills occurring during administration can be managed by temporarily stopping the transfusion, medicating the patient with meperidine intravenously, and then continuing the infusion at a slower rate unless further reaction supervenes. Patients with pulmonary infections or tumors in the lung parenchyma should be observed especially carefully, since untoward pulmonary reactions occur most frequently in this group [36].

CLINICAL USES

Under what circumstances should granulocyte transfusions be used? There are still physicians caring for patients with compromised host defenses, who begin granulocyte transfusions for neutropenia. More disturbing, because it is more widespread, is the use of granulocytes as a substitute for an intelligent approach to the problems of the patient. A patient who is neutropenic and who seems to be deteriorating despite 'broad spectrum' antibiotic therapy must be carefully examined for remediable problems – intravenous cathether infection, abscess, or bronchial inspissation, for example. The possibilities of systemic viral or fungal infections must also be considered. Sometimes antibiograms of offending pathogens are misleading and organisms such as *Staphylococcus epidermis,* although showing disc sensitivity to cephalosporins, may not respond to these in vivo [37]. It is highly likely that many of the 'successful' experiences with granulocyte transfusions in the memory of a practitioner were in actual fact not related to granulocyte transfusions at all, but to marrow recovery, effective antibiotic therapy, or other intercurrent events. Nevertheless, there are clinical situations in which granulocyte transfusions have shown efficacy even in studies reported as 'negative' [39, 42].

Prophylactic use

Random donor granulocyte transfusions are probably not useful to prevent infection in patients undergoing periods of bone marrow aplasia. This is evident not only from clinical studies [38–42], but also from considerations of kinetics; in the absence of infection, granulocytes administered traverse the circulation fairly rapidly and offer 'protection' only during a brief period. Although it is possible that frequent granulocyte transfusions (several times a day) in adequate doses (10^{10} cells or more) could prevent infection, the cost effectiveness and logistics of such an approach make it unworkable. Perhaps the only exception to the rule that prophylactic granulocyte transfusions are of no use would be in the circumstances where granulocytes from a HLA-matched bone marrow donor were used for prophylaxis in the recipient. In fact, Clift's study does indicate that such transfusions are prophylactic [43].

Therapeutic use

A survey of centers treating bone marrow transplant patients and leukemia patients undergoing remission induction therapy does not help in determining when granulocyte transfusions should be administered. Clearly, some centers previously committed to such transfusions now no longer use them, and it is assumed that this would not be the case if definite benefit had been noted. On the other hand, some centers continue to use such transfusions fairly liberally in such patients and one might infer that benefit is perceived by these investigators.

There are several studies in the literature comparing a series of patients treated with granulocyte transfusions with a historical control. Most studies argue that granulocyte transfusions are of benefit [10, 11, 44, 45]. However, an examination of studies in which concurrently treated control groups were also analyzed is instructive.

The first such study was that of Graw, in which patients who had received more than four granulocyte transfusions were noted to have a marked survival advantage when compared to concurrently treated controls in which similar clinical situations had existed [46]. Herzig's later study randomized only patients with neutropenia and septicemia to receive or not receive granulocyte transfusions. Here again, a survival advantage was noted [47]. In Vogler's study, patients with septicemia benefited most by granulocyte transfusions [48]. Our study [49] and that of Alavi [50] also concluded that granulocyte transfusions were effective.

However, other studies did not show benefit. Fortuny's study found no difference in any parameters studied between the treated and control group, although survival rate for his control group was somewhat higher than in the previously mentioned studies and the doses of granulocytes administered were, on the average, somewhat lower than the 'positive' studies [30]. Perhaps the largest study of whether granulocytes benefit infected, neutropenic patients is that of Winston, which suggests no advantage to their use [31]. However, again rather small doses of granulocytes were used to provide a single transfusion and the control group had a very high survival rate.

We believe that granulocyte transfusions are of adjunctive benefit in a proportion of neutropenic febrile patients undergoing therapy with broad spectrum antibiotics, but that equal results might be obtainable by more aggressive and earlier use of other antibiotics than those used in the primary regimen for broad spectrum coverage. Thus, therapeutic recommendations are made with the caveat that administration of granulocyte transfusions in these circumstances is not necessarily the only effective way to manage the problem.

Septicemia. Neutropenic patients with septicemia in the face of effective antibiotic coverage should probably receive granulocyte transfusions. In such patients, the clearest results vis-à-vis their effectiveness have been shown. Furthermore, in the study by Strauss [42] testing the prophylactic value of granulocyte transfusions, the only noticeable benefit was that the transfused patients had significantly less septicemia. Our practice is to institute granulocyte transfusions in these patients as soon as possible, especially in the face of hemodynamic instability. When sufficient doses of granulocytes are given, dramatic responses continue to be seen.

Pneumonitis. Bacterial pneumonia in neutropenic patients, which do not respond to appropriate antibiotic therapy, is also an indication for granulocyte transfusions. Here, it is important to consider bronchoscopy and bronchial washings to identify the suspected pathogen with certainty and also to remedy bronchial obstruction if it exists. Severe pneumonia associated with serious blood gas abnormalities, may respond to granulocyte transfusions, but in our experience, there may be transient worsening of the respiratory problem possibly by the augmented inflammatory response produced. In addition, granulocyte aggregation in the pulmonary vasculature is a well-described phenomenon in alloimmunized patients, and this too may worsen the already percarious pulmonary status.

Other localized infections. Although the migration of transfused granulocytes to sites of localized infection has been demonstrated [51], the risks of granulocyte transfusion should be carefully weighed against the possible benefits. If the infection is not likely to threaten the life of the patient and is likely to clear once marrow recovery takes place, granulocyte transfusions may be helpful, but are not necessary.

Enterocolitis. Severe enterocolitis may complicate marrow ablative chemotherapy and its occurrence is often fatal. We have not seen benefit from granulocyte transfusions in this situation. This is understandable – the life-threatening manifestations are probably the consequence of toxins and localized mucosal injury rather than directly due to the infecting organism, and treatment directed at these problems may be more effective.

Fevers of unknown origin. In febrile, neutropenic patients where the source of infection and the pathogen are not identified, our practice is to introduce granulocyte transfusions if in our opinion the patient is deteriorating. Usually, such patients begin their course with temperatures that seldom increase above 39 °C; patients look well, eat, and ambulate. Increasing temperature associated with rigors, prostration, and other symptoms of worsening can supervene, but often in such circumstances, further diagnostic studies indicate the offending pathogen. When such is not the case, institution of granulocytes empirically may be useful.

Monitoring granulocyte transfusion therapy

Introduction of granulocyte transfusions into a therapeutic regimen requires careful monitoring to determine whether sufficient effective granulocytes are being administered to produce an effect. The number of neutrophils infused should be known as well as the time elapsed from procurement to infusion. Inadequate doses stored for more than 24 hours are useless and often harmful. An immediate or one-hour post-transfusion blood sample should be obtained to determine whether an increment has been produced. Although benefit can be seen without actually producing an increment in the peripheral blood, if benefit does not occur, the lack of an increment may mean that an insufficient number of granulocytes was used. If the patient develops fevers, chills, or other untoward side effects from a granulocyte transfusion, it is probably reasonable to assume that little benefit has been obtained (see below). In such a case. it may be useful to restrict the donor pool for the patient to similar or matched tissue type donors, or alternatively, to premedicate patients with glucocorticosteroids. Fever and chills occurring with centrifuge- or sedimentation-procured granulocytes should probably be attributed to alloimmunization until proven otherwise.

Clinical parameters should be monitored carefully as well. Are the temperature peaks getting lower? Are repeat blood cultures in the patient treated for sepsis now clear? Is the patient feeling better? Although one cannot always attribute such improvements to granulocyte transfusions, lack of improvement should signal the attending physician that the whole therapeutic plan is inadequate. In patients with localized infection, margination, pus formation, and reduction in redness and local edema should follow institution of effective granulocyte transfusion therapy. In patients with pneumonia, regression of the lesion on chest X-ray, increased sputum production, and improvement in clinical condition have the same meaning.

Frequency and duration of granulocyte transfusion therapy

Kinetic considerations suggest that the ideal frequency of granulocyte transfusions should be on the order of every six hours. This is almost never done. Standard practice is to administer a granulocyte concentrate daily. However, we have on occasion increased frequency when daily transfusions were ineffective with good results.

Granulocyte transfusions should be continued for at least five to seven days before judgment is made as to their effectiveness. Patients who show dramatic clinical improvement without resolution of their neutropenia but who still remain febrile, often continue to do well after discontinuing granulocyte transfusions. We normally discontinue transfusions at five to seven days and reinstitute them if deterioration follows.

Complications

General. The use of granulocyte transfusions is not without potentially serious complications. Granulocytes procured using reversible adhesion (filtration leukapheresis) are associated with a reaction rate in recipients of from 15 to 40% [52]. These reactions range from mild fever and chills to wheezing and respiratory distress. Complement activation, release of intracytoplasmic contents into peripheral circulation, and aggregation of damaged cells may account for much of this. With centrifugation- or sedimentation-procured cells, reaction rates are less – 5–15%. In most cases, alloimmunization is probably the reason, although aggregation and complement activation may also occur. Usually these acute reactions can be managed by discontinuing the transfusion and supporting the patient to the degree necessary; such reactions usually resolve in 30–60 minutes. Meperidine 25 mg intravenously may abort chills, and glucocorticosteroids are often useful in the more severe respiratory complications. If reactions are mild and short-lived, the remainder of the granulocytes may be administered at a slower rate, and reactions often do not re-occur.

Alloimmunization. Granulocyte transfusions administered to an alloimmunized donor may cause adverse effects such as fever, chills, and agglutination of granulocytes in the pulmonary capillaries giving rise to transient respiratory distress. The detection of alloimmunization against granulocytes is not easily done in the laboratory. Ungerleider found no predictive value with several different methods of detecting antileukocyte antibodies [53]. However, Appelbaum has shown that animals sensitized to donor granulocytes when given donor granulocytes after being made neutropenic, show lower post-transfusion increments, a poor chemotactic response, and profound thrombocytopenia when compared to unsensitized animals [54]. More clinically relevant perhaps, is the study by Westrick, which demonstrated that dogs previously sensitized to whole blood transfusions did not benefit from granulocyte transfusions compared to those which had not been sensitized. Furthermore, sensitization could not be detected by cytotoxicity assays in most animals [55].

Thus, patients in which alloimmunization is suspected because of previous transfusion history or laboratory studies may not profit from random granulocyte transfusions and may require HLA similar or identical donors.

It should also be pointed out that, in the study by Schiffer of prophylactic granulocyte transfusions, a marked increase in the rate and degree of alloimmunization to other blood products in the treated group was noted [39]. Currently, patients with acute leukemia and other malignant disorders may have to undergo several periods of pancytopenia in the course of their treatment, and indiscriminate use of granulocyte transfusions may impair the effectiveness of future blood product support with potentially serious consequences.

Amphotericin B and granulocyte transfusions. Patients receiving amphotericin B and granulocyte transfusions simultaneously show an increased incidence of serious pulmonary reactions probably due to cell membrane altering effects of the antifungal agent [56, 57]. However, this observation has been disputed [58]. When both are used together, it is our policy to premedicate the patient with steroids before the administration of granulocytes and to administer the granulocytes several hours before or after the amphotericin dose. With this approach, we have not seen pulmonary reactions.

Cytomegalovirus transmission. A number of reports have shown an association between the acquisition of cytomegalovirus infection (or at least serologic conversion) and the administration of granulocyte transfusions [59]. In some randomized studies, other blood product use was similar in both groups and thus granulocyte transfusions were likely the transmitting agent [40–42]. In areas where CMV is endemic among donors, it is probably best to use screened donors for granulocyte procurement. CMV transmission is probably not of great consequence in most patients undergoing standard remission induction therapy for acute leukemia, but is a serious complication in bone marrow transplant patients.

Graft versus host reaction. Granulocyte transfusions have been implicated as a cause of graft vs host reaction, which is usually fatal in this situation [60]. Although the incidence is low, even among susceptible populations (patients with Hodgkin's disease, severely immunocompromised patients, etc.), it is good practice to irradiate granulocytes and other blood products to at least 1500 rads when the equipment is available.

WHY GRANULOCYTE TRANSFUSIONS WORK: A HYPOTHESIS

The most obvious effect of granulocyte transfusion therapy is the clearing of sepsis in the pancytopenic patient. This clearing continues long beyond the transit time of granulocytes in the circulation. The model developed by Epstein in dogs suggests that a single granulocyte transfusion may prolong the appearance of bacteremia for even a few days after the injection of pathogenic organisms [61]. We know that most infections occurring early in the course of neutropenia (which are identified) are due to enteric flora [62]. We also know that the incidence of fevers of unknown origin in patients with drug-induced neutropenia is relatively high – in one large study, 43% of infections [62]. Finally, we know that tissue macrophages persist after chemotherapy or radiotherapy for prolonged periods of time, even after the disappearance of more short-lived phagocytes [63].

Thus, infection in the neutropenic patient may be such that residual host defenses, antibiotic therapy, and pathogen load exist in a precarious balance (Type I infection), and when this is the case, patients may co-exist with their pathogen until marrow recovery. When the balance is in favor of the pathogen, then bacteremia, resultant toxin production and endothelial damage, and other secondary events may result in worsening of the patient's condition (Type II infection). This may be a forme fruste of septic shock (and thus not recognized as such) because it is known that granulocytes enter into the cascade of events responsible for the clinical syndrome [64]. Granulocyte transfusions may act to convert a Type II infection to a Type I infection by shifting the balance in favor of host defenses. Perhaps the prolonged effect of granulocyte transfusions relative to their half-life and the observed efficacy of transfusions prepared by reversible leuko-adhesion (which do not circulate to any great extent) [49] is due to a blood-clearing effect of marginated granulocytes, which continue to ingest organisms long after disappearance from the circulation. In fact, studies with indium oxine labelled granulocytes show that the label persists for as long as 24 to 48 hours after transfusion in liver, lungs, and spleen – the very organs which contain large numbers of macrophages [65].

This hypothesis would explain why granulocytes are not particularly useful as prophylaxis against infection; why their use seldom results in rendering the patient afebrile; and why seemingly small doses of granulocytes can exert an obvious therapeutic benefit.

SUMMARY

The reader may surmise that the author is not enthusiastic about recommending granulocyte transfusions. This was not the intent; rather, an attempt was made to present a balanced perspective. The indications for granulocyte transfusions are fewer than in the past, but used judiciously, they still can rescue patients from otherwise fatal infections. The clinician should continue to be prepared to institute properly prepared transfusions of granulocytes to infected, neutropenic patients who continue to deteriorate despite intelligent and aggressive medical management. Not infrequently, a life will be saved.

REFERENCES

1. Han T, Stutzman L, Cohen E: Effects of platelet transfusions on hemorrhage in patients with acute leukemia. Cancer 19:1937–42, 1966.
2. Higby DJ, Cohen E, Holland JF: The prophylactic treatment of thrombocytopenic leukemia patients with platelets: a double blind study. Transfusion 14(5):440–446, 1974.
3. Tattersall M, Spiers AS, Darrel JH: Initial therapy with combination of five antibiotics in febrile patients with leukemia and neutropenia. Lancet, January 22, 1972, pp 162–165.
4. Preisler HD, Goldstein IM, Henderson ES: Gastrointestinal sterilization in the treatment of patients with acute leukemia. Cancer 26:1076–1081, 1970.
5. Bodey GP, Gehan EA, Freireich EJ: Protected environment-prophylactic antibiotic program in the chemotherapy of acute leukemia. Am J Med Sci 262:138–151, 1971.
6. Levine AS, Siegel SE, Schreiber AD: Protected environment and prophylactic antibiotics: a prospective controlled study of their utility in the therapy of acute leukemia. New Engl J Med 288:477–483, 1973.
7. Schimpff SC, Greene WH, Young VM: Infection prevention in acute non-lymphocytic leukemia. Ann Intern Med 82:351–358, 1975.
8. Yates JW, Holland JF: A controlled study of isolation and endogenous microbial suppression in acute myelocytic leukemia patients. Cancer 32:1490–1498, 1973.
9. Bodey GP, Buckley M, Sathe YS: Quantitative relationships between circulating leukocytes and infection in patients with acute leukemia. Ann Intern Med 64:328–336, 1966.
10. Freireich EJ, Levin RH, Carbone PP: The function and fate of transfused granulocytes from donors with chronic myelocytic leukemia in leukopenic recipients. Ann NY Acad Sci 113:1081, 1965.

11. Bussel A, Benbunan M, Grange MJ, Boiron M, Bernard J: Comparison of clinical results induced by irradiated and non-irradiated chronic myelocytic leukemia cell transfusions and the relationship to in vitro studies. In: Leukocytes: Separation, Collection and Transfusion, Goldman JM, Lowenthal RM (eds). London, Academic Press, 1975, pp 395–401.

12. Freireich EJ, Judson G, Levin RH: Separation and collection of leukocytes. Cancer Res 25:1511–1514, 1965.

13. Djerassi I, Kim JS, Mitrakul C, Suvansri U, Ciesielka W: Filtration leukapheresis for separation and concentration of transfusable amounts of normal human granulocytes. J Med (Basel) 1:358–362, 1970.

14. Mishler JM: Hydroxyethyl starch as an experimental adjunct to leukocyte separation by centrifugal means: review of safety and efficacy. Transfusion 15:449–460, 1975.

15. Mishler JM: The effects of corticosteroids on mobilization and function of neutrophils. Exp Hematol 5 (Suppl 1):15–32, 1977.

16. Nusbacher J, MacPherson JL, Manejias RE, Bennett JM: Leukapheresis: The effect of a single high oral dose of prednisone on granulocyte mobilization, yield and function. Transfusion 13:366, 1973.

17. Mishler JM, Higby DJ, Rhomberg W, Cohen E, Nicora RW, Holland JF: Hydroxyethyl starch and dexamethasone as an adjunct to leukocyte separation with the IBM blood cell separator. Transfusion 14:352–356, 1974.

18. Higby DJ, Salvatori V, Burnett D, Park BH: Improving the quality of granulocytes obtained by filtration leukapheresis. Exp Hematol 7 (Suppl 4):36–41, 1979.

19. Wright DG, Klock JC: Functional changes in neutrophils collected by filtration leukapheresis and their relationship to cellular events that occur during adherence of neutrophils to nylon fibers. Exp Hematol 7 (Suppl 4):11–23, 1979.

20. Nusbacher J, Rosenfeld SI, Leddy J, Kelmperer M, MacPherson JL: The leukokinetic changes and complement activation associated with filtration leukapheresis. Exp Hematol 7 (Suppl 4):31–35, 1979.

21. Duhlke MB, Shah SL, Sherwood WC et al.: Priaprism during filtration leukapheresis. Transfusion 19:482–487, 1979.

22. Wiltbank TB, Nusbacher J, Higby DJ, MacPherson JL: Abdominal pain in donors during filtration leukapheresis. Transfusion 17:159–162, 1977.

23. Wright DG, Kauffman JC, Chusid MJ, Herzig GP, Gallin JI: Functional abnormalities of human neutrophils collected by continuous flow filtration leukapheresis. Blood 46:901–911, 1975.

24. Higby DJ, Henderson ES, Burnett D, Cohen E: Filtration leukapheresis: effects of donor stimulation with dexamethsone. Blood 50:953–959, 1977

25. Djerassi I: Gravity leukapheresis – a new method for collection of transfusable granulocytes. Exp Hematol 5 (Suppl 1):139–143, 1977.

26. Boggs DR: The kinetics of neutrophilic leukocytes in health and disease. Seminars in Hematology 4:359–386, 1967.

27. Craddock CG, Perry S, Lawrence JS: The dynamics of leukopenia and leukocytosis. Ann Intern Med 52:281–293, 1960.

28. Higby DJ: Controlled prospective studies of granulocyte transfusion therapy. Exp Hematol 5 (Suppl 1):57–64, 1977.

29. Strauss RG: Therapeutic neutrophil transfusions: Are controlled studies no longer appropriate? Am J Med 65:1001–1005, 1978.

30. Fortuny IE, Bloomfield CD, Hadlock DC, Goldman A, Kennedy BJ, McCullough JJ: Granulocyte transfusion: a controlled study in patients with acute non-lymphocytic leukemia. Transfusion 15:548–558, 1975.

31. Winston DJ, Ho WG, Gale RP: Therapeutic granulocyte transfusions for documented infec-

tions: a controlled trial in ninety-five infectious granulocytopenic episodes. Ann Intern Med (in press).

32. Lowenthal RM, Grossman L, Goldman JM, Storring RA, Buskard NA, Park DS, Murphy BC Galton DAG: Granulocyte transfusion therapy: a comparison of the use of cells obtained from normal donors with those from patients with chronic granulocytic leukemia. In: Leukocytes: Separation, Collection, and Transfusion, Goldman JM, Lowenthal RM (eds). London, Academic Press, 1975, pp 363–379.

33. McCullough J, Weiblen J, Deinard AR, Boen J, Fortuny IE, Quie PG: In vitro function and post-transfusion survival of granulocytes collected by continuous flow centrifugation and by filtration leukapheresis. Blood 48:315–325, 1976.

34. Price T, Dale D: Neutrophil preservation: The effect of short-term storage on in vitro kinetics. J Clin Invest 59:475–481, 1977.

35. McCullough J, Weiblen BJ, Peterson PK, Quie PG: Effects of temperature on granulocyte preservation. Blood 52:301–310, 1978.

36. Higby DJ, Freeman AI, Henderson ES, Sinks L, Cohen E: Granulocyte transfusions in children using filter-collected cells. Cancer 38:1407–1413, 1976.

37. Christensen G, Bisno AL, Parisi JT, McLaughlin B, Hester M, Luther RW: Nosocomial septicemia due to multiply antibiotic resistant Staphylococcus epidermis. Ann Intern Med 96:1–10, 1982.

38. Ford JM, Cullen MH: Prophylactic granulocyte transfusions. Exp Hematol 5 (Suppl 1): 65–72, 1977.

39. Schiffer CA, Aisner J, Daly PA, Schimpff SC, Wiernik PH: Alloimmunization following prophylactic granulocyte transfusion. Blood 54:766–774, 1979.

40. Winston DJ, Ho WG, Young LS, Gale RP: Prophylactic granulocyte transfusions during human bone marrow transplantation. Am J Med 68:893–897, 1980.

41. Winston DJ, Ho WG, Gale RP: Prophylactic granulocyte transfusions during chemotherapy of acute non-lymphocytic leukemia. Ann Intern Med 94:616–622, 1981.

42. Strauss RG, Connett JE, Gale RP, Bloomfield CD, Herzig GP, McCullough J, Maguire LC, Winston DJ, Ho WG, Stump DC, Miller WV, Koepke JA: A controlled trial of prophylactic granulocyte transfusions during initial induction chemotherapy for acute myelogenous leukemia. New Engl J Med 305 (11):597–602, 1981.

43. Clift RA, Sanders JE, Thomas ED, Williams B, Buckner CD: Granulocyte transfusions for the prevention of infection in patients receiving bone marrow transplants. New Engl J Med 298:1052–1057, 1978.

44. McCredie KB, Hester JP: White blood cell transfusions in the management of infection in neutropenic patients. Clinics in Hematology 5:379–394, 1976.

45. McCredie KB, Hester JP, Freireich EJ: Leukocyte collection and transfusion physiology. Exp Hematol 5 (Suppl 1):33–38, 1977.

46. Graw RG, Herzig G, Perry S, Henderson ES: Normal granulocyte transfusion therapy: treatment of septicemia due to gram-negative bacteria. New Engl J Med 287:367–371, 1972.

47. Herzig R, Herzig G, Graw RG, Bull MI, Ray KK: Efficacy of granulocyte transfusion therapy for gram-negative sepsis: a prospective randomized controlled study. New Engl J Med 296:701–705, 1977.

48. Vogler WR, Winton EF: The efficacy of granulocyte transfusions in neutropenic patients. Am J Med 63:548–555, 1977.

49. Higby DJ, Yates J, Henderson ES, Holland JF: Filtration leukapheresis for granulocyte transfusion therapy. New Engl J Med 292:761–766, 1975.

50. Alavi JB, Root RK, Djerasso I, Evans AE, Gluckman S, MacGregor RR, Guerry D, Schreiber AD, Shaw JM, Koch P, Cooper RA: Leukocyte transfusions in acute leukemia. New

Engl J Med 296:706–711, 1977.

51. Schiffer C, Buchholz DH, Aisner A, Sanel F, Wiernik PA: Clinical experience with transfusion of granulocytes obtained by continuous flow filtration leukapheresis. Am J Med 58:373–381, 1975.
52. Buchholz DH, Houx JL: A survey of the current use of filtration leukapheresis. Exp Hematol 7 (Suppl 4):1–10, 1979.
53. Ungerleider RS, Appelbaum FR, Trapani RJ, Diesseroth AB: Lack of predictive value of antileukocyte antibody screening in granulocyte transfusion therapy. Transfusion 19:90–94, 1979.
54. Appelbaum FR, Trapani RJ, Graw RG: Consequences of prior alloimmunization during granulocyte transfusion. Transfusion 17:460–464, 1977.
55. Westrick MA, Debelak-Fehir KM, Epstein RB: The effect of prior whole blood transfusion on subsequent granulocyte support in leukopenic dogs. Transfusion 17:611–614, 1977.
56. Wright DG, Robichaud KJ, Pizzo PA, Diesseroth AB: Lethal pulmonary reactions associated with the combined use of amphotericin B and leukocyte transfusions. New Engl J Med 304:1185–1192, 1981.
57. Boxer LA, Ingraham LM, Allen J, Oseas RS, Baehner RL: Amphotericin B promotes leukocyte aggregation of nylon wool fiber treated polymorpho-nuclear leukocytes. Blood 58:518–523, 1981.
58. Dana BW, Durie BGM, White RF, Huestis DW: Concomitant administration of granulocyte transfusions and amphotericin B in neutropenic patients: absence of significant pulmonary toxicity. Blood 57:91–96, 1981.
59. Winston DJ, Ho WG, Howell CL, Miller MJ, Mickey R, Martin WJ, Lin Cheng-Hsien, Gale RP: Cytomegalovirus infections associated with leukocyte transfusion. Ann Intern Med 93:671–675, 1980.
60. Von Fliedner V, Higby DJ, Kim U: Graft vs host disease following blood product transfusion: case report and review of the literature. Am J Med (in press).
61. Epstein RB, Waxman FJ, Bennett BT, Anderson BR: Pseudomonas septicemia in neutropenic dogs. I. Treatment with granulocyte transfusions. Transfusion 14:51–57, 1974.
62. EORTC International Antimicrobial Therapy Project Group: Three antibiotic regimens in the treatment of infection in febrile granulocytopenic patients with cancer. J Infect Dis 137 (1):14–29, 1978.
63. Van Furth R: Origin and kinetics of monocytes and macrophages. Seminars in Hematology 7:125–141, 1970.
64. Jacob HS: Granulocyte-complement interaction. Arch Intern Med 138:461–463, 1978.
65. Thakur ML, Lavender JP, Arnot RN, Silvester DJ, Segal AW: Indium-Ill labelled autologous leukocytes in man. J Nucl Med 18:1014–1021, 1977.

5. Nausea and Vomiting Caused by Chemotherapy

ROBERT L. DRAPKIN

INTRODUCTION

Nausea and vomiting is a regulatory response that has evolved in higher animals to maintain the constancy of the cellular environment. Like many other homeostatic regulatory mechanisms, the principles of negative feedback apply. A sensor detects changes from the normal; the sensor signals trigger changes that continue until the normal is again achieved. Nausea and vomiting is deeply rooted in the evolutionary survival of the species and it is not surprising that it is a difficult response to suppress. Today, cancer treatment requires the use of drugs that can cause severe nausea and vomiting. The physician must also treat and study the suffering caused by his treatments. This chapter reviews the physiology of vomiting, the pharmacology of anti-emetic drugs, and the clinical use of anti-emetics.

THE ANATOMY OF THE VOMITING ACT [1–3]

Nausea is the awareness of the urge to vomit. Frequently, nausea precedes vomiting, and during this nausea, duodenal contents reflux into the stomach because gastric tone and stomach peristalsis decrease while jejunal tone and duodenal tone increase. Retching results from the opposition of expiratory contractions of the abdominal muscles and the inspiratory movements of the chest wall and diaphragm (Figure 1). The mouth is closed, the glottis is closed, the upper stomach is relaxed and the antrum contracts. Vomiting occurs as the gastric contents are forcefully expelled out of the mouth. During vomiting, the lower stomach remains contracted, the cardia rises, the abdominal muscles contract, and the diaphragm descends. Retching and vomiting may alternate. Nausea is associated with tachycardia; retching is

Higby, DJ (ed), Supportive Care in Cancer Therapy. ISBN 0-89838-569-5.
© *1983, Martinus Nijhoff Publishers, Boston. Printed in The Netherlands.*

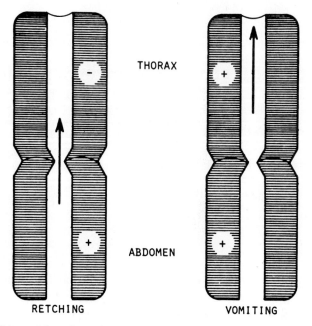

Figure 1. Forceful expulsion of gastric contents out of the mouth.

associated with bradycardia; and vomiting is associated with hypersalivation and defecation.

NEUROANATOMY OF VOMITING [4, 5]

The act of vomiting in man is a complex coordinated and reproducible act under the control of the central nervous system. Electrical stimulation of the dorsal portion of the lateral reticular formation in the medulla can induce vomiting. Vomiting does not occur when this area is ablated with radon needles. This area is the vomiting center (VC) which coordinates all vomiting (Figure 2).

Apomorphine when injected intravenously causes vomiting, which can be eliminated by ablating the VC or the area postrema in the fourth ventricle. The area postrema of the fourth ventricle is an afferent chemoreceptor trigger zone (CTZ) for the vomiting center. When apomorphine is applied to the CTZ, vomiting occurs which is lost when the CTZ is ablated. This area is responsive to chemicals in the blood; electrical stimulation of the CTZ does not cause vomiting. Normally the brain is protected from many chemicals within the blood by the blood brain barrier (BBB). The CTZ is not protected by the BBB [6] and most chemotherapy-induced vomiting is mediated by the CTZ (Figure 2).

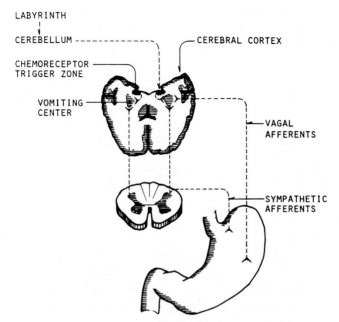

LABYRINTH

CEREBELLUM — — — — — — — — — — —

CEREBRAL CORTEX

CHEMORECEPTOR
TRIGGER ZONE

VOMITING
CENTER

VAGAL
AFFERENTS

SYMPATHETIC
AFFERENTS

Figure 2. A schematic diagram of the anatomy of nausea and vomiting.

Intragastric copper sulfate causes vomiting that can be decreased by ablating vagal and sympathetic afferents, while ablating the CTZ has no immediate effect. Thus, peripheral trigger sites exist in the gastrointestinal tract that cause vomiting. The small intestine appears to be the most sensitive gastrointestinal organ in provoking vomiting by irritation or mechanical stimulation.

The non-auditory labyrinth and the cerebellum play a role in the syndrome of motion sickness through afferents to the CTZ [4]. However, the role of the central nervous system is controversial and apparently complex. Visual, olfactory, and cognitive stimuli may evoke nausea and vomiting. Nausea and vomiting can also become a conditional response. The role of the central nervous system in facilitating vomiting requires further study.

THE MOLECULAR BIOLOGY OF VOMITING: A HYPOTHESIS

Peroutka and Synder postulate that there are 3 separate neurotransmitters involved in the production of nausea and vomiting, and thus, effective anti-emesis requires blocking each of these separate receptors [7]. Nausea and vomiting involve dopamine receptors (D_2); muscarinic cholinergic receptors (MC); and histamine receptors (H_1) [7]. The vomiting center (VC) has sensory input from the tractus solitarius and its nucleus, both containing his-

82

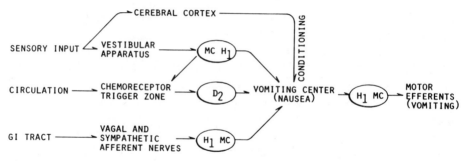

Figure 3. A hypothetic schematic diagram of the pathways and neurotransmitters involved in nausea and vomiting. The muscurinic cholinergic receptors are abbreviated 'MC'; the histamine receptors are abbreviated 'H₁'; the dopamine receptors are abbreviated 'D₂'.

tamine receptors (H_1) [8]. In addition, efferent vagal motor nuclei under the control of the vomiting centers contain muscarinic cholinergic receptors [9]. The lateral vestibular nucleus controlling vestibular input to the vomiting center and/or chemoreceptor trigger zone (CTZ) may contain both muscarinic cholinergic receptors and histamine (H_1) receptors [8, 9]. Dopamine receptors are present in high concentration in the chemoreceptor trigger zone [10]. The hypothetic schema is outlined in Figure 3.

EXPERIMENTAL DESIGN

Anti-emetic properties have been attributed historically to phenothiazines, antihistamines, anticholinergics, steroids, cannabinoids, and miscellaneous agents. The anti-emetic properties of some of these drugs have been established in animal studies using various experimental designs. In some dog studies, apomorphine is given intravenously or intragastrically and the percent of the dogs protected from vomiting by a given dose of the anti-emetic is recorded. Cats, dogs, and ferrets have been used in the laboratory to study vomiting. Attempts to quantify the vomiting act independent of stomach contents have been done by measuring changes in thoracic venous pressure, abdominal venous pressure, and the muscle activity of the diaphragm [11]. In this setting, emesis is characterized by repetitive negative thoracic pressure spikes followed by a single positive spike.

In human experiments, it is possible to study both nausea and vomiting. The subjective experience of nausea can be assessed by having the patient rate the severity of the experience on an arbitrary scale (0–10). Vomiting is usually evaluated in humans by counting the number of episodes of vomiting and measuring the volume of the emesis. These numbers cannot be interpreted correctly unless stomach contents can also be controlled, and this is difficult in human experiments. The subjective rating by the patient may ultimately prove more reliable and less variable.

Patients entered into emetic studies ideally should not have had prior chemotherapy experience. Patients after months of chemotherapy may develop pretreatment emesis. This pretreatment or anticipatory vomiting is triggered by sensory stimuli within the hospital or office setting. Pretreatment vomiting once triggered is refractory to most anti-emetics. This anticipatory behavior appears to be an example of classic Pavlovian conditioning [12]. The incidence of pretreatment vomiting may be as high as 24% [13].

PHENOTHIAZINE COMPOUNDS

This class of anti-emetics acts at the chemoreceptor trigger zone (CTZ) and prevents emesis induced by apomorphine, but fails to prevent emesis due to i.v. or oral copper sulfate. This suggests a diversity of receptors in the CTZ [14]. Phenothiazines are dopamine antagonists. Dopamine is secreted as a synaptic transmitter in certain autonomic ganglia and in certain parts of the brain. The most important side effects of all dopamine antagonists are extrapyramidal syndromes and include: parkinsonism with slow movements (akinesia), mask-facies, rigidity and tremor at rest; akathisia, a compelling need for instant movement; acute dystonia with facial grimacing, torticollis and oculogyric crisis; tardive dyskinesia; and perioral tremor after chronic use of dopamine antagonists. Other side effects of phenothiazines include sedation, orthostatic hypotension, jaundice, blood dyscrasias, photosensitivity, and prolactin elevation. In addition, the anti-emetic properties of phenothiazines are unrelated to their antipsychotic and sedative properties.

Chlorpromazine (thorazine) is the original phenothiazine to which all subsequent agents are compared. There are over 20 phenothiazine derivatives available for use as antipsychotic agents, sedatives, and anti-emetics. Chlorpromazine is used mostly for its antipsychotic properties. The following phenothiazine compounds have been selected for their anti-emetic properties. Triflupromazine (vestrin) is 8 to 10 times more potent than chlorpromazine in preventing apomorphine-induced emesis in dogs and clinically at least 5 times more potent in humans [15, 16]. Prochlorperazine (compazine) has a piperazine side chain and this increases anti-emetic activity. Prochlorperazine is 2 to 6 times more potent than chlorpromazine against apomorphine-induced emesis in dogs [16]. It has desirable features including less hypotension and less adrenergic blockade than chlorpromazine. Thiethylperazine (torecan) has a piperazine side chain like prochlorperazine. It is 4 times more potent against apomorphine and significantly raises the threshold for copper sulfate-induced emesis which is not found with prochlorperazine nor chlorpromazine [16]. Perphenazine (trilafon) has a piperazine side chain and is markedly superior to chlorpromazine at a ratio greater than 20 to 1 [16]. It appears to be more helpful against strong emetic stimuli. Fluphenazine (prolixin) has a piperazine side chain and is the most potent phenothiazine anti-emetic [17]. It is 34 to 124 times more potent against apomorphine when compared to chlorpromazine. This potency is not accompanied by greater sedation nor greater hypotension. Other phenothiazines with slight antiemetic properties include promazine, promethazine, thioridazine, and mepazine. Apomorphine induced vomiting in dogs [16] is the standard by which many of the phenothiazines have been compared. Apomorphine has one site of action at the CTZ. Most phenothiazines have one site of action; however, thiethylperazine and promazine also raise the oral copper sulfate threshold, indicating activity at the vomiting center and 2 sites of action.

ANTIHISTAMINES

Antihistamines theoretically act by competitively blocking released histamines during some biologic event. Dimenhydrinate (dramamine) and the closely related diphenhydramine (benadryl) prevent motion sickness [18]. The mechanism of action is unknown; however, antihistamines have little effect upon apomorphine-induced vomiting, and thus, the CTZ pathway to the VC is intact. Indeed, phenothiazines are less effective in preventing motion sickness. The site of action of antihistamines appears to be vestibular and/or cerebral. The anti-emetic action of antihistamines appears also in the ability of dimenhydrinate and cyclizine (Perazil) to raise the threshold to intragastric copper sulfate [16]. In addition, diphenhydramine can reverse the acute extrapyramidal side effects of phenothiazines, suggesting the clinical utility of using both antihistamines and phenothiazines in combination. The major side effects of antihistamines are sedation and anticholinergic effects. Sedation, antihistaminic action, and motion sickness protection are independent properties. Chlorpheniramine (chlortrimeton) offers no motion sickness protection. In controlled clinical trials antihistamines alone showed no significant anti-emetic effect compared to placebo in treating chemotherapy-induced nausea and vomiting [19, 20].

MUSCARINIC CHOLINERGIC BLOCKING AGENTS

Muscarinic cholinergic blocking agents inhibit the actions of acetylcholine on autonomic postganglionic cholinergic effector nerves and smooth muscles that lack cholinergic innervation. Atropine and scopolamine are the classic models for this group of drugs and both are anti-emetics.

Atropine and scopolamine are ineffective against apomorphine-induced emesis but are similar to the antihistamines in their effect on intragastric copper sulfate [9]. Both atropine and scopolamine have been chiefly used to suppress motion sickness and this activity appears to correlate with their central anticholinergic activity [4]. Side effects are dose dependent and include in order of increasing dose; decreased salivation, bronchial secretion, and sweating; pupil dilatation, loss of visual accommodation, and tachycardia; inhibition of micturition and decreased gastrointestinal secretion and motility. Recently, a new method of drug administration, the transdermal patch, has made scopolamine available by a slow continuous transdermal infusion. This new approach has shown mild anti-emetic activity [21]. Scopolamine is the strongest muscarinic cholinergic blocker and theoretically it may be more useful as an anti-emetic when combined with dopamine and histamine antagonists.

BUTYROPHENONE DERIVATIVES

Butyrophenone derivatives include droperidol (inapsine) and haloperidol (haldol), and like the phenothiazines, are antipsychotic medications. Butyrophenones are also used for anesthetic premedication to provide ataraxia and anti-emesis. Droperidol and haloperidol are possibly the most potent inhibitors of the CTZ [22]. Side effects include sedation and extrapyramidial reactions. Droperidol produces a state of reduced anxiety, quiescence, reduced activity and indifference called neurolepsis. When combined with fentanyl citrate (innovar), a state of neurolept analgesia occurs in which procedures and minor surgery can be performed. Respiratory depression can occur when butyrophenones are combined with any opioid analgesic; however, by themselves, butyrophenones have minimal hypotensive or respiratory effects. Comparative clinical studies have demonstrated that haloperidol is a stronger anti-emetic than prochlorperazine in preventing apomorphine-induced vomiting [23].

SUBSTITUTED BENZAMIDES

Substituted benzamides include two drugs, metoclopramide (reglan) and alizapride; however, the latter drug is not available in the USA. Metoclopramide, though developed from procainamide, has few cardiac effects and little anesthetic action. Metoclopramide is an anti-emetic with potent gastrointestinal tract and CTZ effects. It stimulates directly the orthograde peristalsis of the stomach, thus, accelerating gastric emptying. Metoclopramide has been used to facilitate small bowel intubation and to aid intestinal transit of barium where delayed emptying interferes with radiological examination. More importantly, metoclopramide directly opposes the physiologic events that occur in vomiting as described earlier in this chapter. Metoclopramide is also a dopamine antagonist that acts at the CTZ [24]. The side effects include sedation and extrapyramidal reactions, which occur more frequently in young patients. In dogs given apomorphine, metoclopramide is more effective than phenothiazines or trimethobenzamide [25]. Metoclopramide significantly reduces emesis in patients receiving cis-platinum chemotherapy compared to placebo and is very effective against strongly emetic stimuli [26].

CANNABINOIDS

The plant *Cannibus sativa* L. contains many cannabinoids including delta-9-THC (THC), cannabidiol (CBD), and cannabichromene (CBC). In addition, synthetic cannabinoids have been developed – levonantradol and nabilone.

Sallan et al, were among the first to report the use of oral THC as an anti-emetic [27, 28]. In these studies, an anti-emetic effect was documented with little toxicity in a relatively young population, median ages 29.5 and 32.5 years. The major toxicity was somnolence, occurring in approximately 30%, while less than 2% of these young patients experienced severe dose-limiting toxicities such as dysphoria or hallucinations. In a Mayo Clinic study using older patients, median age 61 years, 35% of the patients had dose-limiting toxicities such as ataxia, hypotension, visual hallucinations and dysphoria [29]. Other side effects include tachycardia, sedation, psychosis, blurred vision, paresthesia, fecal incontinence, and altered mentation. Despite these side effects, THC has anti-emetic efficacy but perhaps only certain subgroups of patients may derive benefit [30].

Presently THC is available from the NCI in capsules which when ingested, give erratic blood levels in patients experiencing nausea and vomiting. Smoking THC provides more predictable blood levels [31].

Levonantradol hydrochloride has been developed in an attempt to modify the THC molecule to separate the anti-emetic and analgesic properties from the 'psychic' properties and the abuse potential [32]. The resulting molecule is a novel synthetic compound structurally distinct from THC and with enhanced analgesic and anti-emetic properties. In a randomized double blind study, levonantradol versus prochlorperazine, early results showed no statistical difference in objective measurements of nausea and vomiting; however, patients subjectively preferred levonantradol to prochlorperazine. The side effects were also greater in the levonantradol group and they included somnolence, dry mouth, dizziness, disorientation, decreased concentration, anxiety, depression, and euphoria [33]. Further evaluation of levonantradol is necessary.

Nabilone is another cannabinoid presently under evaluation to prevent chemotherapy-induced emesis. Nabilone has been compared to prochlorperazine in a double blind study of chemotherapy-induced emesis. Nabilone appeared superior to prochlorperazine for mild nausea; however, it was equal to prochlorperazine against high dose cis-platinum [34]. The side effects from nabilone were dose-limiting drowsiness and dizziness in 25% of the patients. Recently, nabilone has been thought to be nephrotoxic; however, this was a species-specific animal toxicity and studies in humans have been resumed.

CORTICOSTEROIDS

Both dexamethasone and methylprednisolone have anti-emetic properties in patients experiencing chemotherapy-induced nausea and vomiting [35, 38]. One thousand milligrams of methylprednisolone over 24 hours or 50 to 100 milligrams of dexamethasone over 24 hours is effective in reducing nausea and vomiting in patients receiving cis-platinum. The mechanism of action of steroids in reducing nausea and vomiting is unknown. Some authors have speculated upon inhibition of prostaglandin release [37]. Of importance, is the relative lack of toxicity of these brief high-dose steroid treatments. There are few reported adverse side effects and no inhibition of chemotherapy efficacy [36, 38]. In addition, dexamethasone at high doses may be effective without other neuroleptic anti-emetics [38].

The theoretical concern regarding immune suppression and tumor growth with steroids is evident in animal tumor models in which the test tumor has proteins highly antigenic and not normally found in the host animal. In the presence of foreign tumor antigens, the host cellular immune system is called upon to inhibit tumor growth and this can easily be suppressed by corticosteroids resulting in tumor growth. This is not analogous to the spontaneously occurring tumors in humans where strong tumor-specific antigens are difficult to find. More important, is the antitumor effect of corticosteroids in acute lymphoblastic leukemia, malignant lymphoma, breast cancer, and multiple myeloma. Overall, corticosteroids have the fewest side effects of those drugs capable of suppressing the severe nausea and vomiting found with cis-platinum.

CHEMOTHERAPEUTIC DRUGS AS EMETIC STIMULI

In general, nausea and vomiting is a side effect of all chemotherapeutic agents. Drugs vary greatly in their emetogenic properties as do human subjects in their ability to tolerate chemotherapy. Important drug variables include dose, route of administration and duration of treatment. In general, a slow prolonged continuous infusion of chemotherapy is associated with the least nausea and vomiting, suggesting that peak serum concentration determined the emetogenic properties of a given drug. Important individual variables include prior chemotherapy experience and gastric contents at time of treatment. The classical conditioning of vomiting in heavily pretreated patients and the importance of gastric contents have been previously mentioned in the section Experimental design.

Table 1. Chemotherapeutic agents causing nausea in nearly every patient.

1. Mechlorethamine HCL
2. Cis-diamminedichloroplatinum
3. Imidazole carboxamide

There are 3 drugs which produce vomiting in nearly every patient (Table 1). Mechlorethamine HCL (HN_2) may cause severe nausea and vomiting 1 to 3 hours after injection. Emesis may persist for 24 hours and cause severe dehydration. Cis-diamminedichloroplatinum (DDP) produces marked dose-limiting nausea and vomiting 1 to 4 hours after treatment. In some patients, nausea and anorexia may persist from 1 to 7 days after treatment. Both HN_2 and DDP require pretreatment hydration and anti-emetics to combat their side effects. Less nausea is experienced if the DDP is given as a slow 5-day continuous infusion [39]. Imidazole carboxamide (DTIC) induces nausea and vomiting 1–12 hours, and this may disappear during the 5-day schedule, suggesting the development of tolerance. In addition, it is recommended to reduce the first dose of DTIC to lessen toxicity [40].
Table 2 lists those drugs that are associated with nausea and vomiting in the majority of patients. The chlorethyl nitrosoureas and streptozotocin are

Table 2. Chemotherapeutic agents causing nausea in the majority of patients.

1. Chlorethyl nitrosureas (CCNU, methyl CCNU, BCNU)
2. Streptozotocin
3. Actinomycin D
4. Adriamycin/daunomycin
5. Mithramycin
6. Procarbazine

potent emetogenic agents. Treatment with the antibiotic chemotherapeutic agents actinomycin D, mithramycin, adriamycin, and daunomycin, frequently results in severe nausea and vomiting. Procarbazine causes vomiting in 75 to 95% of patients [41]. Other drugs associated with nausea and vomiting include: cytoxan 40–120 mg/kg i.v., high dose methotrexate, 5-fluorouracil 15 mg/kg daily for 5 days, high dose ara-C, and L-asparaginase.

The CTZ is the site of chemotherapy-induced nausea and vomiting. For anti-emetics to be helpful, they should be given prior to chemotherapy and continuously during the treatment period, usually 12–24 hours. Presumably, pretreatment and continuous treatment provides maximum receptor blockade at the CTZ, thus, preventing nausea and vomiting. Many unanswered questions exist as to the precise mechanism of chemotherapy-induced nausea and vomiting.

PRACTICAL GUIDE TO AVAILABLE ANTI-EMETICS

In general, anti-emetic treatment should be given prior to chemotherapy by 3 to 24 hours, and continuously during the chemotherapy treatment period. The patient should be instructed to be on a liquid diet and remain on this diet through the treatment period. Since all anti-emetics have potential side effects, the minimum effective anti-emetic agents should be initiated, and only when judged ineffective, should additions be made. Approximately 10% of patients given DDP can be controlled with the mild anti-emetics, thiethylperazine and hydrozyzine [36].

The phenothiazines are among the safest and most widely available anti-emetics and should be used initially in most patients. Thiethylperazine, prochlorperazine, and fluphenazine are helpful in mild nausea and vomiting. The oral route may be used initially, however, parenteral administration may be required for reliable blood levels if the patient is vomiting. Clinically these drugs cause pain when given by intramuscular injection and suppositories can be substituted despite their less reliable therapeutic benefit.

Antihistamines are not of proven benefit in chemotherapy-induced nausea and vomiting despite theoretical consideration to the contrary. However, it is practical to combine an antihistamine, diphenhydramine, with phenothiazine in order to alleviate some of the side effects of the phenothiazine. Likewise, muscarinic cholinergic agents are not of proven value in chemotherapy-induced nausea and vomiting.

If vomiting is known to be refractory to phenothiazines, high dose steroids can be added. This combination can block the severest nausea and vomiting with few side effects due to the anti-emetics and thus, is a safe next step. If DDP is given with significant volumes of intravenous fluid, dexamethasone at a dose of 50 to 100 mg over 24 hours is recommended owing to its lack of mineralocorticoid activity. However, steroids should not be given to patients with insulin-dependent diabetes mellitus nor with peptic ulcer symptoms.

If patients are refractory to a phenothiazine and high dose steroids, the phenothiazine should be discontinued and replaced with metoclopramide at 2 mg/kg intravenously every three hours for a total of three to five doses. High dose steroids may be used in addition and diphenhydramine added to combat the side effects of metoclopramide (Table 3).

Table 3. Practical guide to available anti-emetics.

---

1. Treat prior to chemotherapy; continuously through treatment period; patient on liquid diet
2. Phenothiazines: prochlorperazine
   thiethylperazine
   fluphenazine
3. Steroids: dexamethasone
   solu-medrol
4. Metoclopramide
5. Butyrophenones: haloperidol
   droperidol

Patients refractory to the above combinations may benefit from a butyrophenone, haloperidol or droperidol. The side effects of the phenothiazines, butyrophenones, and metoclopramide are additive and these 3 groups of drugs are difficult to use at high doses simultaneously. Sedation may also prove beneficial. The best combination of anti-emetics has yet to be discovered. The future belongs to new drugs and the study of the molecular events that occur during nausea and vomiting.

REFERENCES

1. Ingelfinger FJ, Moss RE: The activity of the descending duodenum during nausea. Am J Physiol 136:561, 1942.
2. Lumsden K, Holden WS: The act of vomiting in man. GUT 10:173, 1969.
3. Wolfs: Studies on nausea. Effects of ipecac and other emetics on the human stomach and duodenum. Gastroenterology 12:212, 1949.
4. Wang SC: Emetic and antiemetic drugs. Physiol Pharmacol 11:255, 1965.
5. Wang SC, Borison HL: The vomiting center: a critical experimental analysis. AMA Arch Neurol Psychiat 63:928, 1950.
6. Ganong WF: Review of medical Physiology. Lange Medical Publications, Los Altos, California, 10th ed 1981, p 480.

7. Peroutka SJ, Synder SH: Antiemetics: neurotransmitter receptor binding predicts therapeutic actions. Lancet 1 (8273):658–659, 1982.

8. Palacios JM, Wamsley JK, Kubar MJ: The distribution of histamine H_1 receptors in the rat brain: an autoradiographic study. Neuroscience 6:15–17, 1981.

9. Wamsley JK, Lewis MS, Young WS, III, Kuhar MJ: Autoradiographic localization of muscarinic cholinergic receptors in rat brainstem. J Neurosci 1:176–191, 1981.

10. Stefanini E, Clement-Cormier Y: Detection of dopamine receptors in the area postrema. Eur J Pharmacol 74:257–260, 1981.

11. McCarthy LE, Borison HL, Spiegel PK, Friedlander RM: Vomiting: radiographic and oscillographic correlates in the decerebrate cat. Gastroenterology 67:1126–1130, 1974.

12. Nesse RM, Carli T, Curtis GC, Kleinman RD: Pretreatment nausea in cancer chemotherapy: a conditioned response? Psychosomatic Med 42(1):33–36, 1980.

13. Morrow GR, Arseneau JC, Asbury RF, Bennet JM, Laszlo B: Anticipatory nausea and vomiting with chemotherapy. New Engl J Med 306(7):431–432, 1982.

14. Brand ED, Harris TD, Borison HL, Goodman LS: The antiemetic activity of 10-(γ-dimethylaminopropyl)-2-chlorphenothiazine (chlorpromazine) in dog and cat. J Pharmacol Exp Ther 110:86, 1954.

15. Moyer TH, Conner PK: Clinical and laboratory observations on two trifluoromethyl phenothiazine derivatives. J Lab Clin Med 51:185, 1958.

16. Wyant GM: A comparative study of eleven antiemetic drugs in dogs. Can Anaesthesiol Soc J 9:399, 1962.

17. Laffan RJ, Papandrianos P, Burke JC, Craver BN: Antiemetic action of fluphenazine (Prolixin): a comparison with other phenothiazines. J Pharmacol Exp Ther 131:130, 1961.

18. Gay LN, Carliner PE: The prevention and treatment of motion sickness & seasickness. Bull Johns Hopkins Hosp 84:470, 1949.

19. Moertel CG, Reitemeier RJ, Gage RP: A controlled clinical evaluation of antiemetic drugs. JAMA 186:116–8, 1963.

20. Morran C, Smith DC, Anderson DA, McArdle CS: Incidence of nausea and vomiting with cytotoxic chemotherapy: a prospective randomized trial of antiemetics. Br Med J 1:1323–4, 1979.

21. Longo D, Howser D, Wesley M, Anderson T, Young RC: Randomized double-blind crossover trial of scopolamine vs placebo administered by transcutaneous patch for the control of chemotherapy induced emesis. Proc Am Assoc Cancer Res 22:161, 1981.

22. Edmonds-Seals J, Prys-Roberts C: Pharmacology of drugs used for neuroleptanalgesia. Br J Anesth 42:207–216, 1970.

23. Shields KG, Ballinger CM, Hathaway BN: Antiemetic effectiveness of haloperidol in human volunteers challenged with apomorphine. Anesth Analg 50:1017–1027, 1971.

24. Pinder RM, Brogden RN, Sawyer PR, Speight TM, Avery GS: Metoclopramide: a review of its pharmacological properties and clinical use. Drugs 12:81–131, 1976.

25. Justin-Besançon L, Laville C. Action antiémetique du métoclopromide vis-à-vis de l'apomorphine et de l'hydergine. Cr Soc Biol (Paris) 158:723–727, 1964.

26. Gralla RJ, Itri LM, Pisko SE et al.: Antiemetic efficacy of high-dose metoclopromide: randomized trials with placebo and prochlorperazine in patients with chemotherapy induced nausea and vomiting. N Engl J Med 305:905–909, 1981.

27. Sallan SE, Zinberg NE, Frei E, III: Antiemetic effect of delta-9-Tetrahydrocannabinol in patients receiving cancer chemotherapy. N Engl J Med 293:795–797, 1975.

28. Sallan SE, Cronin C, Zelen M et al.: Antiemetics in patients receiving chemotherapy for cancer. A randomized comparison of delta-9-Tetrahydrocannabinol and prochlorperazine. N Engl J Med 302:135–138, 1980.

29. Frytak S, Moertel CG, O'Fallon JR et al.: Delta-9-tetrahydrocannabinol as an antiemetic for

patients receiving cancer chemotherapy. A comparison with prochlorperamine and a placebo. Ann Intern Med 91:825–830, 1979.

30. Poster DS, Penta JS, Bruno S et al.: A review of oral delta-9-tetrahydrocannabinol clinical antiemetic studies 1975:1980. In: Treatment of Cancer Chemotherapy Induced Nausea and Vomiting, Poster DS, Penta JS, Bruno S (eds). New York, Masson Publishing USA, 1981, pp 55–59.

31. Chang AE, Shiling DJ, Stillman RC et al.: Delta-9-tetrahydrocannabinol as an antiemetic in cancer patients receiving high dose methotrexate. A prospective randomized evaluation. Ann Intern Med 91:819–824, 1979.

32. Milne GM, Johnson MR, Fiese EF, Wolf JS: Selected pharmacological studies with levonantradol. In: Treatment of Cancer Chemotherapy Induced Nausea and Vomiting, Poster DS, Penta JS, Bruno S (eds). New York, Masson Publishing USA, 1981, pp 129–136.

33. Long A, Mioduszewski J, Natale R: A randomized double-blind crossover comparison of the antiemetic activity of levonantradol and prochlorperazine. Proceedings American Society of Clinical Oncology 220:57, 1982.

34. Steele N, Gralla RJ, Braun DW, Young CW: Double-blind comparison of the antiemetic effects of nabilone and prochlorperazine on chemotherapy induced emesis. Cancer Treat Rep 64:219–224, 1980.

35. Drapkin RL, McAloon E, Sokol G et al.: The antiemetic effect of dexamethasone in patients receiving cis-platinum. Proceedings American Association of Clinical Oncology (C-34) 1981, p 419.

36. Drapkin RL, Sokol GH, Paladine WJ et al.: The antiemetic effect and dose response of dexamethasone in patients receiving cis-platinum. Proceedings American Association of Clinical Oncology (C-236) 1982, p 61.

37. Rich WM, Gazi A, DiSain PJ: Methylprednisolone as an antiemetic during cancer chemotherapy – a pilot study. Gynecol Oncol 9:193–198, 1980.

38. Aapro MS, Alberts DS: High-dose dexamethasone for prevention of cis-platin-induced vomiting. Cancer Chemother Pharmacol 7:11–14, 1981.

39. Lokich JJ: Phase I study of cis-diamminedichloroplatinum (II) administered as a constant 5 day infusion. Cancer Treat Rep 64:905–908, 1980.

40. Moore GE, Meiselbaugh D: DTIC (NSC-45388) toxicity. Cancer Treat Rep 60:219, 1976.

41. Stolinsky DC, Solomon J, Pugh RP et al.: Clinical experience with procarbazine in Hodgkin's disease, reticulum cell sarcoma, and lymphosarcoma. Cancer 26:984–990, 1979.

6. Nutritional/Metabolic Support: Parenteral and Enteral

KATHY M. TEASLEY, EVA P. SHRONTS, JOLYNN LYSNE,
NANCY NUWER and FRANK B. CERRA

INTRODUCTION, BACKGROUND AND RATIONALE

The literature is replete with studies and reviews analyzing the effects of nutritional support on patients with various stages of malignancy and undergoing various forms of treatment. Much uncertainty and conflict seemingly exists. The present discussion is designed to place the known data on nutrition and cancer into a working framework, and to proceed from that to a rational, safe and effective application.

The major generalization of the clinical and experimental research to date is that nutritional support is, at best, a poor form of antineoplastic therapy, but is an effective method for controlling the nutritional consequences of malignancy and its various forms of treatment. The efficacy of nutritional support in achieving this control in large part depends on how the malnutrition present was acquired, i.e., as the result of a disorder of nutrition or a reflection of the disordered metabolism that eventually occurs in some patients with cancer.

A nutrition problem is characterized by the setting of not being able to provide sufficient amounts of carbohydrate, fat, and protein at the cellular level. Once there, the nutrient substrate is used normally. The etiologies of the failure to achieve adequate input are primarily those of gastrointestinal tract obstruction, infection (e.g. candida stomatitis or esophagitis), malabsorption or maldigestion. In this setting, the current techniques of nutritional support will control the malnutrition.

The results in nutritional disorders, then, support the concepts that nutritional support in cancer [7-11]: 1) will prevent, correct or effectively support the nutritional disorder; 2) will not alter the clinical course of the tumor per se or the response to chemotherapy, radiation therapy or surgery

Higby, DJ (ed), Supportive Care in Cancer Therapy. ISBN 0-89838-569-5.
© *1983, Martinus Nijhoff Publishers, Boston. Printed in The Netherlands.*

per se; 3) will impact on morbidity and mortality, in as much as that morbidity and mortality is nutritional in origin; 4) will not promote tumor growth at the expense of the host [12–16]; 5) can improve the general quality of life of the patient.

A metabolic disorder is a situation in which substrate utilization is altered at the cellular level, although substrate supply may be adequate. Such disorders are now widely recognized–polytrauma, major general surgery, burns, cirrhosis and sepsis. It also appears as if an altered metabolic state eventually appears in some cancer patients and that that state eventually becomes a primary factor producing death.

The known characteristics of the altered metabolism include: an increased basal energy expenditure in the resting state, increased urinary nitrogen loss, and an increased turnover and utilization of protein and fat. The major changes, however, are in carbohydrate metabolism. These include: hyperglycemia, hyperlactacemia, glucose intolerance, increased recycling of glucose, and increased gluconeogenesis from lactate and alanine [2–8].

As such, these characteristics separate the cancer patient from the resting, fasting patient without cancer. Many of the attributes are reminiscent of the stressed states of surgery, polytrauma and sepsis. These states, however, have many other metabolic characteristics not observed in the altered metabolism of cancer. The neurohumoral response in stress is associated with elevated levels of glucagon, insulin, cortisol, catecholamines and sympathetic tone. Such a profile is not observed in the cancer patient unless that patient also is experiencing the stress of surgery, polytrauma or sepsis. If exogenous glucose is given to the cancer patient with altered metabolism, gluconeogenesis from alanine can be suppressed, nitrogen retention increases, proteolysis decreases, and the plasma levels of triglycerides, free fatty acids and cholesterol fall. Glucose administration during the higher levels of stress and sepsis will not produce these results. When the cancer patient develops sepsis, however, he seems to respond in the same manner as any other septic patient [17–23].

Therefore, in the basal state patients with cancer eventually develop a metabolic disorder that progressively worsens until death. This disorder seems to be primarily one of increased energy demand, increased glycolysis and gluconeogenesis (particularly from alanine), and increased turnover and use of fat and protein.

The end result clinically of this metabolic problem is an inappropriate reduction in lean body mass, i.e., malnutrition. Standard nutritional support does seem to have some impact on this acquired malnutrition as long as the metabolic disorder is not severe and the total calories are increased to approximately 1.5 times the basal energy expenditure. As such, standard nutritional support will induce weight gain, nitrogen retention, stimulate insulin secretion [1, 42], support hepatic protein synthesis, and reverse anergy. It will not, however, alter the course of the tumor or the response to therapy. It may impact on the morbidity and mortality due to the malnutrition and may substantially improve the quality of life for the patient [1, 24–28].

Eventually, however, the metabolic disorder seems to progress so that the acquired malnutrition is no longer compensable by exogenous metabolic support with existing techniques. Progressive cachexia and death usually follow shortly.

As more insight is gained into the altered metabolism of cancer, newer forms of metabolic support or therapy may result; whether branched chain amino acid support or the newer forms of intravenous fat are going to impact on the basal cancer metabolism are currently unknown. The development of metabolic support with a true antineoplastic quality is also conceivable.

The precise origin of the altered basal metabolism in cancer is not currently known. Several hypotheses are available. One such hypothesis is increased energy demand by the tumor. Certainly this can account for some of the increased basal energy need, but tumor burdens are usually not large enough to account for the increases that are routinely observed [29–31]. The glycolysis–gluconeogenic cycle has been thought to contribute because it is basically a futile cycle and generates heat, but not net ATP [6–7]. Whether other futile cycles are present is still unknown. A final consideration is that the tumor is producing some substance that is altering host substrate flow and utilization. Little data is currently available [10].

Thus, the malnutrition of cancer can either be a nutritional or a metabolic problem. The manifestations on routine clinical assessment are the same. The distinction between the two is important therapeutically as one responds well to therapy and one does not. This situation may impact on the decision of whether or not to employ nutritional support therapy.

In large part, the history and physical exam will usually provide a sound base for discrimination. The demonstration of reduced intake in the presence of thrush or an obstructive lesion, or the documentation of maldigestion or malabsorption, would favor a nutritional disorder. The absence of these and/or the presence of true anorexia favor a metabolic disorder. The presence of a high basal plasma lactate in the presence of other laboratory criteria of malnutrition-negative nitrogen balance, e.g., low albumin, low transferrin, or anergy, also favors a metabolic disorder. Ultimately, a test of therapy frequently occurs, as the more sophisticated discriminators (plasma aminograms; isotope studies) are not available for routine bedside use, and current therapy will frequently have some effect in early metabolic disorders. In the absence of other hypermetabolic states, if therapy is appropriately applied and no response is observed in 10–14 days, advanced altered metabolism is usually present.

The issue of whether or not to apply the resources of nutritional support to a given patient, then, depends on the answer to several questions and is ultimately a clinical judgment at the present time.

A. *Is malnutrition present*
  1. If malnutrition is present, is it the result of starvation or from altered metabolism?
  2. Is the problem acute or chronic?

B. *The contemporary therapy*
  1. Is starvation a side effect or a result of the therapy?
  2. Is a positive result expected, such as cure, remission, or control of the disease?

C. *Therapeutic ranking of nutrition*
  The ranking of nutritional support in the therapeutic armamentarium of treating a patient is quite variable and is closely related to the issues presented so far. In addition, the risks of providing the nutritional support must also be considered. To this end, the route of administration is important.

  In current practice, either the gut or central vein must be used. In suitable patients, the nutritional results are the same with either route. The decision, then, becomes one of risk availability and patient tolerance. The intravenous route is generally used when the gut route is not possible. Reasons for this would include severe mucositis, inadequate absorptive capacity, maldigestion, or rapid transit time. Patients in coma or who have a high risk of aspiration for other reasons may require intravenous alimentation. Newer feeding tubes in jejunum, or those that can be passed beyond the pyloris or ligament of Treitz, have markedly reduced the aspiration problem and have facilitated both hospital and home enteral support.

  When present, safely accessible, and tolerated, the use of the gut is still the cheapest and certainly an equally effective route of administration. Each patient must be individualized and assessed. Occasionally, a patient will find one or the other route easier to use. Because of improved compliance, especially in the home setting, one route may have advantages over the other.

D. *Will the quality of life be effected*

Current nutritional support is not antineoplastic therapy. There are, however, several groups of patients who no longer have gastro-intestinal tracts that can sustain useful life either because of the primary disease, e.g., ovarian cancer or colon cancer, or because of the results of therapy or complications, e.g., surgical extirpation of the gut. In either case, remaining organ function (renal, liver, cardiopulmonary, brain) is usually adequate to sustain useful life. In such settings, home enteral or parenteral therapy can provide variable periods of reasonable quality existence, sometimes with return to gainful employment.

The many personal, family, social, ethical and moral problems present in such a setting necessitate an individualized patient approach, usually with the involvement of a multidisciplinary team consisting of a nurse, pharmacist, dietician, social worker and sometimes a psychiatrist or psychologist. Financial coverage, particularly with home intravenous TPN, can sometimes still be a problem. Numerous home delivery services for supplies now exist, minimizing the many problems that can arise e.g., Home Health Care of America or Travacare of Travenol Laboratories, Incorporated.

Using these guidelines, the clinical judgment can be rationally made in an individual patient as to what kind, when, and how long the resources of nutritional support can or should be applied.

PARENTERAL NUTRITION SUPPORT

The components of a nutritional support regimen include a source of carbohydrate, fat, protein, electrolytes, vitamins, and trace elements. All these substrates must be supplied to minimize complications and provide effective support. How much support to supply depends on the existing organ function and level of stress, in addition to the presence or absence of effects due to the tumor itself.

Calories and protein [32–34]

Caloric requirements are based on an estimated basal energy expenditure (Table 1). Low levels of stress generally require 120% of the basal energy expenditure (BEE). Higher levels of stress (burns, sepsis) may require 150–200% of the BEE. Patients with cancer generally require 160% of the BEE. Substrate intolerance (hyperglycemia, hypertriglyceridemia) may develop at higher levels of stress. Substrates should be given only to the extent of tolerance. For example, dextrose in combination with amino acids and intravenous (i.v.) lipid (vide infra) should be given to meet the caloric demand of 150–200% of BEE. Although blood glucose levels may be controlled by larger doses of insulin, the result seems to be an increase in the cellular uptake of glucose, but continued abnormal metabolism of glucose at the mitochondrial level. If glucose intolerance develops (blood glucose persistently >250 mg%), insulin should be administered to a maximum of about two units regular insulin per hour by continuous infusion. If glucose intolerance is not controlled by this level of insulin support, dextrose intake should be reduced until control of blood glucose is achieved. Dextrose intake may be reduced by decreasing the rate of infusion of the dextrose-

Table 1. Equations for calculating estimated basal energy expenditure (BEE).

$$\text{Male: BEE} = 66 + (13.7 \times \text{Wt}) + (5 \times \text{Ht}) - (6.8 \times \text{A})$$
$$\text{Female: BEE} = 655 + (9.6 \times \text{Wt}) + (1.7 \times \text{Ht}) - (4.7 \times \text{A})$$

Ht = height, cm; Wt = weight, kg; A = age, yrs

amino acid solution or by decreasing the concentration of dextrose in the dextrose-amino acid solution. Similarly, i.v. fat emulsions should only be given if a baseline serum triglyceride level is within normal limits. If i.v. lipid is given lipid tolerance should be evaluated by monitoring for serum lipemia and/or remeasuring a serum triglycerides level approximately 8–10 hours following the completion of the i.v. fat emulsion infusion. Elevated serum triglyceride levels and/or persistent lipemia indicate altered fat metabolism and clearance. Lipid administration should be discontinued and lipid tolerance re-evaluated after at least 24 hours. Alternatively, a lesser dose of i.v. lipid (e.g., changing from 20% i.v. fat emulsion to 10% i.v. fat emulsion) may be used if clearance remains adequate.

Protein requirements (as amino acids) during acute stress may be as high as 2.5–3.5 g/kg/day with at least some of the amino acids being preferentially utilized as an energy source. Optimal utilization of protein during acute stress appears to occur when a ratio of approximately 100 non-protein calories (carbohydrate and fat) are provided per gram of nitrogen. Prerenal azotemia may develop and limit the amount of protein which can be administered. The proportion of blood urea nitrogen (BUN) to creatinine should not exceed 20:1 by greater than 20 mg% BUN, e.g., a BUN of 60 mg% with a creatinine of 2.0 mg%. Patients with hepatic failure may manifest a more profound protein intolerance by an abnormal amino acid profile and by the development of progressive hepatic encephalopathy. Patients with cirrhosis should initially be limited to approximately 40 grams of intravenous protein a day (0.5–1.0 g/kg/day). The protein intake may be gradually increased to the desired level of intake for stress. Tolerance is evaluated by monitoring the degree of clinical encephalopathy. If encephalopathy develops, amino acid intake should be reduced.

The nutritional/metabolic requirements of the acutely stressed patient can usually be met by using one of several standardized formulas for parenteral nutrition (Table 2). The non-protein calorie to nitrogen ratio of 100:1 for the acutely stressed patient can be achieved by adjusting the lipid and dextrose proportions of the regimen. In a patient who demonstrated baseline lipid intolerance (hypertriglycerdemia), a fat free regimen should be initiated. Regimen A provides all of the non-protein calories as dextrose. In a patient who demonstrates glucose intolerance, the dextrose intake should be reduced and the calories replaced as fat as in Regimen B. Regimen C also provides calories as a balance of carbohydrate and fat but with a lower proportion of fat than Regimen B. Some patients may demonstrate both lipid and glucose intolerance; Regimen A (no fat) should be used and the rate of infusion adjusted to glucose tolerance. Alternatively, in this setting the dextrose concentration may be decreased or physiologic doses of insulin may be administered. These standardized regimens provide flexibility in

Table 2. Standard formulas for parenteral nutrition (100:1) to provide ~100 non protein calories per gram of nitrogen.

Regimen A – no fat	Regimen B – moderate fat	Regimen C – low fat
TPN Solution:	TPN Solution:	TPN Solution:
Dextrose 20%	Dextrose 10%	Dextrose 15%
Amino acids 4.25%	Amino acids 4.25%	Amino acids 4.25%
Lipid:	Lipid:	Lipid:
None	200 ml of 20% fat emulsion per liter of TPN	200 ml of 10% fat emulsion per liter of TPN
Composition of intake (% of total intake):	Composition of intake (% of total intake):	Composition of intake (% of total intake):
Carbohydrate 80%	Carbohydrate 41%	Carbohydrate 58%
Protein 20%	Protein 19%	Protein 20%
Fat 0%	Fat 40%	Fat 22%
Non-protein kcal: g N = 95:1	Non-protein kcal: g N = 103:1	Non-protein kcal: g N = 99:1

prescribing parenteral nutrition and have the advantage of being less expensive (the ingredients are cheaper and they require less pharmacy time to compound) than specially compounded solutions.

Non-standard solutions can be compounded when special circumstances exist. For example, a more concentrated solution (e.g., dextrose 25% and amino acids 6.25%) may be indicated in a patient with severe fluid restrictions. A less concentrated amino acid solution (e.g., amino acids 2.75%) may be indicated in a patient with severe hepatic failure and protein intolerance.

As the state of acute stress resolves, the patient's ability to metabolize carbohydrate and fat will improve. Caloric requirements will be approximately 150% of BEE, and the proportion of intake of carbohydrate and fat should be increased to provide 150 non-protein calories per gram of nitrogen. Amino acids are being less utilized for energy and protein intake can be reduced to 1.5–2.0 g/kg/day. This level of protein intake seems to be sufficient for wound repair and nutritional repletion in most patients.

In this post-stress period, the standardized formulas for parenteral nutrition can be modified to achieve the desired ratio of 150 non-protein calories per gram of nitrogen (Table 3). A balanced regimen containing both dextrose and lipid is preferred in most patients, as protein utilization appears to be better when both substrates are present. The proportion of carbohydrate and fat which promotes maximum protein utilization is unknown. A regi-

Table 3. Standard formulas for parenteral nutrition (150:1) to provide ~150 non-protein calories per gram of nitrogen.

Regimen D – no fat	Regimen E – moderate fat	Regimen F – low fat
TPN Solution:	TPN Solution:	TPN Solution:
Dextrose 30%	Dextrose 20%	Dextrose 25%
Amino acids 4.25%	Amino acids 4.25%	Amino acids 4.25%
Lipid:	Lipid:	Lipid:
None	200 ml of 20% fat emulsion per liter of TPN	225 ml of 10% fat emulsion per liter of TPN
Composition of intake (% of total intake):	Composition of intake (% of total intake):	Composition of intake (% of total intake):
Carbohydrate 86%	Carbohydrate 58%	Carbohydrate 71%
Protein 14%	Protein 13%	Protein 13%
Fat 0%	Fat 29%	Fat 16%
Non-protein kcal: g N = 143:1	Non-protein kcal: g N = 151:1	Non-protein kcal: g N = 153:1

men containing a lower proportion of carbohydrate ($\leq 50\%$ of calories as dextrose, e.g., Regimen E) is better tolerated in diabetics, patients receiving steroids and others who are glucose intolerant. Regimen D provides all non-protein calories as dextrose. This regimen is indicated in patients who are lipid intolerant.

Essential fatty acids

In addition to providing calories, the fat emulsion is a parenteral source of essential fatty acids. It is estimated that a minimum of 4% of the daily caloric requirement should be provided as essential fatty acids to prevent essential fatty acid deficiency (EFAD). Intralipid® and Travamulsion® (soybean oil) are 64% essential fatty acids (56% linoleic acid, 8% linolenic acid) and Liposyn® (safflower oil) is 77% essential fatty acid (linoleic acid).

The standardized parenteral nutrition regimens (Tables 2, 3) which include the fat emulsion, contain adequate essential fatty acids to meet essential fatty acid requirements. The regimens using only dextrose as the non-protein calorie source may produce essential fatty acid deficiency. If they are continued beyond two weeks, the lipid-free regimens should be supplemented with at least two 500 ml bottles of 10% fat emulsion per week (or one 500 ml bottle of 20% fat emulsion per week) to meet the minimum requirement for essential fatty acids.

Electrolytes in parenteral nutrition

The parenteral nutrition regimen should include sodium, potassium, phosphorus, magnesium, calcium, chloride and acetate as additives to the dextrose-amino acid solution. The usual requirement for these elctrolytes can be met by using two to three liters per day of a standardized electrolyte formula (Table 4). The electrolytes in the standardized formula are added to the amino acid solution by the manufacturer, requires less time to prepare by the pharmacy and are, therefore, less expensive to the patient.

The electrolyte requirements of the critically ill patient may differ from the usual adult requirements because of such problems as renal failure, nasogastric losses, fistula losses, sepsis, and acid–base imbalance. Electrolyte intake via TPN may be adjusted as indicated by the patient's needs. For example, if the patient is in renal failure and has developed hyperphosphatemia and hypermagnesemia, the quantity of phosphorus and magnesium in the parenteral nutrition solution should be reduced to zero. When serum phosphorus and magnesium levels return to normal, these electrolytes should be added to the parenteral nutrition solution in amounts modified for the existing level of renal function.

Acid–base imbalance may be affected by the amount of chloride and acetate in the parenteral nutrition solution. The amino acids are present in the solution as the acetate salts; therefore, all amino acids solutions contain at least acetate as an electrolyte. The amount of acetate present in the amino acid solution is usually sufficient to prevent metabolic acidosis from the metabolism of the amino acids. If acidosis is present or develops, additional acetate may be added as the sodium or potassium salt. If alkalosis is present or develops, increasing the chloride concentration as the sodium or potassium salt and decreasing the acetate concentration may help.

Table 4. Adult electrolyte requirements for parenteral nutrition.

	Usual electrolyte requirement per 24 hours	Standard concentration per liter of TPN
Sodium, mEq	60–100	35
Potassium, mEq	60–100	30
Magnesium, mEq	10–20	5
Calcium, mEq	10–15	5
Phosphorus, mmole	20–45	15
Chloride, mEq	[a]	[b]
Acetate, mEq	[a]	[b]

[a] Varies with acid–base status.
[b] Varies amino acid product use.

If electrolyte deficiencies exist or there is an increased need for replacement (e.g., increased losses via the gastrointestinal (GI) tract), the electrolyte concentrations in the parenteral nutrition solution may be increased as needed. However, it is preferable to use a second i.v. solution, e.g., $D_5 0.45$ NaCl with KCl, to replace GI losses which are not constant as this is a quicker, cheaper means of replacement.

Limitations do exist for calcium, phosphorus and magnesium as their compatibility in the parenteral nutrition solution is concentration dependent. The compatibility of calcium, phosphorus and magnesium is also related to the concentration of amino acids, the temperature of the solution and many other variables. The pharmacy should be consulted to determine compatibility for a given solution.

Vitamins and trace elements in parenteral nutrition

Vitamin and trace element requirements during acute stress are unknown. It is recommended, however, that the usual maintenance doses of vitamins and trace elements be given except in patients with renal failure. In patients with renal failure, the daily trace element intake is given no more than twice weekly to prevent potentially toxic accumulation.

The American Medical Association Nutrition Advisory Group has established guidelines for the daily intravenous intake of vitamins and trace elements. There are numerous multivitamin products for intravenous use which contain different combinations and concentrations of vitamins. MVI-12® (USV Labs), M.V.C. 9+3® (Lypho-Med, Inc.), and Multivitamin Additive® (Abbott) are products currently available which contain all of the essential vitamins (except vitamin K) in appropriate concentrations. The recommended dose of each product is 10 ml daily added to the parenteral nutrition solution as phytonadione (Aquamephyton®); 1 mg daily is sufficient for maintenance requirements.

There are also several multi-trace element products available. All of them contain zinc, copper, manganese and chromium and will meet the American Medical Association Nutrition Advisory Group's recommended intake if the appropriate dose is given. For example, Multi-Trace Metal Additive® (IMS) will provide appropriate amounts of zinc, copper, manganese and chromium (4 mg, 1 mg, 0.5 mg, 10 mcg, respectively) in 1 ml added to the parenteral nutrition solution daily (or twice weekly in patients with renal failure).

Solution administration

Patients who are acutely stressed will generally require a more gradual initiation of the full parenteral nutrition regimen, as their ability to achieve the hormone balance necessary to accept the dextrose load may be com-

UNIVERSITY OF MINNESOTA HOSPITALS & CLINICS

PHYSICIAN'S ORDERS (STANDING ORDERS)

ORIGINATED BY (PHYSICIAN)	ORIGINATED	REVIEWED
Frank B. Cerra	2/82	

PATIENT IDENTIFICATION PLATE

TITLE:

Page 1 of 1

ADULT PARENTERAL NUTRITION MONITORING

Daily weights; I & O

Diabetic urines q6h.

Change tubing, filter and dressing q24h or as per station policy or as per Hospital policy

Calorie/protein counts (notify dietitian)

( ) Routine Lab Screening (for other tests, see "Special Lab Screening" below)

    GNE: qd x 7, then q Mon, Weds, and Fri

    MAD, Mg, Phos, Pre-albumin: day 1 and then q Mon and Thurs

    PT, albumin and transferrin: day 1 and then q Mon

    CBC with diff. and platelets: day 1 and then q Mon

    UUN: 24 hr urine collection on ice 12M to 12M to chemistry at initiation of TPN and q Mon (urinary urea nitrogen for nitrogen balance).

    If patient is on Intralipids: Triglyceride and Cholesterol q Mon (draw before hanging next bottle of Intralipid).

    Special Lab Screening (as indicated)

( ) Skin test battery at initiation of TPN and q14 days - mumps, candida and PPD intermediate strength.

( ) B-OH Butyrate, Acetoacetate, Lactate, Pyruvate: 7cc x 2 grey top on ice to chemistry; CVP or arterial blood.

( ) Aminogram: 10cc green top to Medical Genetics (to Dr. Tsai's lab); draw CVP or arterial blood on ice - amino acids and FFA.

( ) Total Nitrogen: 24 hr. urine collection on ice; 12M to 12M to chemistry.

( ) 3-Methyl-histidine: 24 hr. urine collection on ice to Medical Genetics (to Dr. Tsai's lab).

PSO1-936

PHYSICIANS ORDERS

SIGNATURE OF PHYSICIAN	DATE
M.D.	

21931; JUN 81

ORIGINAL - MEDICAL RECORD · · COPY · PHARMACY

Figure 1. University of Minnesota Hospitals adult parenteral nutrition monitoring.

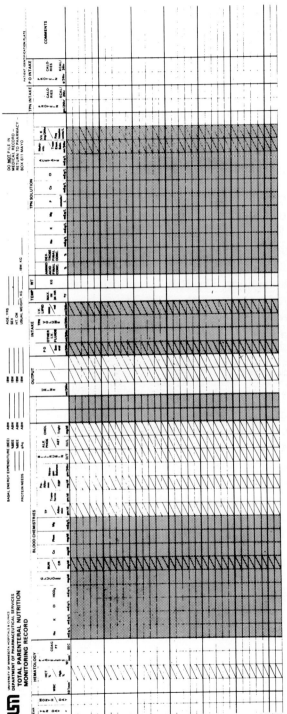

Figure 2. University of Minnesota Hospitals adult TPN monitoring record.

promised. The dextrose-amino acid infusion should be started at an infusion rate of 40 ml/hr and advanced by 50–100% in subsequent 24-hour periods. The maximum desired infusion rate can usually be achieved in 48–72 hours. Blood glucose should be closely monitored as the rate of the infusion is increased. If glucose intolerance develops, the rate should not be further advanced until the hyperglycemia is controlled. Control of hyperglycemia may necessitate decreasing the rate of the dextrose-amino acid infusion or insulin administration.

When parenteral nutrition is no longer required, the dextrose-amino acid solution may be discontinued by reducing the infusion rate to 40 ml/hr for two hours. This will prevent rebound hypoglycemia. If the dextrose-amino acid solution must be stopped abruptly, infuse a 10% dextrose solution at the same rate the dextrose-amino acid solution was infusing.

Intravenous fat emulsions do not require a gradual initiation or tapering. However, the manufacturers usually recommend that an initial test dose of 1 ml/min for 30 minutes be given to observe for any hypersensitivity or other untoward reactions. The 10% fat emulsions should be infused at a rate not to exceed 125 ml/hr, and the 20% fat emulsions should be infused at a rate not to exceed 60 ml/hr. It is not necessary to infuse the fat emulsions at a continuous rate over 24 hours.

MONITORING PARENTERAL NUTRITION [34, 35]

Appropriate monitoring of the parenteral nutrition regimen is critical to its success. Monitoring should include evaluation of the nutritional and metabolic effects of the regimen as well as recognition of potential complications. Monitoring may be facilitated through the use of preprinted physician's orders which identify the parameters to be monitored and the frequency of monitoring (Figure 1). Maintaining a flowsheet on which pertinent data (Figure 2) is recorded daily, will also assist in monitoring the patient's response to the parenteral nutrition regimen.

Assessment of calorie and protein intake

In initiating parenteral nutrition, the patient's calorie and protein requirements are estimated using the guidelines previously discussed. To determine if the patient's actual intake derived from these estimates is adequate, the following parameters should be monitored:

Parameter	Frequency
Weight	QD
Fluid intake and output	Q 24 hours
Calorie/protein count	Q 24 hours
Nitrogen balance	Weekly
Serum proteins: (one or more)	Weekly
albumin	
transferrin	
retinol binding protein	
thyroxine binding prealbumin	

The serum amino acid profile can also be useful in evaluating the patient's tolerance to the particular amino acid solution being infused.

Glucose tolerance

The stressed patient is frequently glucose intolerant. To evaluate the patient's tolerance of the administered dextrose load and response in insulin therapy (if required), monitoring will include:

Parameter	Frequency
Blood glucose	Daily (until stable)
Urine glucose and ketones	Q 6 hours
Blood gases	As indicated
Serum insulin and glucagon	As indicated

Carbohydrate intolerance in the presence or absence of hyperglycemia may also be manifest by an elevated pCO_2. This is due to carbohydrate metabolism which results in a relatively high carbon dioxide production. Insulin resistance may also exacerbate glucose intolerance and can be determined by obtaining serum insulin and glucagon levels.

Lipid tolerance

Lipid metabolism may be abnormal during periods of acute stress. Prior to administration of exogenous lipid, as well as periodically during a course of parenteral nutrition in which lipids are included, lipid tolerance must be evaluated.

Parameter	Frequency
Gross lipemia	Daily
Serum cholesterol/triglycerides	Weekly
Serum free fatty acids	As indicated

During the infusion of an i.v. fat emulsion, the patient will experience a transient lipemia and transient elevation of serum cholesterol and triglycerides. These may persist for several hours after discontinuing the infusion. To allow for normal clearance of the i.v. fat emulsion, lipid tolerance should be evaluated approximately eight hours after completion of the infusion.

Fluid tolerance

As the parenteral nutrition regimen may account for 2–3 liters of fluid intake per day and as the stressed patient frequently has medical problems which may complicate fluid balance, it is important to closely monitor the patient's fluid status.

Parameter	Frequency
Weight	QOD
Fluid intake and output	Q 24 hours
Vital signs	Q 8 hours
Hematocrit	2 times per week
BUN: creatinine	2 times per week
Central venous pressure	As indicated

In addition to the above parameters, the daily physical examination of the patient should include an assessment of fluid status observing for signs and symptoms of dehydration or fluid overload.

Electrolyte and acid–base balance

As the dextrose, lipid and protein are utilized for energy production and tissue synthesis, electrolyte and acid–base balance will be effected. Some electrolytes (e.g., K^+, Mg, Phos) will be transported intracellularly to participate in these processes and others (e.g., H^+) will be generated and released into the extracellular fluid. To assure that the changing demands for all electrolytes in the acutely stressed patient are met and to prevent excesses or deficiencies, close monitoring is required.

Parameter	Frequency
Na, K, Cl, HCO$_3$	Daily until stable
Mg, Phos, Ca	Q 2–4 days
Blood gases	As indicated
Urine electrolytes	As indicated

Electrolyte and acid–base imbalances may also be caused by renal failure, gastrointestinal losses, sepsis and compromised pulmonary function. These factors are frequently present in the acutely stressed patient and emphasize the need for close monitoring to prevent serious complications.

Renal and hepatic function

Renal and hepatic function may influence substrate utilization. Severe impairment of either may necessitate modifications in the parenteral nutrition regimen, especially protein, electrolyte and fluid intake. Hepatic function should also be monitored because of potential toxicity resulting from the parenteral nutrition regimen.

Parameter	Frequency
BUN, creatinine	Twice weekly
SGOT, alkaline phosphatase, bilirubin	Twice weekly

Metabolic status

When necessary, the level of stress can be defined by various indices of metabolic function. The parenteral nutrition will be designed to optimize substrate utilization at each level of stress. To determine when changes in the parenteral nutrition regimen are indicated, metabolic function must be monitored.

Parameter	Frequency
Nitrogen balance	Q 3 days
Glucose intolerance	Daily
Urinary 3-methylhistidine excretion	Q 3 days
Plasma lactate	Q 3 days
Plasma amino acids	Q 3 days

As the patient becomes stabilized and the level of stress is reduced, the frequency of monitoring these parameters can be decreased to once a week.

Infection

The acutely stressed patient may be more susceptible to infection because of many factors including multiple foreign bodies (e.g., foley catheter, subclavian catheter), broad spectrum antibiotic use and prolonged steroids. The development of an infection in the patient receiving parenteral nutrition may cause many serious metabolic complications. Early recognition through appropriate monitoring will facilitate management of the infection and minimize the incidence of subsequent metabolic complications.

Parameter	Frequency
Maximum temperature	Daily
White blood count	Q 3 days
Vital signs	Q 8 hours

COMPLICATIONS OF PARENTERAL NUTRITION

As emphasized in the preceding section, monitoring the patient closely is essential for early recognition and successful management of the complications associated with parenteral nutrition. The critically ill patient may develop sepsis, hepatic failure, respiratory failure, and/or renal failure which may be affected by parenteral nutrition or which may potentiate the complications of parenteral nutrition. Awareness of the factors which frequently predispose the patient to each potential complication will facilitate prevention. The complications associated with parenteral nutrition can be categorized as related to substrate intolerance, electrolyte, fluid and acid–base abnormalities, nutrition, and infection. Each complication will be outlined identifying the predisposing factors and appropriate management.

Substrate intolerance

Problem	Predisposing factors	Management
Hyperglycemia	Stress, corticosteroids, pancreatitis, diabetes mellitus, peritoneal dialysis	↓ dextrose intake: ↓ rate of infusion or ↓ dextrose concentration) and substitute fat calories; insulin infusion

Substrate intolerance (continued)

Hypoglycemia (rare)	Abrupt withdrawal of dextrose, insulin overdose	↑ dextrose intake; ↓ exogenous insulin intake
Excess CO₂ production	Excess dextrose intake	↓ dextrose intake, balance calories as fat and dextrose
Hyperlipidemia (↑ cholesterol, ↑ triglycerides)	Stress, familial hyperlipidemia, pancreatitis	↓ fat intake or discontinue if indicated
Serum amino acid imbalance	Stress, hepatic failure	Modify amino acid intake if possible or ↓ amino acid intake
Abnormal LFTs (↑ SGOT, ↑ alkaline phosphatase, ↑ bilirubin)	Stress, infection, cancer, excess carbohydrate intake, excess total calorie intake, essential fatty acid deficiency	↓ dextrose intake (substitute fat), ↓ total calorie intake, provide essential fatty acids

Fluid, electrolyte and acid–base abnormalities

Problem	Predisposing factors	Management
Hypovolemia	Gastrointestinal fluid losses, osmotic diuresis	↑ fluid intake
Hypervolemia	Renal failure, excess fluid intake	↑ fluid intake, diuretics
Hyponatremia	Gastrointestinal losses, fluid overload, diuretics	(varies with cause)
Hypernatremia	Dehydration	↑ fluid intake
Hypokalemia	Gastrointestinal losses, diuretics, anabolism	↑ potassium intake
Hyperkalemia	Renal failure	↓ potassium intake
Hypophosphatemia	Phosphate-binding antacids, anabolism, phosphate-free dialysate	d/c phosphate-binders, ↑ phosphorus intake
Hyperphosphatemia	Renal failure	↓ phosphorus intake
Hypomagnesemia	Diarrhea, malabsorption, anabolism	↑ magnesium intake
Hypermagnesemia	Renal failure	↓ magnesium intake
Hypocalcemia	Hypoalbuminemia; chronic renal failure	↑ calcium intake (with CFR only)
Hypercalcemia	(Rare)	↓ calcium intake
Metabolic acidosis	Diarrhea, high output fistulae, renal failure; excess amino acid intake	↑ acetate in TPN, ↓ Cl in TPN; ↓ amino acid intake
Metabolic alkalosis	Gastric losses	↑ Cl in TPN, ↓ acetate in TPN

Infection complications

Identifying catheter sepsis in the acutely stressed patient who has multiple potential sources of fever may be difficult. Catheter sepsis is defined as a septic episode in which no other site of infection is obvious, the fever resolves upon catheter removal and cultures of the catheter tip and peripheral blood grow the same organism. The steps to be taken in a patient receiving parenteral nutrition who develops an elevated temperature are:

1. Discontinue the TPN solution, change tubing and administer D_{10} 1/2 NS at the same rate through the same catheter.
2. Culture blood (from CVP and peripherally), sputum, urine as well as other appropriate sites for bacteria and fungi.
3. Monitor vital signs.
4. If the source of infection is found, treat appropriately and reinstitute parenteral nutrition infusion.
5. If no source is found, continue D_{10} 1/2 NS infusion for 12 hours. If temperature then returns to normal, reinstitute parenteral nutrition infusion.
6. If temperature remains elevated, remove catheter and administer fluids peripherally.
7. If the clinical situation warrants it, remove the central line immediately.
8. When the patient has been afebrile 48 hours, parenteral nutrition may be restarted through a new central line.

The incidence of catheter sepsis can be minimized through proper care of the catheter insertion site and by limiting the use of the central line to administration of only the parenteral nutrition solution. Catheter sepsis seldom requires treatment with antibiotics as once the focus of infection has been removed the bacteremia or fungemia will usually clear in two or three days without antibiotics. Exceptions to this generalization include: immunosuppressed patients, immunocompromised patients, and very sick patients. Repeated cultures and the clinical setting will usually clarify the issues.

Nutritional complications

Most of the nutritional complications associated with parenteral nutrition develop after many weeks to months of an inappropriate intake of a particular nutrient. However, in the acutely stressed patient who has a pre-existing condition of malnutrition, nutritional deficiencies may develop earlier in the course of parenteral nutrition if the regimen is lacking in any nutrient. It is therefore important to include essential fatty acids, vitamins and trace elements in at least maintenance doses in all patients receiving parenteral nutrition. If specific deficiencies are identified, replacement doses should be given.

Nutrient toxicities may also develop, but usually are the result of chronic accumulation, particularly of fat soluable vitamins or trace elements. These toxicities result from either excessive intake or reduced elimination. Trace element intake should be reduced in patients with renal failure to prevent potentially toxic accumulation as a result of decreased renal excretion.

HOME PARENTERAL NUTRITION

For those patients where such therapy is required, a 10–14 day training course is usually required. Appropriate line care, pump use, solution use, additive administration, safety, and troubleshooting must be effectively and reliably taught to patients and usually family or friends. The input of nursing, pharmacy, dietary, and social service is usually necessary to establish and implement the necessary protocol, teaching, and follow-up. Many of the existing home care services will also be of some help. However, an interested, trained physician must take the responsibility for the whole process and its follow-up for effective results with a minimum of complications.

ENTERAL NUTRITION SUPPORT

This route of support is the cheapest, eliminates the problems of intravenous support, and does not require sterilized equipment. It does, however, require access to an adequately functioning GI tract. This is particularly so when gastric feedings are done. Here close observation of gastric motility must be done to avoid regurgitation, bloating, vomiting and aspiration. In sick patients gastric motility is usually interferred with early. Generally, routes of administration distal to the pyloris are preferred. Other problems peculiar to tube feeds also occur and will be discussed [36–39].

In many cases where only small or modest calorie/protein deficits exist, oral supplementation can be done. Appropriate monitoring of calorie/protein counts, absorption and effects are necessary to be sure the deficits are being met or to ascertain if a higher level of support is necessary.

The considerations of when to support, how to assess needs and calculate requirements, and the impact of surgical, septic or traumatic stress are also quite applicable to enteral nutrition. To this end, multiple new formulas more appropriate for stress are in testing and will soon be available [38–40].

114

UNIVERSITY OF MINNESOTA HOSPITALS & CLINICS
PHYSICIAN'S ORDERS (STANDING ORDERS)

ORIGINATED BY (PHYSICIAN)	ORIGINATED	REVIEWED
Frank B. Cerra	2/82	

PATIENT IDENTIFICATION PLATE

TITLE:

ADULT ENTERAL FEEDING: PAGE 1 OF 1

ADMINISTRATION AND MONITORING

Formula desired:_____

Aspirate residuals q4h. Call H.O. with _____cc return.
Flush feeding tube with _____cc of _____q4h, after feedings and meds.
Hang fresh feeding q8h.
Check tube placement q shift or before intermittent feeding.
Change feeding bag and tubing q24h.
Elevate HOB 30-45°.
Daily weights; I&O.
Diabetic urines q6h.
Calorie/protein counts (notify dietitian)

Administration of Feedings (choose one)

( ) Continuous Administration

1. Initiate at _____ str. at 50 cc/hr.
2. Increase volume (rate q 12h by 25cc/hr to _____ cc/hr, as tolerated.
3. Increase strength (1/4 to 1/2 to 3/4 to full strength) q 12hr to _____ strength, as tolerated.

( ) Intermittent Administration

1. Initiate at _____ str. at 100cc/fdg. followed by _____cc H_2O q ____h, _____ times a day.
2. On Day 2, increase to _____cc/fdg. (not to exceed 400cc/fdg.), as tolerated.
3. On Day 3, increase to full strength, as tolerated.

( ) Routine Monitoring

1. GNE q d x 3, then Monday and Thursday.
2. MAD, Mg, P Day 1 and then q Monday.
3. PT, albumin, retinol binding protein Day 1 and q Monday.

Special Lab Screening (as indicated)

( ) Nitrogen Balance Study - 24 hour urine collection on ice - 12M to 12M for urea nitrogen, to Chemistry.

( ) Skin Testing - mumps, candida and PPD intermediate strength.

PHYSICIANS ORDERS

PSO2-608

SIGNATURE OF PHYSICIAN	DATE
M.D.	

21931, JUN 81   ORIGINAL - MEDICAL RECORD   COPY - PHARMACY

Figure 3. University of Minnesota Hospitals adult enteral feeding: administration and monitoring.

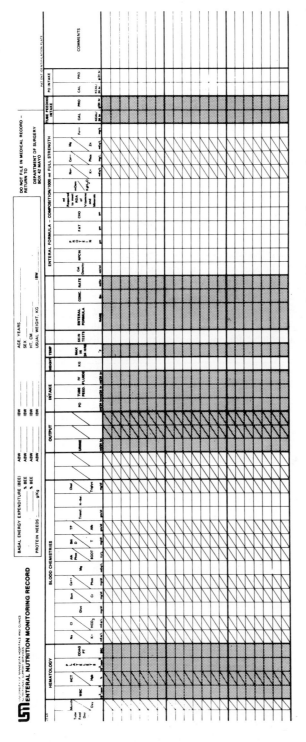

Figure 4. University of Minnesota Hospitals adult enteral nutrition monitoring record.

Having decided route and site, the next issue relates to what formulas are currently available. They are numerous and are grossly categorized into complete or incomplete. Complete formulas contain all 6 necessary components: carbohydrate, fat, protein, vitamins, minerals, and electrolytes. Incomplete formulas do not contain one or more of the 6 components; thus, these may need to be supplemented. The various solutions can then be classified as follows.

A. Blenderized formulas

Definition	— table foods that have been blenderized to liquid form; high in residue
Composition	— intact protein of high biological value (HBV), complex and simple carbohydrates, fiber and long chain fats
Indications	— usually administered to patients whose GI tracts are completely functional but who cannot or will not take food by mouth; particularly ideal for the aged as adequate residue is available to restore or maintain bowel integrity and function
Advantages	— contain all nutrients found in food
Disadvantages	— high viscosity may result in difficulty of passage through small-bore feeding tubes; moderately high in osmolality; may contain lactose; not acceptable for oral supplementation; relatively expensive

Products	Kcal/cc	mOsm/kg	% Kcal as LC fat	gm pro/2000 Kcal	ml. Req. to meet RDA
Compleat B [a]	1	390	36	80	1600
Compleat modified [a]	1	300	31.1	80	1500
Formula 2 [a]	1	435–510	36	75	2000
Vitaneed [a]	1	375	35	69	1470

B. Milk-based formulas

Definition	—	contain protein and nutrients from milk; moderately high in residue
Composition	—	intact protein of HBV; primarily long chain fats, disaccharides, and corn syrup solids
Indications	—	requires a completely functional GI tract; usually administered to patients who cannot or will not take adequate oral nutrition; as a supplement; concentrated source of nutrients; generally not administered via tube
Advantages	—	generally more palatable than milk-free products
Disadvantages	—	contain lactose; high in osmolality

Products	Kcal/cc	mOsm/kg	% Kcal as LC fat	gm pro/2000 Kcal	ml. Req. to meet RDA
Meritene liquid [a]	1	560	30	120	1200
Meritene-powder [a]	1	690	29	138	1040
Sustacal-powder [a]	1	756	22	120	1080
Sustagen [a]	1.7	1100	8.6	133	1050
CIB [a]	1	615–650	25	113	1373
Sport Shake [b]	1.3	NA	33	71	NA

C. Lactose-free formulas

Definition	—	caseinate and soy isolate-based products, lactose free, low in residue
Composition	—	largely intact protein, oligosaccharides; and long chain fats with a limited number containing some medium chain triglycerides (MCT)
Indications	—	in general, require a functional GI tract; may be used as both supplemental or total nutrition via tube or consumed orally
Advantages	—	lactose free; most are moderately palatable and relatively inexpensive to use; free flowing consistency which allows use of small-bore feeding tubes
Disadvantages	—	quality of protein is not as high as that in milk-based or blenderized formulas

Products	Kcal/cc	mOsm/Kg	% Kcal as LC fat	gm pro/2000 Kcal	ml. Req. to meet RDA
Isocal [a]	1	300	30	65	1920
Ensure [a]	1	450	31.5	74	1887
Sustacal HC [a]	1.5	650	34	81	1200
Ensure Plus [a]	1.5	600	32	73	2000
Renu [a]	1	330	36	65	2000
Sustacal [a]	1	625	21	120	1080
Osmolite [a]	1	300	16	74	1887
Magnacal [a]	2	590	36	70	1000
Portagen [a, c]	1	354	5	70	960
Isocal HCN [a]	2	740	39	75	1500
Travasorb [a]	1	488	31.5	74	1900

D. Chemically-defined formulas

Definition	— nutrients are supplied in partially 'predigested' simple forms with minimal residue and lactose free
Composition	— protein composition varies from intact HBV protein to peptide and amino acid mixtures, carbohydrate is supplied as oligo- and disaccharides, in general a minimum of fat is provided mostly as long chain fats
Indications	— designed for patients with limited GI function and/or metabolic abnormalities; may be used as total or supplemental nutrition via tube or orally consumed
Advantages	— requires minimal digestion and absorption for utilization of nutrients (almost totally absorbed in duodenum and proximal jejunum), lactose free; low in viscosity, easily administered via small-bore feeding tube
Disadvantages	— high osmolality may cause GI distress and metabolic derangements (i.e. diarrhea, dehydration, etc.); significantly more expensive than diets composed of intact nutrients; relatively unpalatable in pure form

Products	Kcal/cc	mOsm/Kg	% Kcal as LC fat	gm pro/2000 Kcal	ml. Req. to meet RDA
Precision HN [b]	1	557	1.1	88	2850
Precision Isotonic [a]	1	300	28	58	1560
Precision LR [b]	1	525–545	1.3	52	1710
Citrotein [b]	0.66	500	2	121	NA
Isotein HN [a]	1.2	300	19	114	1800
Travasorb MCT [a, c]	1–2	312–590	6	98	1000–2000
Travasorb Std [a, c]	1	560	5	60	2000
Travasorb HN [a, c]	1	560	5	90	2000
Flexical	1	550	25	45	2000
Vital HN [a, c]	1	460	4	84	1500
Vipep [a, c]	1	520	4	50	2000
Criticare HN [a, c]	1	650	2.8	72	2000

E. Free amino acid formulas (elemental)

Definition	— proteins are supplied in 'predigested' simple forms with minimal residue and lactose free
Composition	— approximately 80–90% of calories as glucose oligosaccharides; amino acids, a minimal amount of long chain fats
Indications	— designed for patients with limited GI function and/or metabolic abnormalities; in general to be used as total nutrition via feeding tube
Advantages	— requires minimal digestion and absorption for utilization of nutrients (totally absorbed in duodenum and proximal jejunum); lactose free; low viscosity, easily administered via small-bore feeding tube
Disadvantages	— high osmolality may cause GI distress and metabolic derangements; relatively expensive; unpalatable

Products	Kcal/cc	mOsm/Kg	% Kcal as LC fat	gm pro/2000 Kcal	ml. Req. to meet RDA
Vivonex [b]	1	550	1.3	41	1800
Vivonex HN [b]	1	810	0.8	84	3000

F. Specialty formulas

Definition	— a product designed for specific organ failure (i.e. liver failure, renal failure)
Composition	— free amino acids, oligosaccharides, short and long chain fats; lactose free
Indications	— designed for patients with specific organ failure; requires some degree of digestion and absorption; may be administered via tube or orally consumed
Advantages	— theoretically, nitrogen balance may be maintained and/or achieved without exacerbating the specific organ failure
Disadvantages	— may have to be supplemented with vitamins, minerals, trace elements, electrolytes, high osmolality may cause GI distress and metabolic derangements; relatively unpalatable; very expensive

Products	Kcal/cc	mOsm/Kg	% Kcal as LC fat	gm pro/2000 Kcal	ml. Req. to meet RDA
Hepatic-Aid [b]	1.6	900	20	54	NA
Amin-Aid [b]	1.9	900	31	20	NA
Travasorb-Hepatic [b, c]	1.1	690	3.5	53	NA
Travasorb-Renal [b, c]	1.35	590	3.5	34	NA

[a] 'Complete' formula, containing all six necessary nutrients: carbohydrates, protein, fat, vitamins, minerals electrolytes.
[b] 'Incomplete' formula missing one or more of the six necessary nutrients.
[c] Contains >2% of Kcal's as LC fat, but may need EFA supplementation.

G. Feeding modules/caloric additives

Definition	— products which supply one single nutrient or combinations of nutrients
Composition	— varies according to product
Indications	— in general, used in specific disease states to alter one or more of the commercial formula or oral diet components; may be combined with other feeding modules to produce a nutritionally complete feeding
Advantages	— allows greater flexibility in tailoring formulas to meet patients special requirements
Disadvantages	— increases amount of labor required to prepare formulas; may need vitamin, mineral, and electrolyte supplementation

CHO source	Polycose and Moducal	— glucose polymers	2 Kcal/cc
	Sumacal	4 Kcal/gm;	2 Kcal/cc
	Sumacal Plus	— maltodextrin	2.5 Kcal/cc
	Hycal	— maltodextrin	2.45 Kcal/cc
		— liquid glucose	
Pro source	Pro Mix	— whey protein hydrolysate	1oz. = 24 gm protein
	Casec	— calcium caseinate	1oz. = 24 gm protein
	Propac	— whey protein concentrate	1oz. = 23 gm protein
Fat source	Lipomul	— corn oil emulsion;	6 Kcal/cc; 54% EFA
	MCT	— fractionated coconut oil;	7.7 Kcal/cc; No EFA
	Microlipid	— safflower oil emulsion;	4.5 Kcal/cc; 72% EFA
CHO and fat source	Controlyte – corn starch, veg. oil; 5 Kcal/gm; 2 Kcal/cc		

Vitamins, minerals, electrolytes: added as necessary

As with the parenteral solutions, appropriate priming must be done to minimize complications. Either continuous or bolus techniques can be used and are summarized as:

1. *Continuous feedings (24 hrs/day)*
    1. Initiate formula at 1/4–1/2 strength, 50 cc/hr
    2. Increase volume (rate) every 12 hours by 25 cc until desired rate is achieved
    3. Increase strength every 12 hours: 1/4 to 1/2 to 3/4 to full strength (FS) as tolerated

2. *Intermittent feedings (4–6 fdgs/day)*
    Day 1: 1/4–1/2 strength at 100 cc/fdg, followed by 50–100 cc water q4-6hrs
    Day 2: Increase to desired volume not to exceed 400 cc formula/fdg, as tolerated
    Day 3: Increase to 3/4 strength and finally FS, as tolerated

The metabolic and nutritional complications are similar to those seen with parenteral alimentation. There are also problems and complications peculiar to tube feeds [39–43].

Gastric retention, vomiting and aspiration are common. Using tubes distal to the pyloris, elevating the head of the bed 30 degrees and using continuous drips with frequent monitoring of residual volume can minimize these risks.

Diarrhea is also a common problem. It is usually not due to osmolality per se, but more often due to high feeding rates or too concentrated a solution. After adjusting these factors by continuous pumped feeds and feeding dilution [37, 38], consideration should be given to the effects of starvation on the GI mucosa, presence of hypoalbuminemia, concomitant use of antibiotic therapy, pancreatic or biliary insufficiency, short gut syndrome, lactose intolerance or contaminated feedings. Antidiarrheals are sometimes useful. If the problem persists, TPN may be necessary.

Monitoring, in addition to those aspects mentioned, is the same as for parenteral (Figures 3, 4). A protocol order sheet is quite useful in facilitating application and minimizing complications and problems. Home enteral nutrition is also now a reality. In general, however, it is usually easier and cheaper than parenteral alimentation.

SUMMARY

Malnutrition as starvation or altered metabolism is a common problem in cancer. Nutritional support is not antineoplastic, but can reduce morbidity and mortality of nutritional complications and can improve the quality of life. Advances in metabolic understanding and improvements in therapy may lead to a true antineoplastic role for this therapy. At the present time, however, the cancer patient at least need not die of starvation.

REFERENCES

1. Brennan MF: Total parenteral nutrition in cancer patients. N Engl J Med 305(7):375–382, 1981.
2. Warnold I, Lundholm K, Schersten T: Energy balance and body composition in cancer patients. Cancer Res 38:1801-1807, 1978.
3. Waterhouse C: Lactate metabolism in patients with cancer. Cancer 33:66–71, 1974.
4. Rudman D, Vogler WR, Howard CH, Gerron GG: Observations on the plasma amino acids of patients with acute leukemia. Cancer Res 31:1159-1165, 1971.
5. Marks PA, Bishop JS: The glucose metabolism of patients with malignant disease and of normal subjects as studied by means of an intravenous glucose tolerance test. J Clin Invest 36:254–264, 1957.
6. Burt ME, Gorschboth C, Brennan MF: A controlled prospective randomized trial evaluating the metabolic effects of enteral and parenteral nutrition in the cancer patient. Cancer 6(44):1092, 1982.
7. Waterhouse C, Heanpretre N, Keilson J: Gluconeogenesis from alanine in patients with progressive malignant disease. Cancer Res 39:1968–1972, 1979.
8. Copeland EM, III, Daly JM, Dudrick SJ: Nutrition as an adjunct to cancer treatment in the adult. Cancer Res 37:2451-2456, 1977.
9. Waterhouse C, Clarke EF, Heinig RE, Lewis AM, Jeanpretre N: Free amino acid levels in the blood of patients undergoing parenteral alimentation. AM J Clin Nutr 32:2423-2429, 1979.
10. Brennan MF, Burt ME: Nitrogen metabolism in cancer. Cancer Treat Rep (in press).
11. Burt ME, Stein TP, Schwade JG, Brennan MF: Effect of total parenteral nutrition on protein metabolism in man. Am J Clin Nutr (Abstract) 34:628, 1981.
12. Buzby GP, Mullen JL, Stein TP, Miller EE, Hobbs CL, Rosato EF: Host–tumor interaction and nutrient supply. Cancer 45:2940-2948, 1980.
13. Steiger E, Oram-Smith J, Miller E, Kui L, Bars HM: Effects of nutrition on tumor growth and tolerance to chemotherapy. J Surg Res 18:455–461, 1975.
14. Goodgame JT, Jr, Lowry SF, Brennan MF: Nutritional manipulations and tumor growth II. The effects of intravenous feeding. Am J Clin Nutr 32:2285-2294, 1979.
15. Popp MB, Morrison SD, Brennan MF: Total parenteral nutrition in a methyl cholathrene-induced rat sarcoma model. Cancer Treat Rep (in press).
16. Brennan MF, Copeland EM: Panel report on nutritional support of the cancer patient. Proceedings of an NIH sponsored conference. Am J Clin Nutr 34(Suppl):1199–1205, 1981.
17. Askanazi J, Carpenteur YA, Michelsen CB: Muscle and plasma amino acids following injury. Ann of Surgery 192:78–80, 1980.
18. Border JT, Chenier R, McMenamy RH: Multiple systems organ failure: muscle fuel deficit with visceral protein malnutrition. Surg Clin of N Amer 56:1147–1150, 1976.
19. Cerra FB, Siegel JH, Border JR. Correlations between metabolic and cardiopulmonary measurement in patients after trauma, general surgery and sepsis. J of Trauma 19:621–626, 1979.
20. Cerra FB, Siegel JH, Border JR: The hepatic failure of sepsis: cellular vs. substrate. Surgery 86:409–503, 1979.
21. Cerra FB, Siegel JH, Coleman B: Septic autocannibalism: a failure of exogenous nutritional support. Ann of Surgery 192:570–574, 1980.
22. Clowes GHA, Heideman M, Lindberg B: Effects of parenteral alimentation on amino acid metabolism in septic patients. Surgery 88:531–535, 1980.
23. Fischer JE, Rosen HM, Ebeid AM: The effect of normalization of plasma amino acids on hepatic encephalopathy in man. Surgery 80:77, 1976.

24. Nixon DW, Moffitt S, Lawson DH et al.: Total parenteral nutrition as an adjunct to chemotherapy of metastatic colorectal cancer. Cancer Treat Rep (in press).

25. Nixon D, Moffitt S, Ansley J et al.: Central intravenous hyperalimentation as an adjunct to chemotherapy in advanced colon cancer. Proc Am Assoc Cancer Res/Am Soc Clin Oncol, Abstract 21:173, 1980.

26. Issell BF, Valdivieso M, Zaren HA et al.: Protection against chemotherapy toxicity by IV hyperalimentation. Cancer Treat Rep 62:1139–1143, 1978.

27. Moghissi K, Hornshaw J, Teasdale PR, Dawes EA: Parenteral nutrition in carcinoma of the oesophagus treated by surgery: nitrogen balance and clinical studies. Br J Surg 64:125–128, 1977.

28. Solassol C, Joyeux H: Artificial gut with complete nutritive mixtures as a major adjuvant therapy in cancer patients. Acta Chir Scand (Suppl) 494:18–187, 1979.

29. Warnold I, Falkheden T, Hylten B, Isaksson B: Energy intake and expenditure in selected groups of hospital patients. Am J Clin Nutr 31:742–749, 1978.

30. Brennan MF: Nutritional support of the patient with cancer. In: Principles and Practice of Oncology, DeVita V, Hellman S, Rosenberg SA (eds). Philadelphia, JB Lippincott (in press).

31. Bozzetti F, Pagnoni AM, Del Vecchio M: Excessive caloric expenditure as a cause of malnutrition in patients with cancer. Surg Gynecol Obstet 150:229–234, 1980.

32. Moore FD, Brennan MF: Surgical injury: body composition, protein metabolism and neuroendocrinology. In: Manual of Surgical Nutrition, Ballinger WF, Collins JA, Drucker WR, Dudrick SJ, Zeppa R (eds). Philadelphia, WB Saunders Company, 1975, p 169.

33. Wilmore DW: Alterations in intermediary metabolism. In: The Metabolic Management of the Critically Ill. New York, Plenum Medical Book Company, 1977, p 129.

34. Cerra FB: Profiles in nutritional management – the trauma patient. Chicago, Illinois, Monograph, Medical Directions, Inc, 1982.

35. DeWijs WD, Kubota TT: Enteral and parenteral nutrition in the care of the cancer patient. JAMA 246:1725–1727, 1981.

36. Heitkemper ME et al.: Rate and volume of intermittent enteral feeding. JPEN 5:125–129, 1981.

37. Herbert JS et al.: Comparison of continuous vs. intermittent tube feedings in adult burn patients. JPEN 5:73–75, 1981.

38. Heymsfield SB, Bethel RA, Ansley JD et al.: Enteral hyperalimentation: an alternative to central venous hyperalimentation. Ann Intern Med 90:63–71, 1979.

39. Kaminiski MV: Enteral hyperalimentation. Surg Gynecol Obstet 143:12–16, 1976.

40. Kaminski MV: Enteral hyperalimentation: prevention and treatment of complications. Nutr Sup Services 1:29–35, 1981.

41. Matarese LE: Enteral alimentation: oral and tube feedings, Part I. Nutr Sup Services 1:41–42, 1981.

42. Matarese LE: Enteral alimentation: administration, Part II. Nutr Sup Services 2:36–37, 1981.

43. Matarese LE: Enteral alimentation: equipment, Part III. Nutr Sup Services 2:48–52, 1981.

7. Problems in Surgical Oncology: The Surgical Approach to Recurrent and Metastatic Cancer

HAROLD O. DOUGLASS, JR.

INTRODUCTION

The discovery of metastatic tumor or the appearance of recurrent primary disease must not be treated as a necessary harbinger of doom. Rather, it is the time for meticulous reassessment and an aggressive attack on the malignant process. For some patients, total cure is still possible. For others, long-term palliation providing a reasonable quality of life remains an achievable goal.

An enlarged liver, a defect on the liver scan, the development of jaundice, intestinal obstruction, a broken bone, or new symptoms of nausea and pain do not always indicate metastatic disease. One must remember that a cancer patient with an abdominal incision is first, a post-operative patient, and second, a patient with cancer. Not all intra-abdominal symptoms are due to malignant disease; patients who have had surgical procedures for non-malignant diseases may also develop post-operative problems. Just as it is easy to assign the appearance of a shower of new lesions in the lung of a cancer patient to metastatic disease (even when they are not of classical configuration) when these may be multiple pulmonary emboli, so the tendency exists to consider all problems in the cancer patient as related to the cancer.

Even hematologically and immunologically impaired patients must not be deprived of an opportunity for palliation requiring surgical intervention. Children with leukemia develop appendicitis. Children and adults with leukemia can develop typhlitis. Both situations are curable surgically. An enlarged liver may represent sepsis. The defect on liver scan may be a fungus ball or a liver abscess.

The first step in the assessment for any of these situations mandates histologic confirmation of disease. The surgeon's hand feeling an unbiopsied lesion is no more accurate than a liver scan, regardless of the expertise of the individual surgeon.

Higby, DJ (ed), Supportive Care in Cancer Therapy. ISBN 0-89838-569-5.
© *1983, Martinus Nijhoff Publishers, Boston. Printed in The Netherlands.*

126

At Roswell Park Memorial Institute experience with patients referred to it with unbiopsied lesions in the pancreas diagnosed as pancreatic cancer showed that of one hundred such patients, twenty did not have cancer. More than another twenty had a cancer, but not a cancer of the pancreas. Rather, they had perivaterian cancers, lymphomas or metastatic cancers from another site and were often candidates for therapy that was either potentially curative or could offer prolonged symptom relief.

Another example of the importance of histologic confirmation comes from an Eastern Cooperative Oncology Group study initiated in 1973 and completed in 1975 [1]. Entered into that study but disqualified were a number of patients who had metastatic lesions in the liver in whom a biopsy of the recurrent carcinoma was not available. The vast majority (87%) of the 524 entered patients treated in this protocol had histologic proof of continuing or recurrent cancer: only one or two remain alive. In contrast, nearly

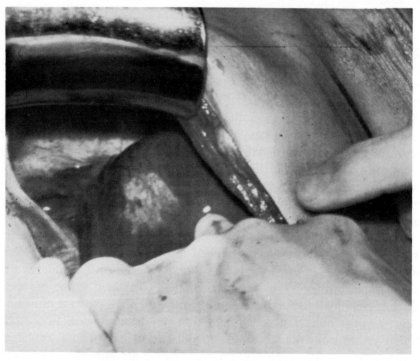

Figure 1. Hepatic nodule thought to be metastatic cancer in patient referred for treatment, but proven on biopsy to be fibrotic sclerosing hemangioma.

twenty percent of the small group (54) of patients who did not have histo-pathologic confirmation appear to be alive and well seven or more years later (Figure 1).

Three basic tenets in the palliative management of the cancer patient must be observed: first, establishment of a diagnosis with histologic confirmation; second, complete assessment of the patient for possible aggressive therapies that may provide long-term palliation or cure; third, evaluation to ensure that the patient's symptomatology is not due to a benign process or secondary complications rather than to recurrent disease.

EXCISION OF METASTASES

The excision of regional metastasis in lymph nodes has long been standard therapy for a number of malignancies. Often these metastatic deposits will be removed at the time of the initial tumor extirpation, but occasionally the lymph node dissection will be deferred. For example, the current trend toward the management of axillary or inguinal lymph nodes in a patient with Stage I, level 1, 2 or 3 melanoma of the extremity would involve observation unless there was clinical evidence of nodal metastases. Should these nodes become enlarged at a later date, they would then be managed by excision. On the other hand, for a patient with a level 4 or 5 or a Stage II melanoma, primary lymph node excision at the time of the initial extirpation of the melanoma is considered by many to be appropriate. Similarly, neck node dissections for carcinoma of the lower lip or small carcinomas of the tongue are often deferred unless node enlargement is noted at the time of the initial operation. Lymphatic resections are part of the local therapy of the tumor, whereas it is the purpose of this chapter to look at the surgical management of patients with distant disease.

Liver metastases

The presence or absence of liver metastases is one of the most significant determinants of survival in the cancer patient. The natural history of histologically confirmed liver metastases suggests a life expectancy averaging five to nine months [2], depending upon the histologic source of the metastatic lesions and the extent of liver involvement. Only a small proportion of patients with liver metastases will survive two years or more. Patients with multiple metastases from colorectal carcinomas usually survive no more than six to eight months, whereas those with tumors that arise in the lung, stomach or pancreas and biliary tracts often expire within two or three months of the diagnosis of metastases. The exception to this rule is the patient with liver metastases from a slowly growing tumor such as an islet cell tumor or carcinoid.

Table 1. Survival following resection of liver metastases.

Primary tumor	Patients	Survival	
		2 year (%)	5 year (%)
Colorectum	259	44	22
Other GI	15	13	7
Melanoma/sarcoma	27	22	7
Other	43	39	19

Results of a nation-wide survey of hepatic resections for liver metastases (after Foster [43]).

Median survivals are even shorter when the metastases involve both lobes of the liver and replace more than 50% of the liver parenchyma, but may extend from sixteen to twenty months when a single or just a few small nodules are present.

For the majority of tumors that metastasize to the liver, systemic chemotherapy is of modest value at best [3]. Among those patients whose tumors arose from sites in the gastrointestinal tract, the rate of objective response to various chemotherapeutic regimens averages no more than 20%. Among metastatic gastric carcinomas, carcinoids and islet cell tumors, a slightly higher response rate can be expected. Radiation therapy may provide pain relief by reducing the discomfort of the enlarged liver caused by the stretching of Glisson's capsule. Unfortunately, the hepatic parenchyma can be damaged by radiation doses in excess of 3,000 rads, while most tumors require 6,000 rads or more before a significant proportion of their contained cells are destroyed. Thus, most tumors that metastasize to the liver are more radioresistant than the adjacent hepatic parenchyma in which they lie. Against this background, an aggressive surgical approach to the management of liver metastasis is seen as rational.

In 1977, Foster surveyed the experience of more than two hundred hospitals evaluating the resection of liver metastases [4]. He was able to identify 259 patients with metastatic carcinoma of the colorectum who had undergone a liver resection. Forty-four percent of this group survived two years, 22% survived five years. However, twelve patients died of recurrence of their carcinoma more than five years following the liver resection (Table 1). Long-term survivals were also seen following resection of liver metastases in patients whose metastases arose from Wilm's tumor, melanoma, sarcoma, pancreatic carcinoma and renal cell tumors.

The analyzed experience at Roswell Park Memorial Institute has been largely confined to metastatic colorectal cancer [5]. Of 34 patients, the excision of the metastatic deposit was done at the time of the primary resection for the colorectal carcinoma in 14 patients, and, at a later date, in 20. Seven patients were found to have more than one metastatic deposit in the excision specimen. Half of the patients treated by excision of the metastases survived two years and most of those patients who survived two years went on to live at least four years following the liver resections.

The margin of normal liver around the tumor mass appeared to be a critical feature in the prolonged survival in the Roswell Park patients [5] for the survival of patients who had margins of normal liver of 2 cm of more.

Reports from the Mayo Clinic emphasize the importance of resection of solitary metastases [6]. Nearly 42% of the patients undergoing resection of solitary metastases survived five years. However, more than one third of these patients subsequently expired of other metastases from the original cancer. On the other hand, no patient from whom multiple metastases were excised lived five years.

Even when not curative, resection of a metastatic deposit in the liver can provide significant palliation for a patient for whom other modalities of therapy are not available. An example of one such patient is a woman with a large liver mass from a carcinoma of the breast (Figure 2). There was no apparent tumor elsewhere. This patient was no longer responsive to hormonal or chemotherapy and had a large, painful mass of tumor replacing most of the right lobe of the liver. In this patient, a hepatic lobectomy was

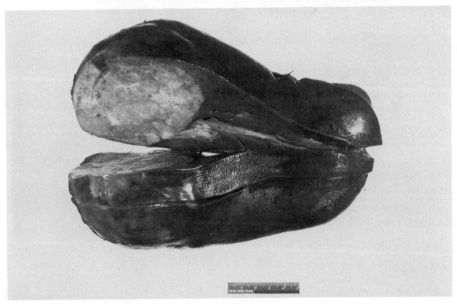

Figure 2. Hepatic lobectomy in a woman with metastatic breast cancer apparently confined to the right lobe of the liver that was no longer responsive to chemotherapy or hormonal manipulation.

130

undertaken as a means of palliating pain and returning the patient to a normally active life, realizing that other metastatic deposits would eventually appear. After a nine month interval during which time the patient was symptom-free, metastatic disease became apparent in bone and in the left lobe of the liver. Whether the survival of this or a similar patient is prolonged by resection can be debated. Nevertheless, the surgical intervention provided an excellent quality of life for much of her remaining existence.

Lung metastases

Metastases largely confined to the lung are frequent in patients with sarcomas of various kinds. They occasionally occur in melanoma and in other

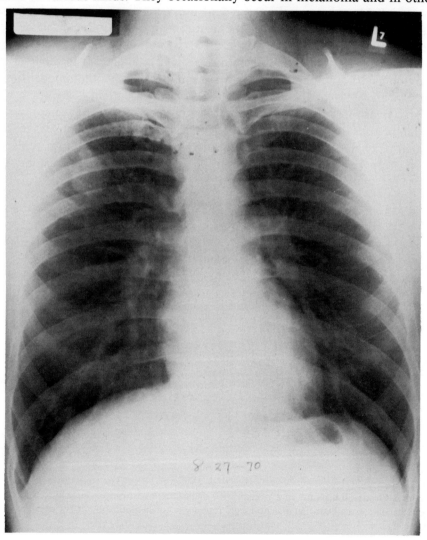

A

tumors, and in association with other resectable sites of metastatic cancer in patients with testicular tumors. Evaluation of possibility of the surgical approach to pulmonary metastases involves a search for disease elsewhere and an assessment of the extent of the pulmonary metastatic disease. Long-term survival and patient cure has followed resection of solitary metastases, resection of multiple metastases, multiple resections for metastases and resection of metastases from both lungs.

Because of the youth of the patients involved, much of the earliest efforts toward aggressive management of pulmonary metastases was aimed at the patients with osteosarcoma. Although in the 1960s, when the five-year survival rate to Roswell Park Memorial Institute patients with osteosarcoma was only 12%, half of those patients who were the long-term survivors had undergone thoracotomy for pulmonary metastases [7]. One such patient, who developed a pulmonary metastasis in the right lobe of the lung one year following amputation for an osteosarcoma of the proximal tibia (Figure 3), was treated by thoracotomy. Ten months later, he was found to have a

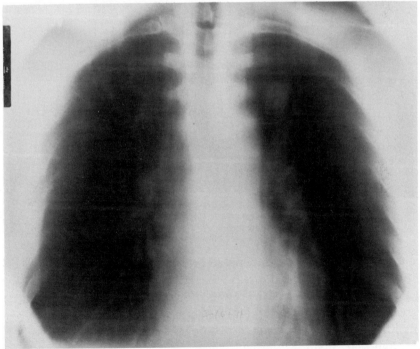

B

Figure 3. Pulmonary metastases from osteosarcoma treated by two thoracotomies six months apart without chemotherapy. The patient remains disease-free eight years later; (A) solitary metastasis in right upper lobe, August 1970; (B) metastasis in right hemithorax has been removed and a new lesion is present in the left upper lobe, March 1971; (C) metastases have been removed and patient is disease-free three years later, April, 1974.

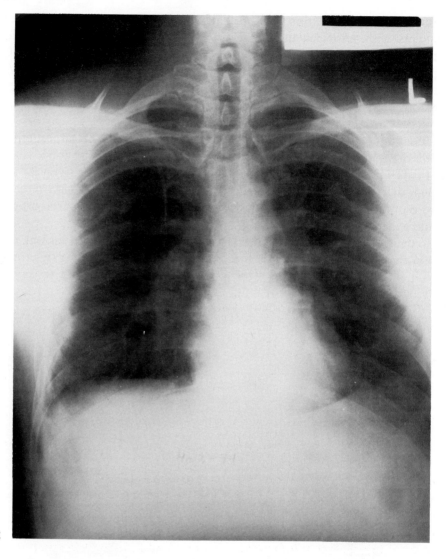

C

second nodule in the opposite lung. Repeat thoracotomy was performed and the patient is now alive and disease-free more than eleven years later, working as a farmer. A review of the results of resection of pulmonary metastases for osteosarcoma indicates that long-term survivals have been reported from Roswell Park, Stanford, the National Cancer Institute, Mayo Clinic and Memorial Sloan Kettering Cancer Center, with two year survivals following pulmonary resections ranging from 30–61% [8–10].

The experience at Roswell Park indicated that there was little difference in the overall survival of patients whose pulmonary metastases appeared within the first year after treatment of the primary tumor, or those whose metastases appeared later [8]. Subsequent to the excision of pulmonary metastases, approximately half of the patients died within two years. A few more died during the third year, but those who lived three years following pulmonary resection were very likely to be long-term survivors.

The number of metastases excised at time of thoracotomy did not significantly affect the outcome, although patients with more than six metastases did less well after the first two post-thoracotomy years, as compared to those who had had five or fewer metastases excised. The latter group had a 40% five-year survival. The unexpected discovery of many small metastases at the time of thoracotomy, not visible preoperatively on X-ray or CT scan, should not discourage the surgeon. One Roswell Park patient had 71 metastases excised by a series of small wedge excisions and is alive and apparently free of disease three years later.

The experience with metastatic sarcomas of all types has been similar to that in osteosarcoma, with 40% surviving five years [11]. Among patients with soft tissue sarcomas, very few who survived the first two years post-thoracotomy subsequently expired. Another group of patients that has done well following thoracotomy and excision of pulmonary metastases are those with testicular carcinomas [12]. Karakousis has demonstrated a 10% five-year survival following excisions of metastases of melanomas from the lung and other sites.

LOCAL RECURRENCE

Recurrences in the operative field may follow excision of a wide variety of neoplastic lesions. Most approachable surgically are local recurrences of gastrointestinal carcinomas, particularly those of the colorectum and the stomach. Close follow-up with frequent endoscopy of patients in whom margins of resection are less than optimal (e.g., 5 cm in the colon and 3 to 6 cm in the stomach) will often permit the finding of recurrent disease at a time when re-resection is still feasible. Sarcomas and head and neck tumors are generally more accessible with recurrences being found earlier.

Anastomotic and regional recurrence of gastrointestinal malignancy

Anastomotic recurrence following resection of large bowel cancers is generally thought to be relatively uncommon, particularly when distal margins of the tumor are in excess of 5 cm as measured by the pathologist in the fresh, unstretched specimen. However, reports of anastomotic recurrences with incidences as high as 10% still appear from major centers. No doubt, some of these recurrences occur because surgeons often take the 5 cm measurement with the bowel on stretch in the operative field when such stretch-

134

ing and traction on the bowel can increase its length by 60% or more. The advent of stapling instruments combined with many reports suggesting that the long-term survival of patients with tumors in the upper rectum treated by anterior resection has been equivalent to that of those treated by abdominoperineal resection, has encouraged surgeons to spare the rectal sphincter, often reducing the margin below the tumor from 5 to 3 cm or even less. The trend toward ever-lower resections saving the rectal sphincter plus the need to preserve more than 2 cm of rectal mucosa to maintain sensation and continence, encourage still further shrinkage of the margins. It is inevitable that the frequency of local recurrence will rise. This change is already being seen at referral centers such as Roswell Park.

When found early enough, anastomotic recurrences are often resectable. Experience dating back more than ten years indicate that a number of patients who undergo a resection of a local recurrence can be cured of their malignancy by the surgical re-resection procedure alone. Such re-resections must, of necessity, be radical. For tumors lower in the pelvis, re-resections mandate abdominoperineal resection, posterior exenteration or possible total pelvic exenteration (Figure 4), occasionally combined with removal of the sacrum. Yet, even with these most radical of operations, the patient can be offered only a 10–20% chance of cure. Assessments as to whether combining these regional resections with radiation therapy can improve the long-term survival and cure rates are currently underway. Preliminary evi-

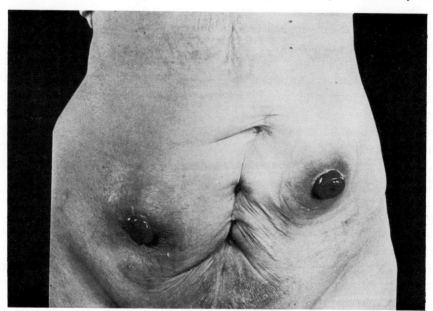

Figure 4. Female patient status post pelvic exenteration five years previously for recurrent colorectal cancer. No adjuvant therapy was given. Patient remains disease-free.

dence would suggest that the symptom-free survival can be prolonged by this combined approach, which can be offered if radiation had not been utilized as an adjuvant to the original excision.

In an attempt to locate these recurrences early and thus avoid the most radical of re-resections, patients with low anterior resections must be closely evaluated by their physicians. In addition to physical examinations and careful taking of a history for symptoms suggesting pelvic recurrence (saddle pain, change in bowel habit, continence problems, dysuria, the sensation of fullness or mass), rectal examination should be accompanied by endoscopic and proctoscopic examination at intervals of two to three months for at least the first three years, since it is the small recurrence that offers the greatest chance for a successful re-resection.

Locally recurrent gastric carcinoma less frequently offers the potential for re-resection. Perhaps no more than 10–20% of these can be re-resected, largely because lesions tend to be far advanced when they are discovered. The risk of anastomotic recurrence appears to be minimized when the distance between the gross tumor and the proximal margin of resection exceeds 6 cm and when the distance between the microscopic edge of the tumor and the margin of resection exceeds 3 cm. Although the group from Memorial Sloan Kettering Hospital in New York City has demonstrated that local recurrence does not universally follow the pathologic finding of tumor at the line of resection [13], these patients do have an approximately 90% chance of developing anastomotic recurrence of their tumor.

When the gastric recurrence is localized and resectable, approximately 10% of these patients can be cured by surgery alone. The success depends more on the extent of the invasion of surrounding tissues such as pancreas and retroperitoneum, extension to lymph nodes and peritoneal dissemination. If the recent report of the Gastrointestinal Tumor Study Group concerning the long-term survival of patients with localized residual disease treated by a combination of radiation therapy plus 5-fluorouracil and Methyl-CCNU is any guide [14], the addition of combined modality therapy following an apparent successful re-resection of a gastric cancer might increase the long-term survival of these patients by another 20% or more.

Sarcomas, head and neck cancers

Two other groups of patients for whom local re-resection of their recurrence offers a potential for cure or long-term survival, particularly when integrated into a combined multi-disciplinary program, are those who have sarcomas or squamous cell carcinomas of the head and neck.

Local recurrence of sarcomas usually indicates the failure of initial adequate excision. When these patients have not had previous irradiation and chemotherapy, the likelihood of successful re-excision, often with limb salvage when the lesion is in the extremity, should exceed 70%. Failures most commonly occur when a vital structure that cannot be sacrificed is involved by the tumor. Such would be the case when the sarcoma extends to the bladder, the sciatic nerve, etc. In circumstances such as these, the addition of radiation therapy when only microscopic tumor remains, may still salvage a significant proportion of the patients. When there is gross invasion, the structures are better sacrificed with the appropriate more extensive operation being performed. Adjuvant chemotherapy reduces the risk of disseminated disease. Current adjuvant programs usually utilize adriamycin and DTIC, either as a two-agent combination or as part of a five-drug program.

Even second and third local recurrences have the potential for surgical cure following re-excision but require ever-widened or radical resectional therapy. There is a tendency for the interval between each subsequence recurrence to be shorter and the need for intensive follow-up in these patients requires that they be seen and evaluated at one to two month intervals.

Local recurrence is the major problem in head and neck tumors, perhaps being responsible for as many as 50% of eventual patient deaths. Life style of the average head and neck patient can make it harder for them to be followed closely post-operatively, but close follow-up and examination is vital for their potential successful management. Any suspicious areas need to be biopsied at the time when first apparent.

Most patients with local recurrence of head and neck squamous cell carcinomas have already had previous radiation therapy. When the recurrence is diagnosed in unirradiated tissue, pre-operative radiation and/or chemotherapy can be followed by wide excision of the entire area originally suspected to contain recurrence, even though repeated biopsies of these areas may show no evidence of tumor following the successful radiation and chemotherapy. Reconstruction of the appropriate delto-pectoral flap or other flap will bring a new blood supply into the irradiated area and promote healing.

REGIONAL THERAPY FOR HEPATIC METASTASES

Hepatic artery ligation

The principles of hepatic artery ligation are based on the unusual anatomy of the liver and the differences in the vascular supply of the normal liver and the tumor. Whereas the normal hepatocyte gets approximately 50% of its oxygen supply via the hepatic artery and 50% via the portal vein, tumor masses get more than 90% of their oxygen supply from the hepatic artery with only the periphery of the metastatic deposit receiving oxygen via the portal vein. Since the hepatocyte can survive a transient period of hypoxia

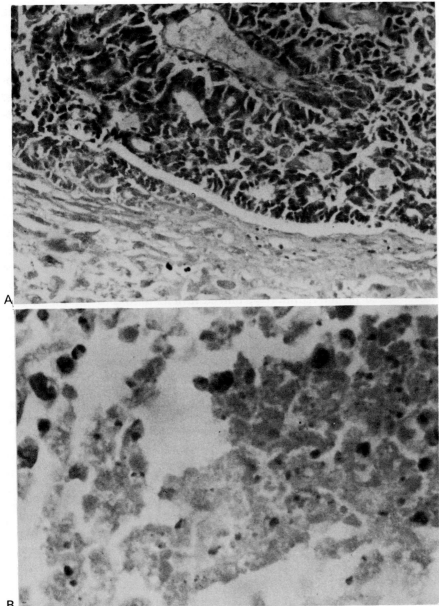

Figure 5. Colorectal liver metastasis treated by hepatic artery ligation; (A) before ligation: cellular adenocarcinoma; (B) after ligation – extensive coagulation necrosis with a few viable tumor cells at the periphery.

following the arterial ligation until collateralization (via the round ligament, triangular ligament, the diaphragm and elsewhere) restores the arterial blood supply (arteriography has shown that the first collaterals can be demonstrated within four days and extensive collateralization is present by two weeks), the logic of ligation of the hepatic artery becomes apparent [15]. The anatomic factors of the distribution of the oxygen to the neoplastic deposit predict an initial massive central necrosis. However, a number of viable cells remain at the periphery of the metastatic lesion (Figure 5). Our experience has shown that the greatest extent of necrosis and the greatest frequency of objective measurable response occurs in tumors that have been angiographically demonstrated to be well vascularized from the hepatic artery. Among the well-vascularized tumors are metastases from sarcomas, carcinoids and islet cell tumors [16].

While metastatic colorectal carcinoma is not well vascularized, patients with colorectal cancers comprise the largest series that have been studied, largely because of the relative frequency of these cancers and of the phenomenon of metastatic colorectal carcinoma with predominant metastases in the liver with little or no tumor apparent elsewhere. One such study performed at Roswell Park Memorial Institute contained 28 patients treated by hepatic artery ligation who were carefully case matched to 28 other patients treated by systemic therapy [17]. Case-matching involved extent of disease, site of primary tumor, histologic differentiation of the tumor and age and sex of the patient. The median survival of patients treated by hepatic artery ligation was in excess of eleven months, whereas those treated by other modalities had a median survival of six and one-half months. The study was then extended to 66 patients with hepatic artery ligation and the median survival was found to exceed a year. Considering that this series carried a low mortality rate and the fever and discomfort that followed hepatic artery ligation usually subsided within two weeks, the benefit of the procedure would seem to be an increased survival by six months or more over conventional modalities. In addition, just under one third of the patients treated by hepatic artery ligation had true objective regression of their tumor masses defined by reduction in the hepatomegaly by 50% or more. Massive tumor necrosis accompanied by abscess formation was not seen in the series of patients with metastatic colorectal cancer treated by hepatic artery ligation, but has been observed following the rapid massive necrosis that results from hepatic artery ligation of angiographically demonstrated highly vascularized tumors [16].

Infusion chemotherapy via the hepatic artery

For 15 years or more, a debate has raged over the value of long-term continuous infusion chemotherapy particularly for localized lesions such as hepatic metastases. It has generally been the feeling of most involved in this therapy that the response rate following regional infusion chemotherapy with 5-fluorouracil was at least twice that which resulted from systemic chemotherapy. Unfortunately, the only randomized study of infusion versus systemic chemotherapy utilized a short-term infusion program and could show no advantage for regional treatment. Nevertheless, current reports of objective regressions of liver metastases by hepatic artery infusion with rates exceeding 75% and median durations of survival extending to a year or more, mandate closer attention to this modality [18].

In order for the catheter to be tolerated for this period of time, it is generally thought wise that it be inserted surgically into the hepatic artery via the gastroduodenal branch, which is ligated [19]. This serves two purposes: it provides a route of access for long-term (6 to 12 months) continuous therapy and prevents the infusion of the 5-fluorouracil into the gastroduodenal artery thereby protecting the duodenal mucosa. At the time of the surgical insertion, the right gastric artery is also ligated, as are numerous small and unnamed branches arising from the hepatic artery and supplying adjacent tissues. In nearly every series of percutaneous hepatic artery infusions, there are reports of a 10–25% incidence of gastrointestinal bleeding, nausea, vomiting and epigastric distress. This most likely is a result of perfusion of the gastric and duodenal mucosa by the 5-fluorouracil administered into the hepatic artery. As a general principle of chemotherapy, the antineoplastic drugs are most effective in destroying rapidly dividing cells. The most rapidly dividing normal cells in the body are those of the duodenal and upper jejunal mucosa, followed by those of the gastric mucosa. Bone marrow cells are less rapidly dividing than the cells of the gastrointestinal lining. With surgical placement of the catheter and ligation of the collateral vessels, these complications occur only rarely, if at all.

PATHOLOGIC FRACTURES

Although the appearance of pathologic fractures may be the first sign of metastatic disease, many patients still have life expectancies of six months to a year or more. While the potential for cure of these patients has been lost, aggressive surgical management provides the best opportunity for pain relief and a return of function. For a patient with a tumor in the lower extremity (the most common site of fracture), internal fixation can lead to a return to an ambulatory status, sometimes completely free of external support [20].

The management of these patients should be aimed primarily towards the early rehabilitation in terms of ambulation and extremity function. One

Table 2. Treatment of pathologic fractures.

	Upper extremity (%)	Lower extremity (%)
Pain relief		
Operative fixation	88	96
Radiation therapy	73	50
Other	29	55
Return of function		
Operative fixation	63	61
Radiation therapy	53	17
Other	28	27

Percent of patients with pain relief and return of function following treatment of patients with pathologic fractures. Others include modalities such as traction, bed rest, cast bracing and amputation.

cannot allow time for the fracture to heal spontaneously or with the aid of radiation and chemotherapy because of the patient's relatively limited life expectancy. Fixation devices must be of sufficient strength to carry the full weight of the patient when the fracture is in the lower extremity, and provide sufficient fixation to eliminate the pain of rotary motion in the upper extremity. The addition of methylmethacrylate after curettage of the bulk of the tumor at the fracture site often provides a more secure repair. Within one to two days, an active rehabilitation program must be undertaken to restore function as completely as possible.

In our experience, upper extremity fixation provides vastly superior pain relief for 88–96% of patients (Table 2) when compared to other modalities of management of the lesion. Patients with fractures in the lower extremity should be ambulatory and able to climb stairs by the time of their hospital discharge. Physiotherapy programs to increase function should extend beyond the period of hospitalization.

JAUNDICE IN CANCER PATIENTS

The appearance of jaundice in a patient with cancer is often felt to represent overwhelming liver metastases and a failure of hepatic function, but the most common cause for jaundice is actually biliary tract obstruction due to metastatic deposits in the liver compressing the right and left hepatic ducts or their junction, or extrahepatic metastases in lymph nodes near the hilum of the liver and along the common hepatic and bile ducts. The advent of percutaneous drainage techniques and ultrasonography to demonstrate dilated bile ducts offers an opportunity to modify the approach to these patients, many of whom are felt to be at the end stage of their disease. Unfortunately, percutaneous drainage techniques do not always return the bilirubin to completely normal levels (Figure 6), thus limiting the potential for chemotherapy by preventing use of full doses of drugs such as adriamycin. Further, the percutaneous drainage techniques and the irrigations that are necessary to keep the catheters open and free from bile encrustations markedly increase the risk of cholangitis. In patients with multiple areas of narrowed ducts due to liver metastases, the resulting edema in the bile duct mucosa due to cholangitis can lead to occlusion of the duct in the region of the metastatic deposit with a resultant abscess forming peripherally to the narrowed area.

A more aggressive approach to these patients is operative drainage [21]. The morbidity and mortality of this procedure can be reduced when temporary percutaneous drainage is established to lower the bilirubin preoperatively while the nutritional status of the patient is being improved by hyperalimentation. The experience at Roswell Park Memorial Institute would indicate that the median survival of patients treated by various intubation techniques is less than four and one-half months, whereas patients who are treated by a Roux-en-Y biliary enteric drainage procedure (hepatojejunostomy or cholangiojejunostomy) have median survivals of ten and

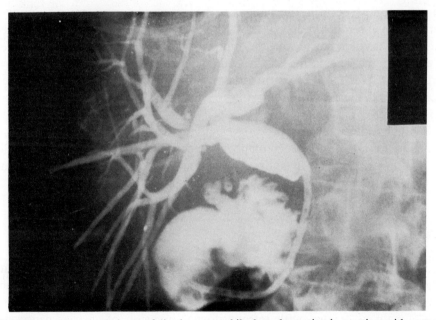

Figure 6. Percutaneous drainage of distal common bile duct obstruction in a patient with metastatic cancer. The percutaneous catheter has been negotiated through the obstruction into the duodenum. Nevertheless, residual dilatation of some bile ducts is noted.

one-half months and far fewer infectious complications, resulting in far fewer days of hospitalization.

The agressive approach to jaundice in the cancer patient has taught us a number of important lessons. First, for the vast majority of patients, jaundice can be relieved because it is obstructive in nature and does not represent a widespread replacement of liver by metastatic disease.

Second, the jaundice is often related to metastatic tumor around the common bile duct or at the hilum of the liver, in the form of lymph node metastases or growth of peritoneal seedlings causing the obstruction. In many patients in whom the external surface of the liver appears to contain multiple metastases, cut sections of the liver will reveal few metastases in the parenchyma. Most of these metastases will have implanted on the liver by the transperitoneal route and are confined largely to the liver surface. This same ingrowth around the bile duct can also result in obstructive jaundice.

Third, a biliary enteric fistula through a defunctionalized loop of small intestine of 25 to 40 cm in length is associated with far fewer infectious complications than are seen following either percutaneous drainage or internal drainage through loops of bowel that are not isolated from the gastrointestinal content and defunctionalized.

Fourth, percutaneous biliary drainage combined with aggressive nutritional support permits the patient to be prepared for an enteric drainage procedure at a much reduced risk. Secondary operations are often prolonged and may involve coring out the hilum of the liver to identify uninvolved ducts for the anastomosis. Cholangiojejunostomy identifying bile ducts within the liver for anastomosis may have to be done in both right and left lobes for satisfactory biliary drainage, but is an alternative when the hilum of the liver cannot be approached.

Finally, biliary bypass procedures in the face of obstructive jaundice, whether or not drained percutaneously, should be handled as potentially contaminated cases with antibiotic coverage including antibiotics that are excreted through the biliary tree.

ABDOMINAL PAIN

Pain, particularly in the upper abdomen, frequently accompanies late stage gastrointestinal and intra-abdominal cancer. There are two situations in which a surgical approach can provide pain relief.

For pain associated with retroperitoneal invasion of gastric, pancreatic and colonic cancer, celiac axis blockade can be of value [22]. Although this procedure can be done percutaneously, the morbidity of percutaneous blockade is not inconsequential. However, if the patient with upper abdominal and back pain due to retroperitoneal invasion is being operated on for other causes, the injection of 5 ml of absolute ethanol into the area of the splanchnic nerves on each side of the celiac axis, can provide significant pain relief for two to four months or more in 50–70% of patients treated. Even when this area has been largely distored by metastatic tumor in lymph nodes, injection of the area with absolute alcohol can provide pain relief for half or more patients so treated.

A second source of pain that is definitely amenable to a surgical approach and deserving of a surgical procedure for that pain, is that associated with obstruction of the pancreatic duct by a malignant process within or metastatic to the pancreas [23]. These patients usually have a dilated pancreatic duct or pseudocyst which is sometimes visible by ultrasonography or CT scanning. Elevations of the urine or serum amylase can also be detected in many of these patients. A therapeutic test of the potential pain relief involves the administration of a prostaglandin inhibitor such as aspirin, which sometimes results in remarkably dramatic pain relief. In these patients, the mechanism of pain is the continued secretion from the pancreatic acini into the pancreatic duct and is relieved by drainage of the pancreatic duct into the intestine. Most commonly utilized is a defunctionalized Roux-en-Y loop to a lateral pancreatojejunostomy. On occasion, these patients will be found to have pancreatic pseudocysts which can be drained in the usual fashion by cystogastrostomy or cystoenterostomy. The morbidity of the procedure is minimal and the patients are often grateful for the relief of a nagging and often severe pain that seldom responds well to opiate derivative therapy.

SUMMARY

The surgical oncologist can offer to the patient with metastatic or recurrent disease an extensive armamentarium of procedures, a number of which have been described in this chapter. In selected situations, local recurrence and limited metastatic disease can be managed by approaches still offering the potential for cure. In other situations, significant prolongation of survival and relief of symptoms can be offered.

Other areas in which the surgical approach may potentially benefit include patients with intestinal obstruction which may be due to adhesions, recurrent tumor, or inflammatory processes. Appendicitis and cholecystitis do occur in patients with cancer. Even the patient with severe leukopenia and thrombocytopenia due to chemotherapy will be benefitted by an indicated appendectomy or cholecystectomy. Typhlitis is a necrotizing process usually occurring in the cecum and right colon in patients with virtual total depletion of leukocytes and thrombocytes, who are usually being treated for hematogenous malignancies. Morbidity and mortality are markedly reduced by removing the necrotic bowel and delaying anastomosis until immunologic competence can be restored. Liver abscesses, often due to fungi, and splenic abscesses, also often of fungal origin, are also seen in immunologically depressed patients. The potential for cure of the infectious process is probably limited to patients in whom the abscesses in the liver are drained and those in the spleen treated by splenectomy.

Continued aggressive utilization of a wide variety of surgical oncologic approaches can provide significant enhancement of survival and palliation in terms of pain relief or improved quality of life.

ACKNOWLEDGMENT

A number of studies reported herein were supported in part by Eastern Cooperative Oncology Group Grant CA 12296 and by the Gastrointestinal Tumor Study Group Contracts N01-CM-43782; N01-CM-43794; N01-CM-07401 and Cooperative Agreement 1-U10-CA-34184.

REFERENCES

1. Douglass HO, Jr, Lavin PT, Woll J, Conroy JF, Carbone PP: Chemotherapy of advanced measurable colon and rectal carcinoma with oral 5-fluorouracil alone or in combination with cyclophosphamide or 6-thioguanine, with intravenous 5-fluorouracil or beta-2′-deoxy-thioguanosine or with oral 3(4 methyl-cyclohexyl)1(2-chloroethyl)-1 nitrosourea. Cancer 42:2538–2545, 1989.
2. Bengmark S, Hafstrom L: The natural course for liver cancer. Progress in Clinical Cancer 7:195–200, 1978.
3. Lavin P, Mittelman A, Douglass HO, Jr, Engstrom P, Klaassen D: Survival and response to chemotherapy for advanced colorectal adenocarcinoma. Cancer 46:1536–1543, 1980.
4. Foster JH: Resection of metastatic cancer from the liver. Contemporary Surgery 12:26–40, 1978.
5. Holyoke ED, Ledesma EL: Prognosis and surgical treatment of colon and rectal cancer. Current Concepts in Oncology 8:3–7, 1982.
6. Adson MA, Van Heerden JA: Major hepatic resections for metastatic colorectal cancer. Ann Surg 191:576–583, 1980.
7. Douglass HO. Jr, Wang JJ, Takita H, Wallace HJ, Friedman M, Mindell E: Improving treatment results in osteogenic sarcoma. Surg Gynecol Obstet 140:693–700, 1975.
8. Huang MN, Takita H, Douglass HO, Jr: Lung resection for metastatic osteogenic sarcoma. J Surg Oncol 10:179–182, 1978.
9. Douglass HO, Jr: Osteosarcoma: Survival gains resulting from multidisciplinary therapy. Progr Clin Cancer 7:83–96, 1978 (Grune & Stratton, NYC).
10. Telander RL, Pairolero PC, Pritchard DJ, Sim FH, Gilchrist GS: Resection of pulmonary metastatic osteogenic sarcoma in children. Surgery 84:335–341, 1978.

11. Huang MN, Edgerton F, Takita H, Douglass HO, Jr, Karakousis C: Lung resection for metastatic sarcoma. Am J Surg 135:804–806, 1978.
12. Takita H, Merrin C. Didolkar MS, Douglass HO, Jr, Edgerton F: The surgical management of multiple lung metastases. Ann Thoracic Surg 24:359–364, 1977.
13. Papachristou DN, Fortner JG: Local recurrence of gastric adenocarcinoma after gastrectomy. J Surg Oncol 18:47–53, 1981.
14. Gastrointestinal Tumor Study Group: A comparison of combination chemotherapy and combined modality therapy for locally advanced gastric carcinoma. Cancer 49:1771–1777, 1982.
15. Bengmark S, Rosengren K: Angiographic study of the collateral circulation to the liver after ligitation of the hepatic artery in man. Am J Surg 119:620–624, 1970.
16. Berjian RA, Douglass HO, Jr, Nava HR, Karakousis C: The role of hepatic artery ligation and dearterialization with infusion chemotherapy in advanced malignancies of the liver. J Surg Oncol 14:379–387, 1980.
17. Evans JT: Hepatic artery ligation in hepatic metastases from colon and rectal malignancies. Dis Colon Rectum 22:370, 1979.
18. Rohde TD, Varco RL, Blackshear PJ: Intra-arterial infusion chemotherapy for hepatic carcinoma using a totally implantable infusion pump. Cancer 45:866–869, 1980.
19. Karakousis CP, Douglass HO, Jr, Holyoke ED: Technique of infusion chemotherapy, hepatic artery ligation and dearterialization in hepatic malignancy. Surg Gynecol Obstet 149:403–407, 1979.
20. Douglass HO, Jr, Shukla S, Mindell ER: Treatment of pathologic fractures of long bones, excluding those due to breast cancer. J Bone Joint Surg 58A:1055–1061, 1976.
21. Karakousis CP, Douglass HO, Jr: Hilar hepatojejunostomy in resection of carcinoma of the main hepatic duct junction. Surg Gynecol Obstet 145:245–248, 1977.
22. Flanigan DP, Kraft RO: Continuing experience with palliative chemical splanchnicectomy. Arch Surg 113:509–511, 1978.
23. Apalakis A, Dussault J, Knight M, Smith R: Relief of pain from pancreatic carcinoma. Ann Royal Coll Surg Engl 59:401–403, 1977.

8. Oral Complications of Cancer Patients Undergoing Chemotherapy and Radiation Therapy

WILLIAM CARL

INTRODUCTION

Systematic chemotherapy, even if for cancer distant from the oral cavity, and radiation therapy for tumors in the head and neck area, precipitate acute and chronic changes in the structures, the function and the physiology of the mouth that may compromise the entire treatment protocol and negatively influence the prognosis of the patient. Physicians, dentists and nurses treating cancer patients must be aware of these effects to provide optimum preventive and supportive oral and dental care.

ORAL MANIFESTATIONS OF CHEMOTHERAPY AND THEIR MANAGEMENT

The development of effective antineoplastic drugs is making cancer chemotherapy an increasingly more popular modality of treatment. However, many chemotherapy agents in use now also have significant oral side effects that require for control specific preventive care and dictate precautions in otherwise routine dental treatment. Myelosuppression and immunosuppression associated with chemotherapy make patients particularly susceptible to infections of pulpal and periodontal origin.

Stomatitis. Stomatitis is an inflammatory reaction of the oral mucosa. It is caused by local or systemic factors and may manifest on the buccal or labial mucosa, palate, tongue, floor of the mouth and the gingival tissues. The oral lesions may be focal or generalized (Figures 1 and 2). Stomatitis often develops when patients are being treated with methotrexate, adriamycin, ara-C, cytoxan, daunomycin, 5-fluorouracil, and bleomycin [1].

Stomatitis, initially precipitated by chemotherapy, may become aggravated by local irritants such as jagged teeth, accumulations of calculus and

Higby, DJ (ed), Supportive Care in Cancer Therapy. ISBN 0-89838-569-5.
© *1983, Martinus Nijhoff Publishers, Boston. Printed in The Netherlands.*

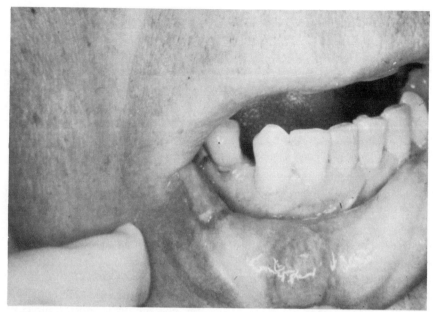

Figure 1. Focal oral mucosal lesions secondary to treatment with adriamycin, cytoxan and vincristine for histiocytic lymphoma.

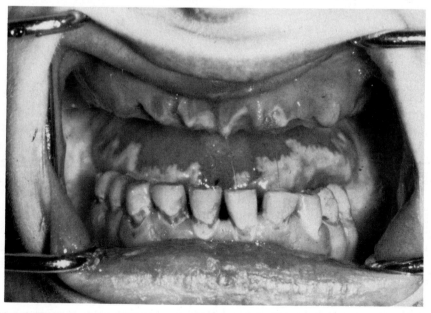

Figure 2. Generalized stomatitis in a patient being treated with adriamycin, vincristine, methotrexate, cytoxan, bleomycin and 5-fluorouracil.

plaque, poorly contoured restorations, and poorly fitting prostheses. The condition frequently becomes very painful requiring analgesics for relief. During the time of acute reaction, patients often are not able to eat properly, thus their nutritional status becomes compromised. In addition, oral hygiene, as it is painful to perform, is neglected. This, in turn, may precipitate a chain reaction of secondary infections and dental pathology because of bacterial accumulation on the teeth and gingiva. Severe stomatitis may at times dictate adjustment of the chemotherapeutic dose [2].

Salivary changes. Quality and quantity of saliva are frequently reduced after administration of chemotherapy. These changes can be observed as early as two days after treatment. Patients complain of dryness of the mouth and accumulation of ropy mucus. Prolonged xerostomia and low salivary pH precipitate dental caries and accelerate periodontal disease as well as monilial infections (Figure 3) [3].

Myelosuppression and immunosuppression. Infection is a constant danger in the severely myelosuppressed and immunosuppressed patient. It has been demonstrated that 70% of patients with acute leukemia and 50% with solid tumors and lymphoma die of infection. The oral cavity is a constant reservoir of microorganisms and potential infection. All oral microorganisms in the compromised patient are potentially lethal [2, 4, 5].

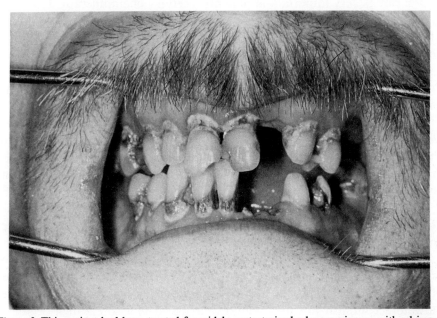

Figure 3. This patient had been treated for widely metastasized adenocarcinoma with adriamycin, mitomycin, 5-fluorouracil and hydroxyurea for three years. During that time he had multiple oral mucosal lesions, xerostomia and ultimately he developed cervical dental caries similar to caries seen in patients who had radiation therapy.

The chemotherapeutic agents that often or always depress the bone marrow at therapeutic doses are methotrexate, daunomycin, cytoxan and other alkylating agents, vinblastine, adriamycin, ara-C, 5-fluorouracil, DTIC, and cis-platinum. Their actions cause thrombocytopenia and leukopenia, disturbing the hematopoietic and immune mechanisms of the patient.

Reduced platelet count in the presence of already existing periodontal disease may lead to spontaneous massive bleeding from the periodontium. The normal platelet count in adults is from $150,000/mm^3$ to $300,000/mm^3$. With intense chemotherapy, this may be reduced below $10,000/mm^3$, especially in the leukemic patient who is being induced into remission or for bone marrow transplantation.

In the myelo- and immunosuppressed patient, previously existing chronic dental pathology may change to an acute stage. Periapical bone lesions may become a source of fever and constant pain; advanced periodontal disease with deep infrabony pockets and defective periodontal attachment may progress to fulminating infection with focal bone necrosis and accelerated alveolar bone loss.

Oral preventive and maintenance measures for patients receiving chemotherapy

Oral care is very important in patients receiving chemotherapy. However, in light of the urgency of a patient's cancer treatment, it is often overlooked. Ideally, pre-chemotherapy dental evaluation and preventive care should become part of a patient's preparatory work-up for treatment. This approach reduces potential complications that may be difficult to control later. Preventive oral care must be shared by the professional staff and the patient.

General oral preventive and dental care. While many of the side effects of chemotherapy are unavoidable, appropriate preventive measures can be practiced with minimal skill, equipment and materials to control infections and maintain comfort and nutrition of the patient [6].

Recognizing the fact that the oral cavity in the compromised patient is a sanctuary for potential pathogens and that most dental pathology is of bacterial origin, the first objective must be to reduce the bacterial activity in the mouth. No medications are required to achieve this. In anticipation of reduced salivary flow and salivary quality and a possible shift in the balance of the oral flora, the mouth must be kept lubricated and clean. The procedures to accomplish this must be uncomplicated to assure a high degree of compliance.

While the patient's medical condition may not allow mechanical debridement of the teeth either with instruments or with toothbrush and floss, there is usually no obstacle to oral irrigations. An effective mouthwash is a solution of 5% sodium bicarbonate used at least four times a day (1 tsp. baking soda, ½ tsp. salt in 16 oz. of lukewarm water). This raises the oral pH and helps prevent overgrowth of aciduric organisms, especially *Candida albicans*. Addition of 2 teaspoons of 3% hydrogen peroxide further reduces the population of anaerobic microorganisms. Unless the mouth is kept lubricated, existing mucus dehydrates and adheres firmly to the epithelium. Mechanical removal may precipitate episodes of bleeding from the underlying tissue. In addition to the irrigation solutions mentioned, artificial saliva may be used to sustain at least some degree of lubrication of the mucous membranes. Vaseline should be used on the lips to prevent accumulation and adherence of blood and mucus (Figure 4).

Irrigation alone, however, does not remove all plaque from the gingival sulci. Patients should continue to use toothbrushes and floss as long as the platelet count allows. Type of toothbrush, position and motion are important factors in achieving good oral hygiene. The Bass technique, using a soft brush with flexible and rounded nylon bristles at a 45° angle in a horizontal direction along the junction of the cervical areas of the teeth and the gingival margin, is most practical and efficient [7]. The technique also meets the requirements of simplicity. The soft bristles follow the contours of the teeth,

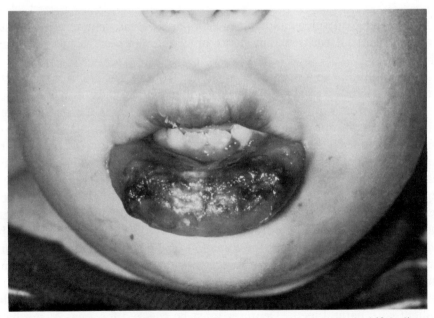

Figure 4. Dehydration and accumulation of mucous and blood can be prevented if the lips and the mouth are kept lubricated. This patient with acute lymphocytic leukemia had developed secondary infection of the lip.

152

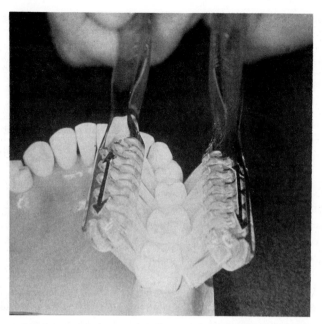

Figure 5. In the Bass technique of oral hygiene a soft bristled brush is placed at an angle of approximately 45° at the junction of the teeth and the gingival margin. The brush is moved in a horizontal direction in short strokes.

enter the gingival sulcus and the interproximal areas, and remove plaque and the bacterial cushion that exists on the surfaces of calculus deposits (Figure 5).

The temptation to discontinue brushing, flossing and other oral hygiene procedures is often great in the face of the patient's other problems. However, a compromised patient with poor oral hygiene runs the risk of developing severe oral infections (Figure 6). In cases where the platelet count is reduced below $20,000/mm^3$, a toothbrush may temporarily have to be replaced by toothets. Toothets have soft foam rubber tips at the end of a handle. They are not as effective as toothbrushes, but they can still be used to good advantage in reducing plaque accumulation. Cotton tips, cotton balls and gauze wrapped around a finger and coupled with vigorous irrigation, are all effective in controlling bacterial activity. Waterpicks must be adjusted to low pressure and the direction of the spray should be horizontally into the interproximal spaces, otherwise laceration of the mucosa and the floor of the mouth can occur.

Oral hygiene for the edentulous patient is as important as it is for the patient with natural teeth. Dentures must be checked for areas of mechanical irritation. If patients lose weight during their therapy, the dentures move on the mucosa and may abrade the surface. Irrigation and lubrication

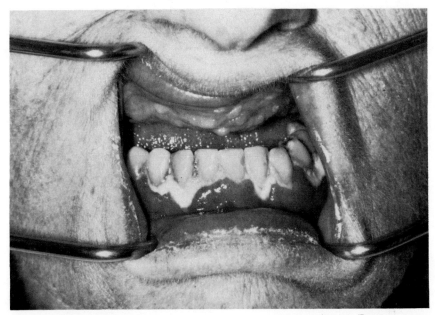

Figure 6. Gingival infection in a patient with acute myelocytic leukemia. Oral hygiene had been completely neglected.

of the mouth coupled with daily cleaning of the dentures using soap and water or a commercial denture cleaner will greatly reduce the risk of secondary oral infections.

Despite all prophylactic measures, the myelo- and immunosuppressed patient does at times require active treatment. It is important to recognize which procedures present a risk and which do not.

Unless a patient has generalized stomatitis, there are usually no contraindications to routine restorative dentistry. As long as the platelet count remains above 50,000/mm^3, scaling of the teeth and even uncomplicated extractions can be performed with minimal risk. To confirm the relative safety level, consultation with the primary physician is necessary. If the platelet count is below 50,000/mm^3, and if extractions, periodontal treatment and biopsies are indicated, arrangements for platelet transfusion should be made.

Management of acute dental emergencies in the myelo- and immunosuppressed patient

Dental problems most often present with active disease and during intensive chemotherapy. The complications frequently occurring are spontaneous bleeding from the gingival tissues, acute periodontal infections, pain precipitated by dental caries or pulp pathology, pericoronitis of partially erupted

154

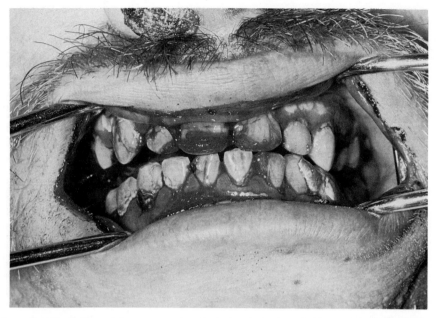

Figure 7. This patient with acute myelocytic leukemia had a platelet count of 500/mm³. In addition he had advanced chronic periodontal disease. Episodes of severe bleeding from the gingival areas occurred several times.

third molars, irritation of tongue, cheeks and gingival tissues by orthodontic bands and wires, and poorly contoured restorations.

Profuse oral hemorrhage in myelosuppressed patients usually occurs from interdental areas that are already weak from existing periodontal disease (Figure 7). The immediate treatment to control the bleeding is irrigation to identify the area, and placement of periodontal dressing (Figure 8). The dressing should be left in place until an improvement in the patient's blood picture is noted. Intermittent bleeding may be controlled with topical thrombin combined with gauze and pressure. Long-term management of this potential complication is treatment of the periodontal condition by removal of plaque and calculus from the gingival pockets and continued good oral hygiene.

Orthodontic bands and wires as well as temporary restorations and copper bands frequently used by dentists become mechanical irritants in myelosuppressed patients (Figure 9). In addition, these appliances are difficult to clean around leading to the accumulation of debris and subsequent infections. It is usually necessary to remove all orthodontic and other prostheses to simplify oral hygiene. At the time of severe myelosuppression, control of oral infections takes precedence over dental esthetics.

Recurrent complications in young patients with leukemia are erupting

155

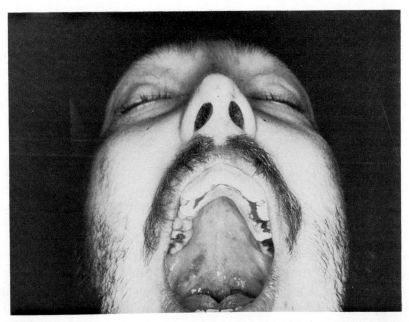

Figure 8. One method of controlling oral bleeding in myelosuppressed patients is by placement of periodontal dressing.

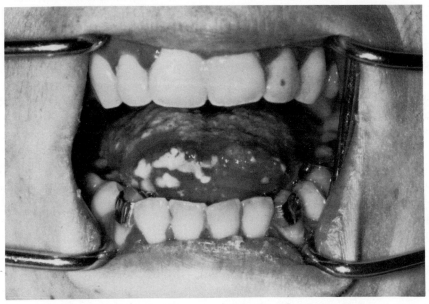

Figure 9. Orthodontic bands and temporary dental restorations often precipitate severe oral infections in myelosuppressed patients. This patient had an anterior mandibular fixed retainer which irritated the tongue and the gingival tissue.

and partially impacted third molars. Severe pericoronitis may be associated with pain and trismus, making proper treatment extremely difficult. Until the patient's systemic condition improves, extractions may be out of the question. To control the infection, the area should be irrigated with a syringe containing warm saline and diluted hydrogen peroxide. In addition, cotton saturated with Betadine should be inserted for 5–10 minutes at a time under the tissue flap. The procedure may have to be repeated for several days until the acute infection resolves. The ultimate solution is extraction of the third molars as soon as the patient's condition allows.

Dental extractions in leukemic patients may precipitate complications of bleeding, infection, osteomyelitis and septicemia. However, if the surgery is done with proper precautions, the risks are acceptable and controllable. Preoperative planning must be done with the support of the primary physician. The surgery should be done only in a hospital. Arrangements for possible blood transfusions have to be made and the patient must be placed on antibiotics until the danger of open wound infection is passed. Penicillin G is the preferred drug unless the patient is allergic to it. While the platelet count is usually a good indicator as to the hemostatic picture of the patient, it cannot always be relied on. Often the count may be near normal, but there may be qualitative defects in the platelets, and abnormal adhesiveness and fibrinolysis may cause prolonged bleeding. A coagulation profile consisting of prothrombin time, partial thromboplastin time, thrombin time, fibrinogen level and template bleeding time should be obtained [8, 9].

The tissue in the immediate area of surgery must be handled as atraumatically as possible. Extraction sites should be closed with sutures; resorbable hemostatic packing should be placed into the sockets.

Postoperative instructions include no smoking, no sucking on straws, and soft diet. No medications that suppress platelet function, such as aspirin, are to be issued. In most cases, the healing time is prolonged and the tissue over the extraction site remains thin and friable for about two weeks.

Complications from existing dental pathology and dental extractions are greatly reduced when patients are in remission. This raises the question as to prophylactic dental extractions of all third molars and questionable teeth when patients are at relatively low risk. This approach may seem radical, but it certainly eliminates many potential complications during a time when the patient is severely myelo- and immunodepressed.

ORAL COMPLICATIONS OF PATIENTS RECEIVING RADIATION THERAPY
FOR CANCER IN THE HEAD AND NECK AREA

As early as 1905, only ten years after Wilhelm Roentgen discovered X-rays, researchers became aware that radiation causes disruption in the development of the teeth that are in the line of the primary beam. It is now generally recognized that radiation therapy precipitates both immediate and long-term tissue and physiologic changes in the oral cavity. The condition of the mouth and the fate of the teeth are therefore matters of considerable concern for both physician and dentist [10, 11].

The reactions of oral and perioral tissues are related to type of radiation, area of exposure, dosage and individual response. They can be generally divided into acute and chronic reactions. Since the advent of mega voltage machines (eight to 50 million electron volts), cancericidal doses now have fewer bone complications than were observed with lower voltage X-ray therapy (150 to 400 kVp). Nevertheless, considerable oral complications still develop even with high voltage irradiation. Fortunately, special care to prevent and control these problems has become an established practice in many treatment centers.

Tissue and physiologic changes associated with radiation therapy

Erythema. The skin of the face and the neck begin to show changes after the patient has been exposed to about 300 to 400 rads. The intensity of the reaction varies with the fractionation of the total dose, the portals being used and the angulation of the beam. The area of erythema resembles a sunburn at first, but as the dosage accumulates, the skin becomes dry and scaly. Loss of hair and loss of gland activity occur within the immediate area of the beam. After therapy the skin remains thin and dry testifying to the absence of internal lubrication.

Mucositis. A most troublesome soft tissue reaction developing during treatment is mucositis. The reaction is characteristic of the type of tissue irradiated, the quality of radiation and the total amount and length of treatment. The first signs of mucositis usually appear after approximately 1,000 rads. The mucosa takes on a whitish appearance and gradually a pseudomembrane forms which eventually sloughs off leaving a reddish and friable underlying epithelium having the appearance of an ulcer. Mucositis may be focal at first but as treatment reaches 2,500 rads, the entire mucosa may become involved. The ulcerated areas are frequently covered by deposits of fibrin (Figure 10). In patients with poor oral hygiene, extensive caries, jagged teeth and poorly fitting prostheses, the problem intensifies because of mechanical irritation.

Pharyngeal tissues are particularly sensitive to radiation and a patient's initial complaint may be about difficulty in swallowing. The intensity of radiation mucositis with associated true inflammation and edema may become so severe that a patient may be unable to take food or even liquids

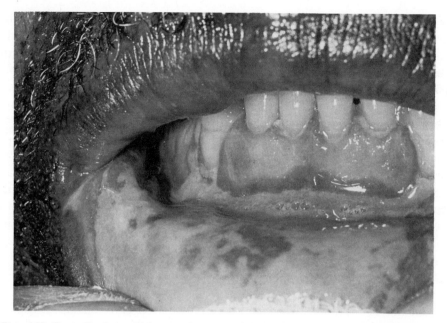

Figure 10. Generalized mucositis secondary to radiation therapy for tumor in the floor of the mouth. Note the pseudomembrane covering the lower lip and the alveolar process.

by mouth. A nasogastric tube to maintain nutritional balance may have to be inserted until the acute reaction subsides.

Intense mucositis as may be seen with radiation treatment for nasopharyngeal tumors, floor of the mouth lesions, or tumors in the retromolar area usually reaches its peak at the 6,000 to 7,000 rads level and persists for two to three weeks after termination of treatment.

Salivary changes. Salivary glands are very sensitive to radiation exposure. The beam passing through them as well as the scatter radiation at the periphery damages the glandular tissues. These changes, coupled with a shift in bacterial population, impair normal function and are very destructive to the teeth.

Salivary changes run parallel with the progression of mucositis, and they are therefore an additional factor in causing discomfort and functional difficulties. The serous acinar cells of the parotid glands are more affected as a rule than the mucinous acinar cells in other areas of the mouth [12]. Because of this shift in salivary gland function, the remaining saliva becomes viscous and ropy. It adheres to the tissues, becomes dehydrated, and the patient has difficulties moving it.

The first signs of xerostomia appear at about 1,500 rads, or within the second week of treatment. Patients may initially complain of dryness at night which improves somewhat during the daytime. As treatment progresses, xerostomia becomes a factor around the clock.

The severity and the chronicity of salivary changes is related to type and dosage of radiation as well as to the area being irradiated and the age of the patient. If the portals include the locations of the parotid and submandibular glands, as is the case in the treatment for nasopharyngeal tumors and tumors in the posterior area of the mouth, salivary function is almost completely arrested causing functional difficulties in eating, speaking and swallowing. Running parallel with this is a loss of taste sensation. Eating becomes a chore for the patient and can only be accomplished with simultaneous drinking of water. Frequently, patients have no desire for food, thus setting up a vicious cycle of nutritional imbalance at a time when the body can least afford it.

Xerostomia seldom reverses in adults. It remains a chronic problem in patients who had radiation treatment above an accumulated dose of 4,000 rads for solid tumors in the mouth or the pharynx. Some improvement usually occurs in young patients who have been treated for Hodgkin's disease.

In addition to the negative quantitative changes, the pH of the remaining saliva gradually decreases from a normal of 6.8–7.0 range to 5.5 and in some cases 5.0. Some investigators have even recorded lows of 4.0 after irradiation of the salivary glands [13].

Dehydration of oral tissues and qualitative negative changes in the remaining saliva precipitate chronic complications. Saliva, normally a buffering and lubricating agent, no longer has that capacity after radiation. In addition, cariogenic organisms, mainly *Streptococcus mutans* and *Lactobacillus* gain at the expense of noncariogenic organisms, *Fusobacterium, Streptococcus sanguis* and *Neisseria* [14].

Radiation caries and periodontal changes. As a result of environmental changes taking place in the mouth, rampant dental caries often occur after radiation therapy to the head and neck. The caries usually develop first in the buccal and lingual cervical thirds of the clinical crowns and on the incisal edges and the cusps of teeth, where natural attrition had worn the enamel.

The carious lesions begin as diffuse demineralization and if left untreated will eventually circle the entire tooth. The tooth eventually breaks off at the gingival margin (Figure 11). Radiation caries gradually undermines the enamel shell and penetrates to the pulp. Decrease of vascularity, atrophic pulp tissues, abnormal formation of osteodentin and odontoblasts after radiation have been reported by various investigators [13, 15, 16].

The fact that teeth develop caries more rapidly after radiation to the head

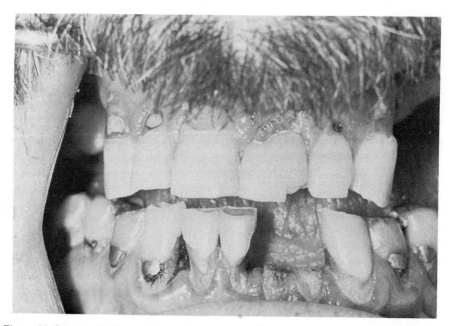

Figure 11. Severe radiation caries in a patient who had been treated with 7,000 rads for lymphoepithelioma of the nasopharynx. Combination of salivary changes and poor oral hygiene led to rampant dental caries.

and neck area whether they were in the direct field of treatment or not, supports the conclusion that environmental changes, primarily xerostomia, low salivary pH and bacterial changes are responsible for radiation caries. Even low dosage and low intensity radiation to the neck and border of the mandible as in the case with Hodgkin's disease, predisposes the teeth to radiation caries in the uncontrolled patient (Figure 12).

The periodontium of teeth directly in the primary beam of radiation also exhibits significant damage. Disorientation of the periodontal ligament fibers in their attachment and direction occurs, as well as thickening of the membrane and loss of vascularity. This reduces the capacity for repair and regeneration of the periodontium. In the presence of already existing periodontal disease, these additional factors influence the decision for pre-radiation extractions.

Edema and trismus. Edema of the buccal mucosa, submental and submandibular areas and the tongue often becomes a significant clinical factor in the post-irradiation period. Tongue and cheek biting in the molar areas may require occlusal alterations of the teeth. Dentures may need alterations in their tooth arrangements. With very severe edema and chronic effects of

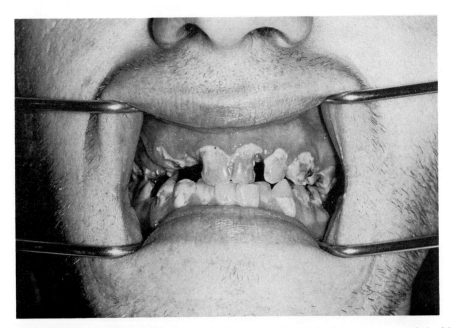

Figure 12. Even relatively low dosage of radiation as for Hodgkin's disease when coupled with poor oral hygiene leads to rampant radiation caries, as in this patient.

mucositis, dentures may not seat at all. In patients who had radical neck dissections, edema becomes particularly troublesome.

Trismus may develop after radiation treatment for nasopharyngeal tumors, tumors in the retromolar areas and the posterior palate. In treating these lesions, the temporomandibular joint and the muscles of mastication are within the primary beam. Trismus becomes particularly severe when surgery and radiation are used as combined treatment, as is the case frequently with rhabdomyosarcoma of the cheeks (Figure 13) [17].

Bone changes associated with radiation therapy. Changes in bone structure and physiology account for much post irradiation morbidity. The most serious complication that may develop is osteoradionecrosis. It is the end stage of progressive and irreversible tissue changes.

The damage that occurs in bone after cancericidal doses of radiation progresses from occlusion, hyalinization and obliteration of small vessels initially to complete devitalization. The effect on the bone itself is a reduction in the number of cells, progressive fibrosis and a negative shift in the osteoblastic–osteoclastic balance. When considering pre-irradiation and post-irradiation dental extractions, these changes must be taken into consideration [12, 18].

Other bone changes, in addition to devitalization, are arrested develop-

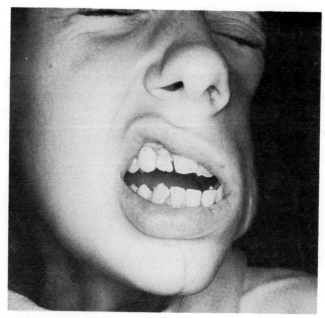

Figure 13. Severe trismus in a young patient who had been treated with radiation and surgery for rhabdomyosarcoma of the left cheek.

ment of the maxilla and mandible and incomplete development of teeth if very young patients are treated with radiotherapy. The mandible fails to expand fully anterior-posteriorly and superior-inferiorly and the teeth fail to form roots (Figure 14) [19].

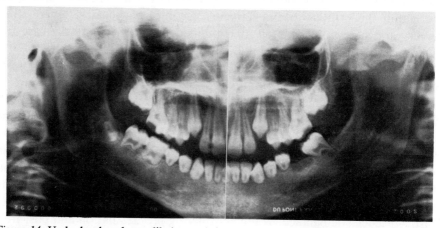

Figure 14. Underdeveloped mandibular teeth in a ten-year old patient who had been treated with 5,000 rads of radiation for rhabdomyosarcoma in the submandibular area when she was four years old. The teeth erupted fully but the roots did not form. (Reprinted from Carl, W. and Wood, R. [19].

Other effects of radiation. Any interference, be it by surgery, radiation or chemotherapy, in the normal function of part of the body, effects the entire patient physically, mentally and emotionally. After surgery most patients recover; after chemotherapy tissues, at least, return to a degree of normalcy. But radiation, especially in the head and neck area, permanently disrupts functions that are basic determinants in the quality of life. Except in young patients, where the powers of recovery and regeneration of tissues often survive despite elevated doses of radiation, the loss of taste, chronic dryness of the mouth, and pain in swallowing will be companions for the duration of life. Hand in hand with these side effects go loss of appetite, nausea, chronic malaise and loss of weight.

The effects of radiation are progressive and irreversible. The patient is faced with an unending chain of oral complications. Continued medical, dental and dietary support must become a natural extension of an irradiated patient's primary treatment.

Oral and dental care for the irradiated patient

Many effects of radiation treatment on the clinical level can be modified with specific care, patience and awareness. Such care not only involves the physician, the dentist and the nurse, but it also requires the participation of the patient him/herself. Increasing a patient's awareness of the implications of radiation treatment and the penalties associated with neglect, can only be achieved through repeated instructions and frequent follow-up. On the other hand, the dentist treating the irradiated patient must realize that he is faced with a chronic situation that requires his constant supervision.

Preparing a patient for the side effects of radiation therapy and placing the mouth in a relative state of dental health should be done before treatment is even started [11]. Oral hygiene is the determining factor in gaining and maintaining control over dental pathology. This applies to patients with natural teeth as well as to patients wearing dentures. A number of factors dictate the course of dental treatment that should be taken.

Despite all preventive measures that exist now, there are definite indications for pre-irradiation dental extractions. Factors in favor of pre-irradiation extractions are poor motivation in oral hygiene, advanced decay and advanced periodontal disease, and teeth that cause mechanical irritation of bone and soft tissue (Figure 15). Existing dental pathology, especially periodontal disease, is difficult to control in the altered environment of the irradiated patient and impossible to manage in a patient with low dental awareness or with inability to practice good oral hygiene. Advanced periodontal disease greatly increases the risk of osteoradionecrosis.

In cases where teeth with a questionable prognosis are located in the primary beam of radiation, an aggressive extraction policy is indicated. An

164

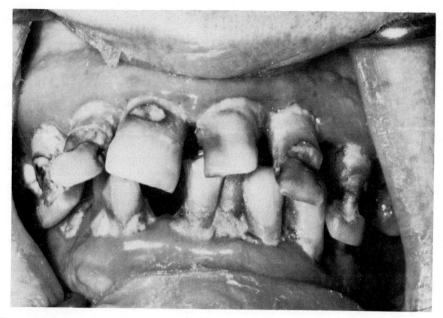

Figure 15. Advanced dental pathology and poor oral hygiene are definite indications for pre-irradiation dental extractions as in this patient who is scheduled for radiation therapy for an intraoral tumor.

edentulous area is easier to keep clean than an area with defective soft tissue attachment to teeth.

Oral hygiene is the most important factor in maintaining control over dental pathology. Unless there is compliance on the part of the patient, the dentition gradually deteriorates. The patient should be informed in simple terms of the changes that will take place as radiation progresses and the consequences of neglected oral care. As with chemotherapy, it is important to keep the oral mucous membranes moist and the bacterial activity low. This can be accomplished with repeated irrigations using mild saline, peroxide solutions, and solutions of baking soda. These solutions alleviate discomfort from mucositis and dissolve ropy mucous from accumulating. In addition, irrigation with these solutions eliminates aciduric and anaerobic organisms and reverses the acidity of the remaining natural saliva.

The Bass technique of brushing and flossing is probably the most effective method for controlling the onset of cervical caries and gingivitis. Its application has been described above in detail. Brushing should be coupled with flossing, daily irrigations and daily topical fluoride applications to the teeth either by mouthwash or in a custom-made tray.

In the last few years, saliva substitutes have been developed by a number of manufacturers. Glandosane, Salivart, and Ora-lube are some products available now. All have as major components carboxymethylcellulose, sorbital, minerals and buffering agents. Most are applied in spray form when needed. Their purpose is to provide lubrication, buffer acid saliva and aid in deglutition. They are only a partial and temporary solution to the problems of xerostomia.

Other instructions to the patient are to reduce alcohol intake and stop smoking. Commercial mouthwashes must be avoided; as most of them contain alcohol, they tend to dry out the mucous membranes even more. Dental examinations every two to three months are necessary.

Changing habits of a lifetime is a most difficult process. Many patients soon forget the implications of their treatment and continue as before. On the other hand, experience has demonstrated that these preventive measures, if carried out as explained, reduce the unfavorable side effects of radiation to a tolerable level. To be sure, even the best oral hygiene will probably not eliminate radiation caries entirely, but it provides a measure of control for the dentist in maintaining oral health.

Dental extractions after radiation therapy have long been regarded as being the main cause of osteoradionecrosis. To prevent it, many clinicians have in decades past advocated extraction of all teeth before radiation.

The potential complications can be reduced to a minimum if certain factors are considered. These are: the amount of radiation; location of the tumors; was radiation therapy combined with surgery; is there preexisting bone pathology from pulpal or periodontal disease; the manner in which the extractions are done; and the time span between radiation and extraction [20].

Patients who received 5,000 rads or more and who had tumors in the floor of the mouth or in a location where the mandible was in the primary beam, are at high risk as to developing osteoradionecrosis. Patients who in addition to radiation had surgery, constitute another high risk category. In many cases surgery includes a radical neck dissection. The vascularity of the region is even more compromised. In the routine radical neck dissection, the external maxillary artery and its cervical and facial branches are sacrificed. The cervical branches, ascending palatine, tonsillar, glandular, submental and muscular arteries, provide much of the blood supply to the mucosal lining and periosteum of the mandible. At the connection of the periosteum to bone by Sharpey's fibers, relatively large blood vessels enter the bone. Where the periosteum is loosely connected, attachment to the bone is largely maintained by small blood vessels that pass from the external layer through the canals of Volkmann to the Haversian system [21]. If the major source of blood supply to an area is surgically removed, the area then has to rely on collateral circulation from other small vessels which are more vulnerable to the effects of radiation.

When extractions after radiation therapy have to be performed, the patient should be covered prophylactically with antibiotics starting the day before oral surgery and continuing for at least two days post-operatively. The antibiotic of choice is Penicillin K, 250 mg every 6 hours. The surgery itself should be as atraumatic as possible. Sharp bony edges must be carefully contoured, and the extraction site must be sutured without tension on the tissue flap. This may require mobilization of mucosa from the lingual or the buccal. To avoid overtaxing the already limited blood supply, the number of extractions should be limited to two or three teeth at any time.

Radiation-induced tissue changes are in most cases irreversible and progressive. This must also be kept in mind when considering dental extractions. The patient having extractions long after radiation therapy is at a greater risk because of more progressed bone changes. On the other hand, the patient having oral surgery during radiation therapy or shortly after seems to heal with minimal complications.

SUMMARY

Supportive care for the cancer patient to insure the highest possible quality of life is as important as primary care. The mouth reflects many tissue and physiologic changes associated with radiation and chemotherapy. Physicians, dentists and nurses must be aware of these complications and the management of them.

REFERENCES

1. Carl W: Oral and dental care for cancer patients receiving radiation and chemotherapy. Quint Intern 12:861–869, 1981.
2. Hickey AJ, Toth BB, Lindquist S: Effect of intravenous hyperalimentation and oral care on the development of oral stomatitis during cancer chemotherapy. J Am Dent Assoc 47:188–193, 1982.
3. Carl W: Dental management and prosthetic rehabilitation of patients with head and neck cancer. Head and Neck Surg 3:27–42, 1980.
4. Rodriguez V: Acute infections in cancer patients. University of Texas System Cancer Center Newsletter 23:4, 1978.
5. Dreizen S, Brodey GP, Rodriguez V: Oral complications of cancer chemotherapy. Postgrad Med 58:75, 1975.
6. Lindquist S, Hickey AJ, Drane JB: Effect of oral hygiene on stomatitis in patients receiving cancer chemotherapy. J Prosthet Dent 40:312–314, 1978.
7. Bass CC: The optimum characteristics of toothbrushes for personal oral hygiene. Dental Items of Interest 70:696–718, 1948.
8. Carl W: Dental treatment for patients with leukemia. Quint Intern 9:9–14, 1978.
9. Segelman AE, Doku HC: Treatment of the oral complications of leukemia. J Oral Surg 35:469–477, 1977.

10. Desjardins AU: Osteogenic tumors: growth injury of bone and muscular atrophy following therapeutic irradiation. Radiology 14:296–308, 1930.
11. Carl W, Schaaf NG, Chen TY: Oral care of patients irradiated for cancer of the head and neck. Cancer 30:448–453, 1972.
12. Beumer J, Curtis T, Harrison RE: Radiation therapy of the oral cavity: sequelae and management. Head and Neck Surg 1:301–312, 1979.
13. Frank RM, Herdly J, Philippe E: Acquired dental defects and salivary gland lesions after irradiation for carcinoma. J Am Dent Assoc 70:868–883, 1965.
14. Brown LR, Dreizen S, Handler S et al.: The effect of radiation-induced xerostomia on human oral microflora. J Dent Res 54:740–750, 1975.
15. Gowgiel JM: Experimental radio-osteonecrosis of the jaws. J Dent Res 39:176–197, 1960.
16. Koppang HJ: Studies on the radiosensitivity of the rat incisor. Odont T 75:413–450, 1967.
17. Carl W, Sako K, Schaaf NG: Dental complications in the treatment of rhabdomyosarcoma of the oral cavity in children. Oral Surg 38:367–371, 1974.
18. Solomon H, Marchetta F et al.: Extraction of teeth after cancericidal doses of radiotherapy to the head and neck. Am J Surg 115:349–351, 1968.
19. Carl W, Wood R: Effects of radiation on the developing dentition and supporting bone. J Am Dent Assoc 101:646–648, 1980.
20. Carl W, Schaaf NG, Sako K: Oral surgery and the patient who has had radiation therapy for head and neck cancer. Oral Surg 36:651–657, 1973.
21. Bloom W, Fawcett DW: Bone. In: A Textbook of Histology, Bloom W, Fawcett DW (eds). Philadelphia, WB Saunders Co, 1962 (8th ed), pp 162–163.

9. Hematopoietic Dysfunction Resulting from Antineoplastic Therapy: Current Concepts and Potential for Management

ROSS A. ABRAMS

INTRODUCTION

As is well known, the systemic administration of chemotherapeutic agents or the application of large field irradiation results in cytotoxic effects. Specifically, this cytotoxicity is seen earliest and most clearly in rapidly proliferating tissue, whether normal or neoplastic. Although the bone marrow is not the only rapidly proliferating normal tissue, cytotoxic effects in the bone marrow are easily quantified since declines in circulating levels of granulocytes, platelets, and reticulocytes are easily measured and more often than not directly reflect the extent to which any antineoplastic therapy has acutely impaired the ability of the bone marrow to function. In practice, hematologic toxicity as defined by declines in hemoglobin, leukocytes, granulocytes, platelets, and to a lesser degree reticulocytes has become the dose limiting clinical parameter for guiding the administration of systemic antineoplastic therapy [1].

Recent advances in our understanding of hematopoiesis, interaction of antineoplastic therapies with hematopoiesis, pharmacology, and cell cryopreservation hold promise that the hematopoietic consequences of antineoplastic therapies may be both better understood and diminished. In this chapter, following a review of our current understanding of hematopoiesis and the interaction of antineoplastic agents with hematopoiesis, we will examine currently available results that have been achieved with efforts aimed at diminishing hematopoietic toxicity. Remarks regarding bone marrow transplantation have been confined to auto-transplantation, leaving the large and complex field of allogeneic transplantation for separate discussion.

Higby, DJ (ed), Supportive Care in Cancer Therapy. ISBN 0-89838-569-5.
© *1983, Martinus Nijhoff Publishers, Boston. Printed in The Netherlands.*

CONCEPTS OF HEMATOPOIESIS

The formed elements of the blood have known half-lives in the circulation ranging from weeks (red cells) to days (platelets) or hours (granulocytes). In spite of these finite survivals and the need for constant resupply, under normal circumstances the circulating levels of these formed elements are held relatively constant by resupply from the bone marrow. Examination of bone marrow aspirate and core biopsy sections reveals an impressive array of cellular proliferation among erythroid, granulocytic, and megakaryocytic lines. Current understanding of these coexistent findings of extensive heterogeneity and apparently balanced cellular proliferation and loss has been greatly augmented by the development of both suitable technical methodologies for studying hematopoiesis and the concomitant formulation of appropriate physiologic concepts specifically relevant to the field of hematopoiesis (Tables 1, 2). Utilizing these methodologies and concepts it is now possible to formulate a more rational understanding regarding both acute and chronic hematologic toxicity.

Table 1. Methods for studying hematopoiesis.

Method	Reference
Bone marrow histology and ultrastructure	[2]
Spleen colony assay	[3, 4]
In vitro soft gel cultures	[5–7]
In vitro liquid cultures	[8, 9]
Intraperitoneally implanted diffusion chambers	[10]
Animal models of defective hematopoiesis	[11]

As listed in Table 2 one can now identify at least five basic concepts which, when taken together, can be utilized to provide an integrated understanding of hematopoietic activity. Central to this construct is the availability of totipotent hematopoietic stem cells capable of self renewal, differentiation, extensive proliferation when needed, and external control (Table 3) [12]. Although based on currently available in vitro and in vivo assay

Table 2. Hematopoiesis – fundamental concepts.

1. Stem cell – progenitor cell populations
2. Stem cell niche
3. Microenvironmental regulation
4. Humoral regulation
5. Marrow-blood barrier

Table 3. Stem cell characteristics.

1. Self renewal
2. Extensive proliferative capacity
3. Differentiated progeny
4. Subject to regulation

techniques (vide infra), one can demonstrate the presence of and identify a variety of discrete hematopoietic progenitors (that is, cells morphologically and biophysically similar to the totipotent hematopoietic stem cell, but which are no longer totipotent nor necessarily capable of self replication and which may have undergone a variety of alterations in surface membrane markers) [13, 14] (Figure 1). It is likely that these proposed 'discrete' identities merely represent stopping points on a series of branched continua. When further augmented by the refining concepts of nutrient niches specific to the bone marrow, microenvironmental regulation, humoral regulation and specific mechanisms for regulating cellular egress from the bone marrow (marrow-blood barrier), the hematopoietic stem cell – progenitor cell concept integrates well with a great deal of experimental data and provides a resilient construct for the formulation and testing of new hypotheses related to hematopoiesis [15].

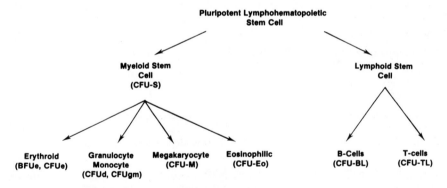

Figure 1. Proposed phylogeny of lymphohematopoietic cells.

METHODOLOGIES AND RESULTS CONFIRMING THIS CONSTRUCT
OF HEMATOPOIESIS

A. Hematopoietic stem cells and hematopoietic progenitor cells
The seminal observations regarding the identity and existence of pluripotent hematopoietic stem cells were made in mice by Till and McCulloch [3].

These workers observed splenic nodules 8–10 days following the administration of large doses of systemic irradiation and injection with syngeneic bone marrow cells. These nodules were observed to contain granulocytic, erythroid, and megakaryocytic elements either singly or in combination. Extensive subsequent studies have revealed that each nodule appears to derive from a single cell ('clonality') [4], that these colonies in turn appear to contain more hematopoietic stem cells (self renewal capacity), and that at least in some cases lymphoid and myeloid elements may be derived from a common stem cell [16]. This assay has become commonly known as the CFU-S assay.

Following rapidly upon the development of the CFU-S assay, has been the development of a number of purely in vitro assay systems (Table 4). These systems typically consist of a semisolid matrix such as agar or methylcellulose, supplemented nutrient media, and either a source of colony stimulating activity, erythropoietin, or both. Using these systems it is now possible to grow granulocyte-monocyte precursors (CFUc, CFUgm, CFUeo), erythroid precursors (CFUe, BFUe) megakaryocytic colonies (CFUm), and mixed colonies (CFUgemm, CFUmix) [5–7, 17–21]. In addition to these purely hematopoietic colonies, lymphoid colonies have also been grown [22]. The mixed colonies are of particular interest since it would be highly desirable to have a direct in vitro assay for the pluripotent hematopoietic stem cell. While this would represent a modest technical advance in mice where the CFU-S assay can already be performed, in man this would represent a breakthrough since at the current time there is no direct assay for (pluripotent) hematopoietic stem cells per se and the relationship of other hematopoietic progenitors to the hematopoietic stem cell may vary substantially based on the conditions of study and the prior clinical expe-

Table 4. In vitro short-term assays for human hematopoietic progenitors.

Cell type	Stimulator
Granulocyte-monocyte	CSA
Eosinophilic	CSA
Erythroid colonies (CFUe)	EPO
Erythroid bursts (BFUe)	EPO, BPA
Mixed colonies	EPO, PHA-LCM
Leukemic colonies	PHA-LCM
T cell	
B cell	
Lymphoma	

CSA = colony stimulating activity; EPO = erythropoietin; BPA = burst promoting activity; PHA-LCM = media condition by lymphocytes in the presence of phytohemagglutinin.

riences of the patient with respect to antineoplastic therapy and/or illness. Fauser and Messner, who have pioneered in man the study of the CFU-gemm, have suggested a possible relationship between this in vitro assay and the pluripotent hematopoietic stem cell based on their observations that the mixed colonies contain granulocytic, erythrocytic, megakaryocytic, and T cell lymphoid elements and appear to have some low potential for self renewal [19]. However, this area remains controversial and in mice the currently available data suggest that cells harvested from mixed colonies grown in vitro contain very little potential for developing splenic colonies when utilized in the CFU-S assay [21]. Consequently, Metcalf has suggested that in the physiologic continuum that ranges from truly pluripotent hematopoietic stem cells to unipotent progenitor cells incapable of self renewal, the mixed colony assay may represent the physiologic state of a progenitor cell capable of multipotential differentiation with little to no potential for self replication [21].

These assays have provided increased understanding of altered physiology in a number of hematopoietic disease states and have provided additional insight to the relationship between hematopoietic toxicity and systemic and regional antineoplastic therapy. Subsequent off-shoots of the development of hematopoietic stem cell assays have been the development of assays in vitro for leukemic and tumor stem cells [23, 24]. Especially with regard to the tumor stem cell assay the opportunity to investigate the extent to which antineoplastic agents interfere with in vitro growth may enable physicians to refine their treatment decisions regarding the utilization of systemic antineoplastic therapy by identifying agents which are more likely to be effective in specific, individual cases based on results with the patient's own tumor cells [25, 26].

B. The hematopoietic microenvironment and the concept of the nutrient niche

Wolfe [27] has recently reviewed the data which attest to the high probability of microenvironmental influences upon hematopoietic stem cell behavior.

1. Hematopoiesis is an organ-specific process in higher animals. This observation of itself suggests the possibility of stromal or microenvironmental influences being required for hematopoietic stem cell proliferation. This possibility is further supported by the observation that in the mouse the transplantation of cell-free hematopoietic stroma obtained from either the marrow or the spleen to typically nonhematopoietic organs can be followed by full hematopoiesis at such sites once the transplanted stroma has become revascularized.

2. It can be shown by karyotypic analysis that when limiting numbers of

hematopoietic stem cells are injected into lethally irradiated mice both lymphoid and myeloid lines may be reconstituted from a single precursor. Yet, lymphopoiesis and hematopoiesis occur simultaneously but predominantly in different anatomic regions. That is, CFU-S colonies do not contain lymphoid cells and thymic glands do not reveal hematopoiesis.

3. Within the spleen there is geographic variation with regard to the types of hematopoietic colonies (erythroid vs granulocytic) that predominate. Similarly, while the murine spleen is essentially an erythroid organ, the murine marrow is essentially a myeloid (i.e. granulocytic) organ. If a small fragment of bone marrow is transplanted into the spleen it can be observed that granulocytic colonies spilling out of the transplanted marrow stroma into the spleen abruptly become erythropoietic upon entering the splenic stroma.

4. Genetically transmitted hematologic defects are observed in mice (Table 5). Two such examples are the W/W^v mouse and the Sl/Sl^d mouse. In both strains the hematologic abnormality consists primarily but not exclusively of macrocytic anemia. When hematopoietic stem cells are transplanted from the W/W^v mouse into the Sl/Sl^d mouse no improvement in hematopoiesis occurs in the recipient animal. In contrast, when hematopoietic stem cells are transplanted from the Sl/Sl^d into a W/W^v recipient normal hematopoiesis results. Based on these observations and others it would appear that the W/W^v mouse has a defective hematopoietic stem cell (CFU-S) and a normal hematopoietic stroma. In contrast it seems that just the reverse is true with the Sl/Sl^d mouse; namely, this mouse contains a defective stroma but a normal CFU-S population.

Table 5. Animals models of hematopoietic interest.

W/W^v – stem cell defect
Sl/Sl^d – microenvironmental defect

5. Finally, the development of long-term in vitro cultures capable of supporting hematopoiesis for weeks by Dexter and his colleagues [28] clearly underscores the importance of microenvironmental and stromal influences on hematopoiesis. When marrow cells are flushed into small tissue culture flasks containing nutrient media and incubated under appropriate laboratory conditions, hematopoiesis does not occur. However, tissue culture flasks which are flushed with marrow do develop upon incubation a population of cells adherent to the inner surface of the flask. If additional marrow cells are then introduced, and appropriate

care taken to prevent excessive build-up of cells and depletion of nutrients, proliferation of murine CFU-S will occur. It can be shown that the stromal elements involved in support of hematopoiesis consist of macrophages, endothelial cells, and fat cells. The results and findings obtained with the Dexter colony assay system lend support to the possibility of nutrient niches as suggested by Schofield [16, 29]. In this construct it is proposed that specific cellular compartments are required to promote hematopoietic stem cell renewal and under adverse circumstances prevent stem cell depletion. Further data supporting this view derived from the use of Dexter flasks studies have been recently summarized by Bentley [30].

C. Humoral regulation

Specific stimulators for erythroid (erythropoietin), granulocytic (colony stimulating activity – CSA), and megakaryocytic (thrombopoietin) proliferation appear to be involved at the systemic level in effecting humoral promotion of hematopoiesis. It would also appear that there are specific inhibitors of hematopoiesis, especially for granulocytic and erythroid cell lines. Additionally, hematopoietic cells are, at least in vitro, known to be sensitive to the effects of glucocorticoids, androgens, estrogens, thyroxine, and various beta adrenergic agents. These observations have been extensively reviewed [13, 31–34] and will not be elaborated further in this discussion.

D. The blood-marrow barrier

As reviewed by Tavassoli [35] it would appear that the emergence of cells from the bone marrow is a selective process which occurs transcellularly rather than intracellularly. This transcellular phenomenon results in nuclear sequestration as erythrocytes leave the marrow. The appearance of circulating, nucleated red blood cells can be taken as suggestive evidence of disruption of the normal marrow-blood barrier.

IN VITRO INSIGHTS TO CLINICALLY OBSERVED HEMATOPOIETIC TOXICITY FOLLOWING ANTINEOPLASTIC THERAPY

The acute hematologic toxicity of antineoplastic therapy is the usual dose limiting toxicity in the management of patients with neoplastic disease. This well-known observation has recently been reviewed in detail, especially with regard to timing, extent, predominant cell line affected (granulocyte vs platelet), and relationship to classical cell cycle kinetics [36]. In fact, even beyond this acute clinical toxicity clinicians are aware of delayed and cumulative effects following cytotoxic therapy. Even though these effects are widely appreciated at the clinical level, their mechanisms are poorly understood. There is, however, appreciation that 'bone marrow reserve' may vary substantially from patient to patient and that second neoplasms may occur as a consequence of cytotoxic therapy. Using the methodologies and concepts described above, additional insights into these subacute and chronic hematopoietic effects of systemic and regional antineoplastic therapy are being obtained.

For example, as reviewed by Marsh [37], it is possible to demonstrate proliferative suppression of hematopoietic progenitors using any of a wide variety of assay techniques. In reviewing 205 reports he observed that extent of hematopoietic progenitor cell suppression could be related to drug dose, schedule, and route of administration, as well as the proliferative state and cell cycle state of the target cell. Although quantitative correlation of these results with observed clinical toxicity is difficult, there have been a variety of other interesting observations and correlations. DeWys and colleagues [38] have observed in mice that the sequential administration of two large intraperitoneal doses of cyclophosphamide produces maximal animal mortality when the second dose is timed to coincide with CFU-S recovery and substantially less mortality if the second dose is administered prior to the onset of CFU-S recovery. Other studies reviewed by Marsh [37] have shown that the concomitant administration of more than one cytotoxic agent over brief time periods may result in either additive, synergistic, or impaired cell kill as compared to single doses of either agent administered alone. For example, studies of CFU-S survival following the administration of ara-C and daunorubicin as well as cyclophosphamide and vincristine reveal only additive cell death when the drugs are administered within 24 to 36 hours of each other. Leukemic cells, on the other hand, are synergistically killed by the combined administration of these agents. In contrast, the combined administration of methotrexate and ara-C or methotrexate and vinblastine results in less cell kill than would be expected from using the same dose of either agent alone.

If, following the administration of cytotoxic agents, hematopoietic stem cell and hematopoietic progenitor cell behavior were simply parallel to the behavior of more conventionally measured hematologic parameters (leukocytes, granulocytes, and platelets), there would be little insight added to our understanding of hematology by the use of these functional assays except perhaps for kinetic insights into the best way of combining drugs as noted in the preceeding paragraph. If this were the case, then measurement of hematopoietic stem cells (CFU-S) and hematopoietic progenitor cells would offer no insight into the occurrence of late hematologic complications following systemic antineoplastic therapy. These complications include the development of persistent cytopenias, inability to tolerate subsequent systemic antineoplastic therapy, and the occurrence of second neoplasms. It is particularly of interest that the persistence of cytopenias is not a prerequisite for the development of either of the other two complications, nor is the absence of persistent cytopenia a guarantee that the other two complications will not occur.

Several groups have now shown that the administration of either radiation therapy or various alkylating agents such as busulfan, BCNU, and cyclophosphamide may be associated with cumulative hematopoietic damage reflected either at the level of the pluripotent hematopoictic stem cell and its descendants or in the stromal compartment or both [39–47]. Morley and co-workers [39–41] have described a particularly elegant model of chronic and cumulative hematopoietic damage induced by repeated administration of busulfan to mice. In this model acute hematopoietic toxicity resolves rather nicely and 60 days following the cessation of busulfan about 60% of the animals have normal blood counts and 35% have normal marrow cellularity. In the remaining animals the cytopenias in the blood and marrow are relatively mild. Even so, by 240 days 80% of the mice become ill and die either as a consequence of marrow aplasia or in a minority of mice the development of leukemia. Measurement of routine blood counts in mice containing latent hematopoietic injury (that is those mice who ultimately go on to develop aplasia) reveals essentially no decline in hematocrit, reticulocyte count, or platelet count and only minor declines in neutrophil and lymphocyte counts as compared to controls. The most striking decline during the latent period was observed in monocyte numbers. These workers subsequently demonstrated that this latent bone marrow failure was associated with well defined abnormalities in both CFU-S and CFUc hematopoietic compartments. Using a modification of the classic CFU-S assay, they found that marrow cells from mice pretreated with busulfan produced delayed and deficient hematopoietic recovery (as reflected by CFU-S, CFUc, and nucleated cells per tibia) when injected into normal mice exposed to high doses of whole body irradiation. Interestingly they also observed in the reverse experiment where normal marrow cells were infused into busulfan treated mice without additional radiation that though there was a substantial recovery of CFU-S and CFUc levels, the recovery was not complete. This latter observation suggested that part of the latent marrow damage involved the stromal element of the marrow in addition to the hematopoietic stem cells per se. These workers have also shown that while BCNU produces evidence of residual damage similar to that found with busulfan, other agents such as cyclophosphamide, 5-fluorouracil, 6-mercaptopurine, methotrexate, and vinblastine are in their model not associated with evidence of residual marrow damage.

Botnick et al. [42, 43] have also focused attention on stem cell failure after alkylating agent therapy. They hypothesize that cellular proliferation among normal stem cells has a finite limit and that for vital organs such as the bone marrow or gastrointestinal tract this limit is not exhausted during the lifetime of normal animals. In contrast, in nonvital organ systems such as those of the hair or hair color, stem cell function may be depleted as reflected by baldness or graying. They further propose that the stress of repeated cytotoxic injury whether induced by radiation therapy or alkylating agents can under some circumstances exhaust the proliferative potential of vital stem cells.

They have tested these hypotheses using busulfan, L-phenylalanine mustard, and cyclophosphamide in mice. In order to test the proliferative capacity of pluripotential hematopoietic stem cells following exposure to alkylating agent therapy, serial bone marrow transfers were utilized. Specifically, mice were exposed at weekly intervals to five or six doses of individual alkylating agents. Then, at intervals ranging from 10 to 95 weeks following the last administration of drug, bone marrow cells from treated animals were transfused into irradiated normal hosts. Fourteen days later these secondary animals were sacrificed, marrow cellularity determined, and the cells harvested for injection into tertiary animals. This process was repeated until the hematopoietic system was exhausted.

Among animals receiving alkylating agent therapy evidence of stem cell damage beyond that in the hematopoietic system was evaluated by examination for early graying of the fur, cataract formation in the lens, and ability of the animals to respond to immunization with sheep red blood cells.

The results are of interest in that they showed different effects among the three agents tested (busulfan, L-phenylalanine mustard, and cyclophosphamide). For example, busulfan use was associated with early graying, decreased response to immunization with sheep red cells, increased frequency of cataract formation, and permanent damage in bone marrow proliferative capacity as tested by the serial transplantation technique described above. In contrast, L-phenylalanine mustard use was associated with a less severe defect in hematopoietic proliferation but an increased frequency of leukemia and also of tumors in the harderian glands. Finally, the use of cyclophosphamide was associated only with an impaired immunologic response to sheep erythrocytes but no damage in hematopoiesis was noted.

The impact of the hematopoietic lesion induced by busulfan has also been studied by Hays et al. in the long-term, Dexter colony system [44]. Following repeated exposure of mice to busulfan, animals were sacrificed and their cells utilized to initiate long-term in vitro marrow cultures. Results with cells from busulfan-treated animals were compared to results with cells from control animals. They found that in cultures from busulfan-treated animals the production of CFU-S and CFUc occurred at markedly reduced levels as compared to controls and that there was a defect in stromal cells that were derived from busulfan treated mice as well.

Several elements of the studies described by Morley et al. and Botnick et al. should be of concern to clinicians involved in the management of patients with cancer. Specifically: 1) the development of second neoplasms in a minority of animals treated following exposure to some but not all of the alkylating agents used; 2) the fact that the latent hematopoietic injury which appears following the expected acute decline in blood counts is rather hidden, and if manifested at all, is manifested primarily by mild to moderate reductions in granulocyte and monocyte counts and in bone marrow cellularity; 3) in the studies of Morley et al. many animals developed overt aplasia following the period of latent injury.

This last concern is of special relevance given the frequency with which alkylating agent therapy is utilized as an adjuvant among patients with potentially long-term disease-free intervals and survival.

A number of clinical observations and studies suggest that these models may have substantial clinical relevance. For example, Penn [48] has reviewed 106 reports describing second neoplasms following either radiation therapy, chemotherapy, or combined modality therapy with both. He confirms that there is a striking increase in the frequency of second neoplasms, especially and predominantly acute leukemias, among patients treated with chemotherapeutic regimens that include alkylating agents or combined modality therapy. Einhorn et al. [49] have recently reported on 51 women who received a minimum of 300 mg of melphalan for ovarian cancer and survived for at least three years. In 12 cases the amount of melphalan administered exceeded 800 mg. Six of these 51 women subsequently developed acute leukemia from three to six years after the initiation of treatment with melphalan. In five cases the leukemia was heralded by the development of pancytopenia. Finally, Lohrmann et al. [50] have serially studied patients with breast cancer undergoing adjuvant therapy with cyclophosphamide and adriamycin. In a detailed study involving all aspects of granulopoiesis, they have clearly demonstrated that following six cycles of adriamycin and cytoxan (at conventional doses) there is a long-lasting decline in the number of circulating granulocyte-monocyte precursors as well as mild declines in circulating numbers of neutrophils and in the number of neutrophils contained in the marrow. The potential parallel in this study between a relatively subclinical defect in granulopoiesis and the busulfan model developed by Morley et al. is striking. Further follow-up studies of this patient population will be of interest.

In summary, hematopoiesis can be viewed as consisting of three distinct but interrelated compartments. The first of these compartments contains the pluripotential hematopoietic stem cell. The second compartment contains the intermediately differentiated, unipotential hematopoietic progenitor cells, and the third compartment contains the morphologically recognizable precursors of the formed elements of the blood. Data now exist which demonstrate that there may be significant hematopoietic injury present in either the first or the second compartment with only minimal manifestations in the third compartment. These concepts have been nicely developed in animal models which appear to have substantial possibility for clinical relevance to patients treated with systemic antineoplastic therapy.

EFFORTS AIMED AT OVERCOMING THE ACUTE MYELOSUPPRESSION ASSOCIATED WITH SYSTEMIC ANTINEOPLASTIC THERAPY

In the immediately preceding discussion our focus of attention was the cumulative effects of systemic antineoplastic therapy on hematopoiesis and the potential for both predicting and studying this phenomenon utilizing current hematopoietic concepts and available methodologies.

However, the fact remains that it is the acute toxicity of systemic antineoplastic therapy which is both most predictable and frequently most frustrating in the management of patients with malignancy. In fact, although there are many organ system toxicities associated with the administration of systemic antineoplastic therapy (e.g. cardiac, pulmonary, renal, and gastrointestinal), it is hematopoietic toxicity – as reflected by alterations in peripheral blood counts — that remains as the usual dose limiting toxicity. The ability to overcome acute hematopoietic toxicity would, in addition to decreasing patient morbidity, also have the potential for permitting the use of increased dosages of chemotherapeutic agents. Such a development might in turn improve our ability to manage various types of malignant disease. Several methodologies aimed at overcoming acute hematopoietic toxicity following the administration of antineoplastic therapy are under study. Some of the techniques that will be discussed are still in their experimental stages and others have not yet entered into clinical trials; however, their discussion seems justified based on their future potential for clinical applicability or because they indicate possible directions for future research.

PHARMACOLOGIC AND CYTOKINETIC EFFORTS AT OVERCOMING ACUTE HEMATOPOIETIC TOXICITY

Hematopoietic protection by the use of a specific antidote

Methotrexate, as is well known, is a potent antineoplastic agent which is cell cycle phase specific and produces its primary effect through the inhibition of dihydrofolate reductase. Due to this unique mechanism of action its toxicity can be overcome by supplying adequate amounts of reduced folates in the form of calcium leucovorin. This method of utilizing methotrexate has been extensively studied both preclinically and clinically. Although it remains unclear that the use of high doses of methotrexate with leucovorin offers any increased tumoricidal efficacy over more conventional doses of methotrexate, it is clear that the concomitant use of calcium leucovorin provides effective protection and rescue from the otherwise myelosuppressive and gastrointestinal toxicities associated with the use of this drug [51].

Hematopoietic protection by augmenting granulopoiesis

One method currently available for augmenting granulopoiesis and granulocyte counts following the administration of cytotoxic, systemic chemotherapy involves the administration of lithium carbonate [52, 53]. Following observations that the administration of this drug to patients with manic depressive disorders was on occasion associated with the development of granulocytosis, trials were undertaken to explore both the mechanism of this granulocytosis as well as its potential application in preventing or reversing the granulocytopenia which predictably results from the administration of systemic chemotherapy. These studies have indicated that the effect of lithium carbonate on granulopoiesis most likely results from augmentation of endogenous colony stimulating activities. When used clinically the drug can definitely be shown to be associated with statistically significant increases in granulocyte levels following the administration of chemotherapy [54]. However, even though these statistically significant increases in granulocyte levels have been demonstrated in settings frequently associated with severe granulocytopenia such as the management of patients with small cell carcinoma of the lung or acute nonlymphocytic leukemia, as pointed out by Greco [55] these statistically significant findings are frequently of clinically marginal value, may occur in only a minority of patients, do not necessarily permit an increase in the amount of drug administered, and have not consistently been associated with decreased incidence of infection or increased rate of response to chemotherapy. Additionally, there are many potential toxicities associated with the use of lithium, only some of which are dose related. The potential for severe gastrointestinal (nausea, vomiting, diarrhea), central nervous system (seizures, confusion, coma), renal (nephrogenic diabetes insipidus-like syndrome), and cardiovascular (arrhythmias, hypotension) toxicity coupled with the rather limited magnitude of the overall clinical benefit has argued against the routine use of this drug among patients receiving cytotoxic chemotherapy. The possibility should be left open that in the future it will be possible to identify selected subsets of patients who may predictably benefit from the use of lithium. In addition, it should be noted that there have been reports of clinical benefit from the use of lithium in patients with neutropenia of other causes such as patients with idiopathic neutropenia and patients with Felty's syndrome [56, 57].

Hematopoietic protection by chemotherapeutic 'priming'

A third mechanism for ameliorating both acute hematopoietic and gastrointestinal toxicity following the administration of either high dose whole body irradiation or high dose systemic melphalan or busulfan involves the administration of a 'priming' dose of cyclophosphamide several days prior to the administration of the ablative, cytotoxic insult. Millar and Huddspith and their co-workers have demonstrated in mice that the prior administration of a moderate dose of cyclophosphamide can substantially ameliorate the lethality associated with whole body irradiation, high dose busulfan, high dose cyclophosphamide or high dose melphalan [58–60]. The precise mechanism of this protection remains unclear, but seems to be related to an accelerated rate of hematopoietic recovery following the ablative insult rather than a decreased sensitivity of the hematopoietic stem cells to the ablative insults per se.

A limited study of the potential of this effect in man was subsequently undertaken by Hedley et al. [61]. These workers administered 500 mg of cyclophosphamide seven days prior to the administration of 140 mg/M^2 of intravenous melphalan to seven patients. They compared the hematopoietic effects of the cyclophosphamide–melphalan combination to the administration of lower doses of melphalan (60–125 mg/M^2) to four patients who did not receive cyclophosphamide priming. In both groups the nadir of leukocytes and granulocytes were the same, but the patients who had received the cyclophosphamide priming recovered their leukocyte count to a level of 1,000/μl earlier than the patients who had not had cyclophosphamide priming (day 18 vs day 24, $p = 0.01$). This observation is of some importance since high dose melphalan is now being utilized with increased frequency in studies involving the treatment of patients with malignancy refractory to conventional therapy. In these studies, which have been accomplished with the adjunctive use of autologous cryopreserved marrow infusions, it has been observed that dose-limiting toxicity is gastrointestinal. It may be hoped based on animal data that gastrointestinal toxicity may also be ameliorated by the administration of a priming dose of cyclophosphamide.

An additional mechanism for protecting against hematopoietic and other toxicities following irradiation or systemic chemotherapy is the use of 'radioprotectors' such as the experimental agent WR2721. As discussed in detail by Yuhas [62], radioprotectors are sulfhydro compounds which appear to exert their protective effect through a mechanism involving the scavenging of free radicals. This effect which might be anticipated to occur in settings involving the use of alkylating agents as well as in settings involving the use of radiotherapy can be clearly demonstrated in mice in terms of radiation dose required to produce 50% mortality at 30 days ($LD_{50/30}$) as well as radiation dose required to produce a standard amount of skin ulceration. Based on considerations of intracellular differences in enzymes, differential drug absorption with respect to the radioprotecting agent, differential drug availability with respect to the radioprotecting agent, and the potential for differential response of hypoxic and well-oxygenated cells, it may be anticipated that normal tissues might experience radioprotection in the absence of radioprotection of tumor tissues. This hypothesis is based in part on the fact that radioprotecting agents which have shown effect in mice are agents which require in vivo activation by normal tissues. Subsequent studies in mice have demonstrated substantially greater protection of normal tissues than of tumors by WR2721 among a broad range of tumors studied including a mammary carcinoma, a lung adenoma, and the KHT sarcoma. WR2721 has entered Phase I and Phase II clinical trials [63]. It has been demonstrated that single doses of WR2721 of 600 mg/M^2 and multiple doses of 100 mg/M^2 can be given with clinical safety. At the current time, however, it remains unclear whether the clinical use of this agent provides any significant protection against the hematopoietic or other toxic-

Table 6. Therapeutic efforts aimed at overcoming acute chemotherapy-related hematopoietic toxicity without using stem cell infusions.

Concept	Example	Clinical trial	Clinical efficacy demonstrated
1. Specific pharmacologic rescue	Calcium leucovorin following methotrexate	Yes – extensive	Yes
2. 'Radio protectors'	WR 2721	Yes – Phase II	Uncertain
3. Cytokinetic manipulations			
a. 'Priming'	Low dose cytoxan 1 week prior to high dose melphalan	Yes	Limited
b. Hematopoietic stem cell inhibitors	Protection of murine CFU-S from 1B-D-arabinofuranosylcytoxine	No	–
4. Hematopoietic stimulators	Lithium to augment granulopoiesis	Yes	Yes – but effect marginal
5. Encourage stem cell proliferation away from a specific hematopoietic path	Hypertransfusion with red cells to discourage erythropoiesis and augment granulopoiesis	Yes – limited	No

ities associated with radiation therapy or the systemic administration of cyclophosphamide or other chemotherapeutic agents [63–65].

Some of the methodologies which have been studied in an effort to minimize hematopoietic toxicity following the administration of systemic antineoplastic therapy are summarized in Table 6. One effort noted there which has not yet entered clinical trial has been the use of hematopoietic stem cell inhibitors to protect from the acute hematopoietic toxicity of a cycle-specific agent [66]. The use of transfusions to direct stem cells away from erythropoiesis toward granulopoiesis, although promising in mice, did not in a single small study of patients with acute lymphoblastic leukemia demonstrate convincing efficacy [67].

The use of infusions of autologous hematopoietic stem cells
as an adjunct to the management of patients with neoplasia

In view of the limitations imposed on systemic antineoplastic therapy by the consequences of acute hematopoietic toxicity, it would be desirable to be able to prevent or reverse this therapeutically limiting toxicity. A logical way of seeking this end would be to infuse viable hematopoietic stem cells following the administration of systemic antineoplastic therapy. In theory, stem cells infused at that time would not have been exposed to the toxic effects of therapy, and would thus immediately begin to renew hematopoiesis. In the 1960s and early 1970s the ability to rescue animals from treatment-related, hematopoietic death was accomplished through the administration of infusions of hematopoietic stem cells. Following this demonstrated preclinical efficacy, from the mid 1970s to the present there have been numerous clinical studies of the use of infusions of autologous hematopoietic stem cells in association with intensive antineoplastic therapy [68]. These studies have clearly demonstrated that infusions of autologous cryopreserved marrow are capable of rescuing patients from potentially lethal

Table 7. Use of autologous hematopoietic stem cells for hematopoietic reconstitution – clinical issues.

1. What does the availability of hematopoietic stem cell collections accomplish?
2. What is the rationale for ablative levels of therapy?
3. What is the hematopoietic consequence of an autologous collection?
4. When is therapy sufficiently intense that hematopoietic reconstitution is advised or necessary?
5. When is bone marrow collection and ablative therapy optimally utilized in a patient's course?
6. For which diseases should ablative therapy with autologous hematopoietic rescue be considered?
7. What is the hematological consequence of ablative therapy with hematopoietic rescue?
8. Future directions.

hematopoietic damage following ablative levels of therapy and that the administration of such therapy can, at least in some cases, be associated with durable complete responses not achievable by other means [69]. In spite of this, there are many questions that confront the physician who contemplates the use of autologous hematopoietic stem cell infusions and who seeks to integrate rationally the use of this technique into the management of his patients. Some of these questions are listed in Table 7. In addition to these clinical issues there are also several technical issues relating to how marrow is processed and frozen in the laboratory and some of these are summarized in Table 8. A discussion aimed at providing perspective and overview regarding these issues seems in order.

Table 8. Use of autologous hematopoietic stem cells for hematopoietic reconstitution – technical issues.

1. How long can marrow be stored without cryopreservation per se?
2. How is cryopreservation accomplished?
3. What are the risks of cryopreservation?
4. How is marrow processed prior to cryopreservation?
5. Can one identify tumor contamination?
6. Can one reliably monitor marrow following cryopreservation for viability?
7. Can tumor cells be selectively removed or destroyed in vitro from marrow collections?

The essential point of storing and infusing autologous hematopoietic stem cell collections is to effect post treatment hematopoietic recovery or reconstitution that could not otherwise reasonably be expected to occur. Viewed in isolation, the availability of such stem cell collections by themselves has no immediate purpose. Thus, the value of these stem cell infusions lies in their permitting the administration of therapies which would otherwise be hematopoietically lethal or crippling and which are substantially more tumoricidal than other less hematopoietically damaging therapies. In fact, the vast majority of cytotoxic therapies do not produce irreversible hematopoietic damage, even when designed to produce severe lowering of peripheral blood counts. For example, induction therapies used in the management of acute nonlymphocytic leukemia typically eventuate in granulocyte counts that approach zero and platelet counts that may hover in the range of 5,000 to 20,000/µl for as long as one to three weeks and then be followed by excellent and resilient hematopoietic recovery (if the leukemic infiltrate is eradicated). In practice, the design of chemotherapeutic regimens which are truly hematopoietically ablative and yet associated with acceptable levels of nonhematopoietic toxicity has proved to be quite difficult. The ability of bone marrow to tolerate and recover from cytotoxic insult is probably generally underestimated. There are several distinct indicators as to when a therapy is not hematopoietically ablative. These include failure to achieve a granulocyte count of 100/μl or lower, failure to achieve a platelet count of 20,000/μl or lower, and the onset of hematopoietic recovery prior to 14 to 21 days following the time of infusion of the transfused hematopoietic stem cells. Although in theory the issue of whether a specific therapy requires hematopoietic reconstitution could be easily resolved by doing the appropriate prospective controlled trial, in practice investigators are confronted with a severe ethical dilemma that mitigates against the use of such trials. Specifically, since hematopoietic stem cell infusions are believed to be effective in producing an accelerated rate of hematopoietic recovery following ablative levels of therapy, it is difficult, if not impossible, to deny patients the potential benefit of this form of supportive care when the consequences of hematopoietic failure are well known and include a significant risk of mortality. In practice, therapy incorporating high doses of whole body irradiation, large doses of nitrosoureas, and large doses of some but not all alkylating agents (specifically busulfan and melphalan) have been felt to be sufficiently myelosuppressive to justify the use of autologous hematopoietic stem cell infusions. In this context four facts, however, deserve emphasis:

1. Very large doses of nitrosoureas – either alone or in combination chemotherapy regimens – are not necessarily hematopoietically ablative [70] and may be associated with nonhematopoietic, dose-limiting toxicity [71, 72].

2. Hematopoietic reconstitution–whether allogeneic, syngeneic, or autologous appears to occur only after an obligatory period of profound cytopenia when truly ablative preparative regimens are utilized [73–75]. This period of 14–21 days seems to reflect the interval required for infused pluripotent stem cells and their progeny to undergo sufficient self renewal and proliferative maturation to repopulate the marrow. In fact, it is likely that the difference between therapies that require exogenous hematopoietic reconstitution and those that do not hinges on the extent to which the self renewal properties of endogenous pluripotent stem cells have been eliminated. The depth of granulocyte and platelet nadirs alone do not necessarily give insight regarding this issue.

3. It is necessary to undertake cryopreservation if the interval between stem cell collection and re-infusion exceeds 48–72 hours. Cryopreservation and its attendant processing steps are associated with some risk of losing cell viability. However, there is no direct methodology for assessing pluripotent hematopoietic stem cell content in vitro. Consequently clinical investigators are confronted with an ethical dilemma between using therapies which are not ablative (reconstitution not required) and ablative therapies (reconstitution required but cannot be guaranteed).

4. At ablative levels of therapy nonhematopoietic toxicity may be sub-

stantial and clearly dose limiting. In fact, toxicity involving cardiac, pulmonary, and gastrointestinal organs may on occasion be so severe as to obviate the value of any brief or limited clinical response achieved [69, 71, 72, 76–78].

Patients frequently enquire of the hematopoietic consequences of collecting enough bone marrow to permit subsequent hematopoietic reconstitution. The amount of bone marrow collected is of the order of magnitude of 2×10^8 nucleated bone marrow cells/kg. The total amount of bone marrow available in the body of a normal person is estimated to be approximately $3\text{–}4 \times 10^9$ nucleated bone marrow cells/kg. Consequently, the amount of bone marrow collected is probably 10% or less of total body bone marrow. Such collections are associated with essentially no hematopioetic sequelae; that is, there is no persistent effect on peripheral blood granulocyte or platelet counts. However, the aspirated marrow fluid is rich in red cell hemoglobin, and the collection of the required amount of marrow aspirate results in a hemoglobin loss equivalent to the hemorrhage of one to two units of whole blood. In otherwise well individuals, such as those donating bone marrow for purposes of allogeneic transplantation, this hemoglobin loss is of little practical consequence, particularly if iron losses are replaced. In the autologous setting, in contrast, patients are frequently anemic prior to bone marrow collection and marrow recovery may be limited by subsequent therapy. Consequently, the hemoglobin losses attendant to autologous bone marrow collection usually need to be replaced by transfusion of appropriate amounts of packed red blood cells.

The timing of bone marrow collection and the integration of ablative therapy into the patient's overall management represent complex issues. Logically, bone marrow collection is preferably undertaken when the patient is in the best possible physiologic condition for undergoing the rigors of a general anesthetic and also when the chance of tumor stem cell contamination of the marrow is minimized. For neoplasms that frequently metastasize by hematogenous routes both of these conditions are best satisfied when the patient is in a complete remission or has achieved the best remission possible within the limitations of currently available standard therapy. This posture leaves open the possibility that some patients who have obtained a complete clinical remission will undergo a bone marrow storage without ever requiring ablative therapy or bone marrow reinfusion. However, with an awareness of the patient's pretreatment characteristics with respect to tumor type, clinical stage, and expected tumor response to available therapies one can eliminate from further consideration patients for whom the risk of relapse is so small that the collection of bone marrow during complete remission will seem unwarranted. For example, in the management of patients with Burkitt's lymphoma it is well known that patients who present with disease limited to one site outside of the abdomen or patients who present with abdominal disease such that >90% can be surgically resected, are at a relatively low risk for relapse once complete remission has been achieved with conventional chemotherapy [79, 80]. Bone marrow collection in these patients would not seem warranted. In contrast, patients with Burkitt's lymphoma who present with disease on both sides of the diaphragm or who present with intra-abdominal disease that is not amenable to surgical resection are at a much higher risk of relapse even if they achieve complete remission [80]. In these patients the collection of bone marrow at a time of complete remission is more attractive. The alternative to collecting bone marrow relatively early in the patient's course (at a time of good clinical remission), is to try to collect bone marrow at times of obvious relapse. There are many difficulties associated with this approach. Specifically, there are invariably some time delays involved in confirming the relapse and restaging the patient's disease; it is extremely difficult to predict the rate at which clinical situations will deteriorate once tumor progression has been observed; organ system dysfunction may preclude the possibility of general anesthesia at such times; and the opportunity to collect bone marrow free of contaminating tumor stem cells may be lost.

Determining the optimal timing of intensive or ablative levels of therapy following bone marrow collection must also take into account the precise nature of the patient's tumor, clinical stage, and response to prior therapy. In situations where even complete responses are known to be nondurable (e.g. patients presenting with extensive small cell carcinoma of the lung) one might wish to consider the administration of ablative therapy shortly after complete response has been obtained. Such an approach would be predicated on the rationale that intensive therapy will have its greatest effect and produce its most durable result when applied at a time of minimal tumor burden. This is the approach currently being taken in the management of patients with acute nonlymphocytic leukemia who undergo allogeneic transplantation shortly after the achievement of complete remissions [81]. Such timing runs the risk of compromising good quality life that the patient might otherwise have experienced prior to relapse; it can be justified only if the risks of morbidity and mortality following treatment and autologous transplantation are sufficiently low in each clinician's own institution to warrant risking the otherwise available benefit of the current remission. Thus, for institutions initiating their experience with autologous bone marrow reconstitution, it would seem prudent to avoid this adjuvant intensive setting until adequate institutional experience has been obtained to permit an accurate assessment of the on-site risks and benefits involved for each patient. For patients who have already relapsed following initial therapy, it is frequently the case that second line therapies are unable to produce complete remissions and that the more frequently occurring partial remissions are of limited value. In these situations it seems reasonable to offer patients the possible benefits of therapeutic intensification in the hope of achieving a more complete and durable remission. This approach has been utilized in patients with non-Hodgkin's lymphoma, small cell carcinoma of the lung, neuroblastoma, acute leukemia, melanoma, testicular cancer, breast cancer, gliomas, and sarcomas [68, 75, 82–93]. For tumors that are known to have significant responses to conventional therapy it does not seem logical to use bone marrow collection and ablative therapy at the time of initial presentation. In many respects such an approach is analogous to collecting bone marrow at times of relapse. The disadvantages of that approach have been discussed above. In the setting of small cell carcinoma of the lung, attempts at collecting bone marrow and using ablative therapy as initial therapy have not been promising [94].

Certain malignant diseases have characteristic courses which make the integration of ablative therapy into their management attractive. These features are: 1) the occurrence of significant remissions followed by the occurrence of relapse; 2) a clinical 'window' in time for collecting marrow at times of good performance status and minimal risk of tumor involvement; 3) a predictable course in which the occurrence of protracted disease-free intervals following initial therapy is known to be unlikely; 4) occurrence in a patient population that is not severely restrained by concomitant non-neoplastic disease and/or age.

Situations which fulfill these criteria can be found among patients with lymphomas, sarcomas, neuroblastoma, small cell carcinoma of the lung, certain subsets of malignant breast tumors, testicular carcinoma, and perhaps advanced stage epithelial ovarian malignancies. In these settings the use of autologous hematopoietic reconstitution in association with ablative therapy may be regarded as a form of Phase III clinical study aimed at augmenting or extending other currently available and efficacious therapeutic options.

Intensive therapy trials supported by autologous hematopoietic reconstitution have also been undertaken in settings where currently available standard therapeutic options are substantially lacking in efficacy. To date such trials have involved large single doses of drugs such as BCNU (72), L-pam (88), mitomycin C (95), m-AMSA (96), and VP-16 (97); and have been undertaken in patients with metastatic melanoma, gliomas, non-small cell lung cancer, and other tumors refractory to less intensive forms of intervention. Trials such as these are essentially Phase I/II studies aimed at finding encouraging clinical responses in association with acceptable nonhematopoietic toxicity. The value of these studies remains to be determined. However, it is possible that they may in time permit a rational development of hematopoietically ablative combination chemotherapy regimens and provide increased ability to anticipate overall nonhematopoietic effects.

The ability to effect hematopoietic reconstitution following ablative levels of therapy may have implications for long-term management. For example, in a small group of patients with Ewing's sarcoma treated with intensive combined modality therapy, hematopoietic reconstitution was associated with both accelerated hematopoietic recovery and increased tolerance to subsequent maintenance chemotherapy [98].

The desirability of using autologous hematopoietic stem cell reconstitution would be greatly enhanced if it were possible to definitively eliminate contaminating stem cells following bone marrow harvesting. Recent reports suggest that both immunologic methodologies utilizing specific monoclonal antibodies in the presence of complement and in vitro chemotherapeutic manipulations may be feasible for this approach [99–101]. When further refined, these approaches may greatly enhance and expand our ability to apply ablative levels of therapy with autologous hematopoietic reconstitution to patients with acute leukemia, lymphoma, and therapeutically responsive solid tumors involving the bone marrow.

In the future it may also be possible to collect hematopoietic stem cells for purposes of reconstitution from the peripheral blood [102]. It is well known that hematopoietic progenitor cells (granulocyte monocyte precursors, burst forming units, and mixed hematopoietic progenitors) circulate in the peripheral blood [102]. In fact, among patients with chronic phase, untreated, chronic myelogenous leukemia (CML) there is extensive amplification of these circulating hematopoietic progenitor cell numbers, and this amplification is proportional to the degree of leukocytosis. Using this naturally occurring phenomenon, Goldman and co-workers have demonstrated the feasibility of autologous hematopoietic reconstitution using cryopreserved cells collected from the peripheral blood of patients with CML [103]. We have shown that in non-CML man, in the unperturbed state, circulating hematopoietic stem cell numbers do not appear to be adequate for effecting hematopoietic reconstitution [104]. However in both dogs and man a significant expansion of circulating hematopoietic progenitors occurs during hematologic recovery following conventional chemotherapy [105, 106]. In dogs this expansion of hematopoietic progenitor numbers is associated with increased potency on a cell for cell basis for hematopoietic reconstitution [106]. Pending further studies to define the clinical frequency of this type of hematopoietic progenitor expansion as well as confirmation in the clinical setting of the reconstitutive potency of hematopoietic stem cells collected from the circulation, it seems feasible that in the future non-CML patients undergoing treatment with conventional levels of chemotherapy will be able to have hematopoietic stem cells collected through the use of pheresis techniques. This would avoid the need for conventional bone marrow harvesting under general anesthesia.

Technically, the logistics and results associated with currently used methodologies of cryopreservation seem sufficiently well defined that the cryopreservation of bone marrow per se need no longer be considered experimental. Using properly controlled freezing techniques it seems clear that hematopoietic reconstitution occurs reliably with the use of autologous cryopreserved marrow stem cells [75, 92, 98]. These techniques involve the use of controlled rate freezing and the use of a cryoprotectant, preferably dimethylsulfoxide. The optimal freezing rate remains controversial, but appears to be between 1 and 3 °C/minute [107–110]. The primary risk of cryopreservation is the loss of stem cell viability. At the current time there is no completely agreed upon technique for monitoring loss of viability following cryopreservation; whether the measurement of granulocyte monocyte precursors or alternatively the measurement of burst forming units or mixed hematopoietic progenitors before and after freezing will be useful for this purpose is a matter of ongoing investigation. The primary technical hurdle to be overcome in this sphere is the incompletely explained variability in post cryopreservation measurement of these hematopoietic progenitors. These difficulties may relate to the release following freezing and thawing of inhibitory substance into the culture milieu, loss of stimulation by non-stem cell marrow cells which do not necessarily survive the process of cryopreservation, or to cryoinjury per se and are compounded by our inability to measure directly pluripotent hematopoietic stem cells. However, it seems likely that these difficulties are at least in part technical, rather than fundamental, since the cryopreservation techniques utilized have already been shown to be efficacious in multiple animal models [107] and clinically [75, 92, 98].

The processing of marrow prior to cryopreservation has been variable. Investigators have utilized minimal processing, separation of red cells by simple centrifugation, or density–gradient separation [75, 108]. Effective hematopoietic reconstitution has been claimed using all three methodologies. Potential advantages of selectively isolating bone marrow mononuclear cell populations (containing the hematopoietic progenitor and stem cells) include a reduction in the number of contaminating granulocytes and red cells which are known not to survive the process of cryopreservation, a reduction in the amount of 'cellular debris' that will be thus reinfused in the patients following the thawing of the frozen marrow, and perhaps an increased ability to detect small populations of contaminating tumor stem cells. Future methods of selectively isolating hematopoietic progenitors may involve the use of counter-flow elutriation techniques and immunologic marking [111–114].

The absolute duration of viability following cryopreservation of bone marrow cells is not known with certainty. However, hematopoietic stem cell collections from the peripheral blood of patients with chronic granulocytic leukemia have been shown to retain viability as measured both by in vitro granulocyte monocyte determinations as well as reconstitutive potency when reinfused several years after the time of collection and cryopreservation [103].

SUMMARY

The ultimate role of autologous hematopoietic reconstitution in the management of patients with malignant disease remains to be defined. This role will increase as methodologies for guaranteeing reconstitutive efficacy are improved, suitable settings and regimens are more completely defined, and techniques for selectively eliminating contaminating tumor cells are developed. To date the intensification of therapy permitted by autologous hematopoietic reconstitution has been shown to be of substantial value in patients with lymphoma refractory to conventional therapy – some of whom appear to have been cured – and excellent palliative value among patients with acute leukemia refractory to primary therapy. Objective tumor responses have been obtained in a number of solid tumor settings. It would appear that future studies aimed at rationally integrating ablative and standard therapies are now in order for appropriate patient populations. Such efforts combined with in vitro and clinical investigation aimed at collecting hematopoietic stem cells from the peripheral blood and identifying and selectively eliminating tumor cell populations are likely to result in a better defined and growing role for autologous hematopoietic reconstitution techniques.

REFERENCES

1. Rubin P, Scarantino CW: The bone marrow organ: the critical structure in radiation–drug interaction. Int J Rad Oncol Biol Phys 4:3–23, 1978.
2. De Bruyn PPH: Structural substrates of bone marrow function. Semin Hematol 18: 179–193, 1981.
3. Till JE, McCulloch EA: A direct measurement of the radiation sensitivity of normal mouse bone marrow cells. Radiation Res 14:213–222, 1961.
4. Becker AJ, McCulloch EA, Till JE: Cytological demonstration of the clonal nature of spleen colonies derived from mouse marrow cells. Nature 197:452–454, 1963.
5. Metcalf D: Detection and analysis of human granulocyte. monocyte precursors using semi-solid cultures. Clinics in Hematol 8:263–286, 1979.
6. Ogawa M, Parmley RT, Bank HL, Spicer SS: Human marrow erythropoiesis in culture I. Characterization of methylcellulose colony assay. Blood 48:407–417, 1976.

7. Gregory CJ, McCulloch EA, Till JE: Erythropoietic progenitors capable of colony formation in culture: state of differentiation. J Cell Physiol 81:411–420, 1973.

8. Dexter TM, Spooncer E, Hendry J, Lajtha LG: Stem cells in vitro. In: Hematopoietic Cell Differentiation, Golde DW, Cline MJ, Metcalf D, Fox CF (eds). New York, Academic Press, 1978, pp 163–174.

9. Dicke K, Spitzer G: Introduction to liquid cultures of hematopoietic cells. In: Hematopoietic Cell Differentiation, Golde DW, Cline MJ, Metcalf D, Fox CF (eds). New York, Academic Press, 1978, pp 213–230.

10. Gordon MY: Changes in human bone marrow colony-forming cells following chemotherapy using an agar diffusion-chamber technique. In: Experimental Hematology Today, Baum SJ, Ledney GD (eds). New York, Springer-Verlag, 1977, pp 233–237.

11. Harrison DE: Use of genetic anemias in mice as tools for haematological research. Clinics in Hematol 8:289–262, 1979.

12. Lajtha LG: Stem cell concepts. Differentiation 14:23–34, 1979.

13. Quesenberry P, Levitt L: Hematopoietic stem cells. N Engl J Med 301:755–760, 819–823, 868–872, 1979.

14. Fitchen JH, Foon KA, Cline MJ: The antigenic characteristics of hematopoietic stem cells. N Engl J Med 305:17–24, 1981.

15. Lajtha LG (ed): Cellular Dynamics of Haemopoiesis. Clinics in Hematol 8:2, London, WB Saunders Ltd, 1979.

16. Schofield R: The pluripotent stem cell. Clinics in Hematol 8:221–237, 1979.

17. Mazur EM, Hoffman R, Bruno E: Regulation of human megakaryocytopoiesis. J Clin Invest 68:733–741, 1981.

18. Vainchenker W, Bouguet J, Guichard J, Breton-Gorius J: Megakaryocyte colony formation from human bone marrow precursors. Blood 54:940–945, 1979.

19. Messner HA, Fauser AA: Culture studies of human pluripotential hematopoietic progenitors. Blut 41:327–333, 1980.

20. Ash RC, Detrick RA, Zanjani ED: Studies of human pluripotential hematopoietic stem cells (CFU-GEMM) in vitro. Blood 58:309–316.

21. Metcalf D, Johnson GR: Mixed hemopoietic colonies in vitro. In: Hematopoietic Cell Differentiation, Golde DW, Cline MJ, Metcalf D, Fox CF (eds). New York, Academic Press, 1978, pp 141–152.

22. Wilson JD, Dalton G: Human T lymphocyte colonies in agar: a comparison with other T-cell assays in healthy subjects and cancer patients. Aust J Exp Biol Med Sci 54:27–34, 1976.

23. Buick RN, Till JE, McCulloch EA: Colony assay for proliferative blast cells circulating in myeloblastic leukaemia. Lancet i:863–864, 1977.

24. Hamburger AW, Salmon SE: Primary bioassay of human tumor stem cells. Science 19:461–463, 1977.

25. Salmon SE, Hamburger AW, Soehnlen B et al.: Quantitation of differential sensitivity of human-tumor stem cells to anticancer drugs. N Engl J Med 298:1321–1327, 1978.

26. Alberts DS, Salmon SE, Chan HSG et al.: In vitro clonogenic assay for predicting response of ovarian cancer to chemotherapy. Lancet ii:340–342, 1980.

27. Wolf NS: The haemopoietic microenvironment. Clinics in Hematol 8:469–500, 1979.

28. Dexter TM, Allen TD, Lajtha LG: Conditions controlling the proliferation of haemopoietic stem cells in vitro. J Cell Physiol 91:335–344, 1977.

29. Schofield R: The relationship between the spleen colony forming cell and the haemopoietic stem cell. Blood Cells 4:7–25, 1978.

30. Bentley SA: Bone marrow connective tissue and the haemopoietic microenvironment. Br J Haematol 50:1–6, 1982.

194

31. Cline MJ, Golde DW: Controlling the production of blood cells. Blood 52:157–165, 1979.
32. Greenberg HM, Parker LM, Newburger PE et al.: Corticosteroid dependence of continuous hemopoiesis in vitro with murine or human bone marrow. Hematol Blood Trans 26: 289–293, 1981.
33. Beran M, Spitzer G, Verma DS: Testosterone and synthetic androgens improve the in vitro survival of human marrow progenitor cells in serum-free suspension cultures. J Lab Clin Med 99:247–253, 1982.
34. Golde DW, Cline MJ: Hormonal interaction with hematopoietic cells in vitro. Transplantation Proceedings 10:95–97, 1978.
35. Tavassoli M: The marrow-blood barrier. Br J Haematol 41:297–302, 1979.
36. Hoagland HC: Hematologic complications of cancer chemotherapy. Sem Oncol 9:95–102, 1982.
37. Marsh JC: Effects of cancer chemotherapeutic agents on normal hematopoietic precursor cells: a review. Cancer Res 36:1853–1862, 1976.
38. DeWys WD, Goldin A, Mantel N: Hematopoietic recovery after large doses of cyclophosphamide: correlation of proliferative state with sensitivity. Cancer Res 30:1692–1697, 1970.
39. Morley A, Blake J: An animal model of chronic aplastic marrow failure I. Late marrow failure after busulfan. Blood 44:49–56, 1974.
40. Morley A, Trainor K, Blake J: A primary stem cell lesion in experimental chronic hypoplastic marrow failure. Blood 45:681–688, 1975.
41. Trainor KJ, Morley AA: Screening of cytotoxic drugs for residual bone marrow damage. J Natl Cancer Inst 57:1237–1239, 1976.
42. Botnick LE, Hannon EC, Hellman S: A long lasting proliferative defect in the hematopoietic stem cell compartment following cytotoxic agents. Int J Rad Oncol Biol Phys 5:1621–1625, 1979.
43. Botnick LE, Hannon EC, Hellman S: Multisystem stem cell failure after apparent recovery from alkylating agents. Cancer Res 38:1942–1947, 1978.
44. Hays EF, Hale L, Villarreal B, Bitchen JH: Stromal and hemopoietic stem cell abnormalities in long term cultures of marrow from busulfan-treated mice. Exp Hematol 10:383–392, 1982.
45. Boggs DR, Boggs SS, Chervenick PA, Patrene KD: Murine recovery from busulfan induced hematopoietic toxicity as assessed by three assays for colony-forming cells. Am J Hematol 8:43–54, 1980.
46. Fried W, Barone J: Residual marrow damage following therapy with cyclophosphamide. Exp Hematol 8:610–614, 1980.
47. Wathen LM, Knapp SA, DeGowin RL: Suppression of marrow stromal cells and microenvironmental damage following sequential radiation and cyclophosphamide. Int J Rad Oncol Biol Phys 7:935–941, 1981.
48. Penn I: Second neoplasms following radiotherapy to chemotherapy for cancer. Am J Clin Oncol (CCT) 5:83–96, 1982.
49. Einhorn N, Eklund G, Franzen S et al.: Late side effects of chemotherapy in ovarian cancer. Cancer 49:2234–2241, 1982.
50. Lohrmann H-P, Schreml W, Lang M et al.: Changes of granulopoiesis during and after adjuvant chemotherapy of breast cancer. Br J Haematol 40:369–384, 1978.
51. Dorr RT, Fritz WL (eds): Cancer Chemotherapy Handbook. New York, Elsevier North-Holland, 1980, pp 523–537.
52. Barrett AJ: Haematological effects of lithium and its use in treatment of neutropenia. Blut 40:1–6, 1980.

53. Stein RS, Howard CA, Brennan M, Czorniak M: Lithium carbonate and granulocyte production: dose optimization. Cancer 48:2696–2701, 1981.
54. Rossof AH, Robinson WA (eds): Lithium Effects on Granulopoiesis and Immune Function, Adv Exp Med Biol, New York, Plenum Press, 1980, pp 167–399.
55. Ibid, pp 275–279.
56. Gerner RH, Wolff SM, Fauci AS, Aduan RP: Lithium carbonate for recurrent fever and neutropenia. JAMA 246:1584–1586, 1981.
57. Gupta RC, Robinson WA, Syth CJ: Efficacy of lithium in rheumatoid arthritis with granulocytopenia (Felty's Syndrome). Arthritis Rheum 18:179–184, 1975.
58. Millar JL, Huddspith BN: Sparing effect of cyclophosphamide pretreatment on animals lethally treated with γ-irradiation. Cancer Treat Rep 60:409–414, 1976.
59. Millar JL, Huddspith HN, Blackett NM: Reduced lethality in mice receiving a combined dose of cyclophosphamide and busulfan. Br J Cancer 32:193–198, 1975.
60. Millar JL, Clutterbuck RD, Smith IE: Improving the therapeutic index of two alkylating agents. Br J Cancer 42:485–487, 1980.
61. Hedley DW, McElwain TD, Millar JL, Gordon MY: Acceleration of bone marrow recovery by pre-treatment with cyclophosphamide in patients receiving high dose melphalan. Lancet ii:966–968, 1978.
62. Yuhas JM: On the potential application of radioprotective drugs in solid tumor radiotherapy. In: Radiation-Drug Interactions in the Treatment of Cancer, Sokol GH, Maickel RP (eds). New York, John Wiley & Sons, 1980, pp 113–136.
63. Kligerman MM, Blumberg AL, Glick JH et al.: Phase I trials of WR2721 in combination with radiation therapy and with the alkylating agents cyclophosphamide and cis-platinum. Cancer Clin Trials 4:469–474, 1981.
64. Woolley PV, Ayoob M, Smith FP, Dritschlo A: A controlled trial of the effects of radioprotector WR2721 on the toxicity of cyclophosphamide (abstract). Proceedings AACR 23:136, 1982.
65. Glick JH, Glover D, Weiler C et al.: Phase I trial of the chemoprotector WR2721 with cyclophosphamide, nitrogen mustard, or platinum (abstract). Proceedings ASCO 1:24, 1982.
66. Guigon M, Jean-Yves M, Enouf J, Frindel E: Protection of mice against lethal doses of 1B-D-arabinofuranosylcytosine by pluripotent stem cell inhibitors. Cancer Res 42:638–641, 1982.
67. Toogood IRG, Ekert H, Smith PJ et al.: Controlled study of hypertransfusion during remission induction in childhood acute lymphocytic leukemia. Lancet ii:862–864, 1978.
68. Deisseroth A, Abrams RA: The role of autologous stem cell reconstitution in intensive therapy for resistant neoplasms. Cancer Treat Rep 63:461–471, 1979.
69. Deisseroth A, Abrams R, Bode U et al.: Current status of autologous bone marrow transplantation. In: Biology of Bone Marrow Transplantation, Gale RP, Fox CF (eds). New York, Academic Press, 1980, pp 145–158.
70. Foon KA, Haskell CM: Inadvertent overdose with lomustine (CCNU) followed by hematologic recovery. Cancer Treat Rep 66:1241–1242, 1982.
71. Appelbaum FR, Strauchen JA, Graw RG, Jr et al.: Acute lethal carditis caused by high-dose combination chemotherapy. Lancet i:58–62, 1976.
72. Herzig GP, Phillips GL, Herzig RH et al.: High dose nitrosourea (BCNU) and autologous bone marrow transplantation: a Phase I study. In: Nitrosoureas – Current Status and New Developments, Prestayko AW et al. (eds). Academic Press, London, 1981, pp 337–342.
73. Thomas ED, Buckner CD, Banaji M et al.: One hundred patients with acute leukemia treated by chemotherapy, total body irradiation, and allogeneic marrow transplantation. Blood 49:511–533, 1977.

196

74. Fefer A, Buckner CD, Thomas ED et al.: Cure of hematologic neoplasia with transplantation of marrow from identical twins. N Engl J Med 297:146-148, 1977.
75. Herzig GP: Autologous marrow transplantation in cancer therapy. In: Progress in Hematology, Vol XII, Brown E (ed). Grune & Stratton, New York, 1981, pp 1-23.
76. Lazarus HM, Gottfried MR, Herzig RH et al.: Veno-occlusive disease of the liver after high dose mitomycin-C therapy and autologous bone marow transplantation. Cancer 49:1789-1795, 1982.
77. Gottdiener JS, Appelbaum FR, Ferrans VJ et al.: Cardiotoxicity associated with high dose cyclophosphamide therapy. Arch Int Med 141:758-763, 1981.
78. Glode LM: Dose limiting extramedullary toxicity of high dose chemotherapy. Exp Hematol 7(Suppl 5):265-278, 1979.
79. Magrath IT, Lwanga S, Carswell W, Harrison N: Surgical reduction of tumour bulk in management of abdominal Burkitt's lymphoma. Br Med J 11(May):308-312, 1974.
80. Ziegler JL, Deisseroth AB, Appelbaum FR, Graw RG, Jr: Burkitt's lymphoma – a model for intensive chemotherapy. Semin Oncol 4:317-323, 1977.
81. Thomas ED, Buckner CD, Clift RA et al.: Marrow transplantation for acute nonlymphoblastic leukemia in first remission. N Engl J Med 301:597-599, 1979.
82. Phillips G, Herzig G, Herzig R et al.: Cyclophosphamide, total body irradiation, and autologous bone marrow transplantation for refractory malignant lymphoma (abstract). Blood 58(Suppl 1):175a, 1981.
83. Graze PR, Wells JR, Ho W et al.: Successful engraftment of cryopreserved autologous bone marrow stem cells in man. Transplantation 27:142-144, 1979.
84. Dicke KA, Zander A, Spitzer G et al.: Autologous bone marrow transplantation in relapsed adult acute leukaemia. Lancet i:514-517, 1979.
85. August CS, Serota FT, Koch PA et al.: Bone marrow transplantation for relapsed Stage IV neuroblastoma (abstract). Proceedings AACR 23:122, 1982.
86. Pritchard J, McElwain TJ, Graham-Pole J: High dose melphalan with autologous marrow for treatment of advanced neuroblastoma. Br J Cancer 45:86-94, 1982.
87. Blijhan G, Spitzer G, Litam J et al.: The treatment of advanced testicular carcinoma with high dose chemotherapy and autologous marrow support. Eur J Cancer 17:433-441, 1981.
88. McElwain TJ, Hedley DW, Burton G et al.: Marrow autotransplantation accelerates haematological recovery in patients with malignant melanoma treated with high dose melphalan. Br J Cancer 40:72-80, 1979.
89. Cornbleet MA, Corringhan RET, Prentice HG et al.: Treatment of Ewing's sarcoma with high dose melphalan and autologous bone marrow transplantation. Cancer Treat Rep 65:241-244, 1981.
90. Lazarus H, Herzig R, Herzig G et al.: A Phase I study of high dose melphalan and autologous bone marrow transplant for refractory malignancies (abstract). Proceedings ASCO 1:190, 1982.
91. Spitzer G, Dicke KA, Litam J et al.: High dose combination chemotherapy with autologous bone marrow transplantation in adult solid tumors. Cancer 45:3075-3085, 1980.
92. Douer D, Champlin RE, Ho W et al.: High-dose combined-modality therapy and autologous bone marrow transplantation in resistant cancer. Am J Med 71:973-976, 1981.
93. Ekert H, Ellis WM, Waters KD, Taurd GP: Autologous bone marrow rescue in the treatment of advanced tumors of childhood. Cancer 49:603-609, 1982.
94. Spitzer G, Farlla P, Valdivieso M et al.: High dose chemotherapy with autologous bone marrow transplantation in untreated small cell bronchogenic carcinoma (abstract). Exp Hematol 10(Suppl 11):19, 1982.
95. Sarna GP, Champlin R, Wells J, Gale RP: Phase I study of high dose mitomycin with autologous bone marrow support. Cancer Treat Rep 66:277-282, 1982.

96. Zander AR, Spitzer G, Legha S et al.: High dose AMSA and bone marrow rescue in patients with solid tumors. Cancer Treat Rep 66:385–386, 1982.

97. Wolff SN, Fer C, McKay J et al.: High dose VP-16 and autologous bone marrow transplantation for advanced malignancies – a Phase I study (abstract). Proceedings AACR 23:134, 1982.

98. Abrams RA, Glaubiger D, Simon R et al.: Haemopoietic recovery in Ewing's sarcoma after intensive combination therapy and autologous marrow infusion. Lancet ii:385–389, 1980.

99. Netzel B, Rodt H, Haas RJ et al.: The concept of antileukemic, autologous bone marrow transplantation in acute lymphoblastic leukemia. In: Immunobiology of Bone Marrow Transplantation, Thierfelder S, Rodt H, Kold HJ (eds). Springer-Verlag, Berlin, 1980, pp 297–307.

100. Ritz J, Sallan SE, Bast RC et al.: Autologous bone marrow transplantation in cALLA-positive acute lymphoblastic leukaemia after in vitro treatment with J5 monoclonal antibody and complement. Lancet ii:60–63, 1982.

101. Kaizer H, Stuart RK, Fuller DJ et al.: Autologous bone marrow transplantation in acute leukemia: progress report on a Phase I study of 4-hydroperoxycyclophosphamide incubation of marow prior to cryopreservation (abstract). Proceedings ASCO 1:131, 1982.

102. Abrams RA, Deisseroth AB: Prospects for accelerating hematopoietic recovery following myelosuppressive therapy by using autologous, cryopreserved hematopoietic stem cells collected solely from the peripheral blood. Exp Hematol 7(Suppl 5):107–115, 1979.

103. Goldman JM, Catovsky D, Hows J et al.: Cryopreserved peripheral blood cells functioning as autografts in patients with chronic granulocyte leukaemia in transformation. Br Med J (May 19):1310–1313, 1979.

104. Abrams RA, Glaubiger D, Appelbaum FR, Deisseroth AB: Result of attempted hematopoietic reconstitution using isologous peripheral blood mononuclear cells: a case report. Blood 56:516–520, 1980.

105. Abrams RA, Johnston-Early A, Kramer C et al.: Amplification of circulating granulocyte-monocyte stem cells numbers following chemotherapy in patients with extensive small cell carcinoma of the lung. Cancer Res 41:35–41, 1981.

106. Abrams RA, McCormack K, Bowles C, Deisseroth AB: Cyclophosphamide treatment expands the circulating hematopoietic stem cell pool in dogs. J Clin Invest 64:1392–1399, 1981.

107. Schaefer UW: Bone marrow stem cells. In: Low Temperature Preservation in Medicine and Biology, Ashwood-Smith MJ, Farrant J (eds). Baltimore, University Park Press, 1980, pp 139–154.

108. Wells JR, Ho WG, Graze P et al.: Isolation, cryopreservation, and autotransplantation of human stem cells. Exp Hematol 7(Suppl 5):12-20, 1979.

109. Lowenthal RM, Park DS, Goldman JM et al.: The cryopreservation of leukaemia cells: morphological and functional changs. Br J Haematol 34:105–117, 1976.

110. Turner AR, McGann LE, Allalunis MJ, Turc J-M: Optimum cooling and warming rate for the cryopreservation of autologous hematopoietic stem cells (abstract). Proceedings ASCO/AACR 21:440, 1980.

111. Rubin P, Wheeler KT, Keng PC et al.: The separation of a mixture of bone marrow stem cells from tumor cells: an essential step for autologous bone marrow transplantation. Int J Rad Oncol Biol Phys 7:1405–1411, 1981.

112. Jemionek JF, MacVittie TJ, Byrne PJ et al.: Fractionation of mammalian bone marrow by counterflow centrifugation-elutriation using a continuous albumin gradient: analysis of granulocyte-macrophage colony-forming units. Br J Haematol 50:257–267, 1982.

113. Linker-Israeli M, Billing RJ, Foon KA, Teraskaki PI: Monoclonal antibodies reactive with acute myelogenous leukemia cells. J Immunol 127:2473–2477, 1981.

114. Netzel B, Haas RJ, Rodt H, Kolb HJ, Thierfelder S: Immunological conditioning of bone marrow for autotransplantation in childhood acute lymphoblastic leukaemia. Lancet i:1330–1332, 1980.

10. Medical Management of Chronic Pain Caused by Cancer

ROBERT B. CATALANO

INTRODUCTION

The patient with cancer may experience a number of distressing symptoms, the most common being that of pain. The generalization that pain is an inevitable consequence of cancer usually stems from an experience of having known someone with cancer who has suffered excruciating pain. In truth, most patients do not need to suffer pain. Successful palliation of patients with cancer pain is possible in 95–99% [1–3]. Nevertheless, for many cancer patients pain relief is far from optimal because of both inadequate knowledge and improper application of current knowledge.

Marks and Sachar found that medical in-patients were almost universally undertreated with narcotic analgesics [4]. Even experienced clinicians hesitate to prescribe adequate doses or administration schedules of narcotic analgesics for terminal cancer patients, often because of a fear of 'addiction'. Saunders and others have found, however, that significant addiction develops very infrequently [5, 6–17].

Counterproductive attitudes in the management of cancer pain stem primarily from a failure to allow sufficient priority to the principles of supportive care, which is primarily an attempt at palliation of symptoms with optimization of the quality of life remaining. 'Rescue-mode' and 'palliative-mode' therapy are best seen as overlapping rather than exclusive, of course.

In the management of pain, the major emphasis is placed on the evaluation and control of a symptom rather than on control of the disease causing the symptom. Cancer pain is hard to quantify or study, surrounded as it is by folklore and emotion. Yet, it represents a prime goal of health care: 'To heal sometimes, to relieve often, and to comfort always' (Trudeau).

Higby, DJ (ed), Supportive Care in Cancer Therapy. ISBN 0-89838-569-5.
© *1983, Martinus Nijhoff Publishers, Boston. Printed in The Netherlands.*

GENERAL CONSIDERATIONS

Pain can be considered as acute or chronic. Acute pain is the most common complaint of patients seeking care. This is the type of pain which most physicians are accustomed to treat and which is most often studied. It is linear (begins and ends), usually reversible, and serves as a warning of underlying pathology. Initially, all complaints of acute pain should lead to a search for a treatable cause. Efforts to control pain should then be directed primarily towards the elimination of the cause. This concept applies to the management of pain in malignant disease also. Unfortunately, the pain of cancer is complex. While the incidence of severe pain in advanced cancer is relatively low, there are many instances where the tumor is refractory to specific antineoplastic therapy, thus necessitating the use of symptomatic treatment with analgesics. This pain then takes on the characteristics of chronic pain.

Chronic pain, then, differs from acute pain in that it no longer is protective, and has become an object of treatment in itself. The chronic pain of cancer has been experienced by few practicing physicians and thus it is difficult for them to understand the meaning of this problem to the patient. The experience of pain is complex, involving sensation, expression and environment. The sensation of pain, on the other hand, involves relatively simple neural mechanisms. The expressive component of pain, called suffering, is the action elicited by the sensation. Suffering, which is what is perceived by the observer, depends on the patient's background, fear of underlying disease, fear of the significance of the pain, past experience of pain, and the level of support from significant others. Since these factors are extremely variable from patient to patient, and even in a single patient over time, objectively measuring pain remains a problem. From a clinical standpoint, a definition of pain can be given: 'pain is whatever the experiencing person says it is, and exists whenever he says it does, and to the severity he has determined'.

INCIDENCE OF CANCER-RELATED PAIN

The incidence and severity of cancer pain can be inferred from the data provided by several surveys. It is variable depending on the primary site as well as the stage of the disease [24] (Table 1). More severe complaints of pain are experienced more often in advanced states of cancer, but complaints of moderate to severe pain have been experienced in about one third of patients with intermediate stages of the disease [1–7].

Using the patient's assessment of frequency and severity of pain and

Table 1. Incidence of cancer-related pain in relation to primary disease and stage [24].

I. *Stage of disease*	*c/o Pain (%)*
Regional only (Stage II/III)	30
Advanced disease (Stage IV)	60–80
II. *Site of primary disease*	*c/o Pain (%)*
Cervical cancer	82
Gastric cancer	75
Rectal cancer	60
Breast cancer	52
Lung cancer	45
Lymphoma	20
Leukemia	5

attempting to correlate this with how the pain subsequently impacts on daily life, Dant and Cleeland surveyed 650 patients being treated at a comprehensive cancer center [8]. At a given severity, pain impacts on quality of life in proportion to the patient's perception of the cause of pain. When the pain was thought to be due to cancer, quality was affected more than when another cause was implicated. Patients with cancer and pain due to other reasons may profit from simply knowing that the pain is not cancer-related.

Oster evaluated the degree of pain experienced by dying patients with and without cancer [9]. Patterns of analgesic administration and medical records demonstrated that patients dying with cancer had significantly more pain than those dying without cancer. Of the 90 patients evaluated, 75 % of those with cancer endured various degrees of pain in their terminal days [10, 11].

Table 2 summarizes several studies regarding the incidence of cancer-related pain and suggests that 60 to 80 % of patients with cancer will expe-

Table 2. Incidence of cancer-related pain [1].

Investigator	No. of patients	Incidence of pain
Wilkes [12]	300	58 %
Twycross [13]	500	80 %
Foley [24]	540	52–85 %
Bonica [14]	387	Early disease = 38 %
		Terminal phase = 80 %
Pannuti [15]	290	64 %
Parker [16]	400	In-patients = 59 %
		At home = 71 %

rience pain [12–16]. Based on 1982 incidence statistics [18], 450,000 to 600,000 patients each year will experience some sort of pain associated with their cancer. Thus, chronic pain in cancer is a major concern and warrants a thorough understanding on the part of the physician regarding methods of evaluation and treatment.

EVALUATING PAIN

Despite the poor prognosis associated with advanced malignancies, selection of appropriate therapy for pain can be accomplished only after consideration of several parameters, all of which contribute to the total pain picture [19–20]. These include: 1) location, 2) mechanism, 3) physical and mental condition of the patient, 4) nature of the cause, and 5) availability and suitability of various pain control methods.

In the cancer patient there is a tendency to attribute all complaints of pain to the patient's primary disease. The non-malignant causes of pain may be overlooked. Since pain symptoms are debilitating and therapy is dependent on the correct diagnosis, the need for differential diagnosis is obvious.

The pain evaluation should seek to identify certain characteristics of the pain that point to its underlying pathology [21–23]. These include:

1. Site: pain may be demonstrated in one site or several, and may be stationary or radiating. Body diagrams may be helpful in delineating and recording the distribution.
2. Intensity: pain control requires reliable and repeatable pain measurement to evaluate effectiveness of therapy. Several scales have been designed including the five-point scale, the visual analogue scale, and the McGill-Melzack pain questionnaire. These all allow some quantitation of perceived pain and are all quite useful.
3. Quality: different pains are described by patients in consistent ways, e.g., *boring,* associated with visceral pain; *crushing,* associated with angina; *burning,* associated with esophageal ulceration or reflux.
4. Variation: pain most commonly varies according to time, position, and activity, and may be constant, spasmodic, or periodic. Pain may be most severe at night when there is less diversion. Pain can be affected by body position, breathing, eating, urination, defecation, etc.
5. Response to prior therapy: this may provide useful information for both differential diagnosis and for selection of agents to be used.

In a general cancer patient population, pain is caused by tumor in approximately 75% of patients, by therapy in 20%, and by other causes in 5% [23] (Table 3).

Table 3. Pain syndromes in patients with cancer [24].

I.   Pain associated with direct tumor involvement
    A.   Tumor infiltration of bone
        1. Base-of-skull metastases
            A.   Jugular foramen
            B.   Clivus
            C.   Sphenoid sinus
        2. Vertebral-body metastases
            A.   Subluxation of the atlas
            B.   C-7-T-1 metastases
            C.   L-1 metastases
            D.   Sacral metastases
    B.   Tumor infiltration of nerve
        1. Peripheral neuropathy
        2. Brachial, lumbar, sacral plexopathy
        3. Meningeal carcinomatosis
        4. Epidural spinal-cord compression
    C.   Tumor infiltration of hollow viscus
II. Pain associated with cancer therapy
    A.   Pain occurring postsurgery
        1. Postthoracotomy pain
        2. Postmastectomy pain
        3. Postradical neck pain
        4. Phantom-limb pain
    B.   Pain occurring postchemotherapy
        1. Peripheral neuropathy
        2. Postherpetic neuralgia
        3. Steroid pseudorheumatism
        4. Aseptic necrosis of bone
    C.   Pain occurring postradiation
        1. Radiation fibrosis of the brachial plexus and lumbar plexus
        2. Radiation myelopathy
        3. Radiation-induced peripheral nerve tumors
III. Pain unrelated to cancer or cancer therapy
    A.   Diabetic neuropathy
    B.   Cervical- and lumbar-disc disease
    C.   Rheumatoid arthritis

PSYCHOLOGIC ASPECTS OF PAIN

Psychological variables play an important role in the perception of chronic pain, and depending on the emotional state of the patient, this may vary considerably. Patients with cancer manifest fear, anxiety, apprehension, and depression, all of which may accent the painful stimulus. Long standing pain may become an overwhelming problem that completely dominates life. Patients with chronic pain often seem increasingly more sensitive and seem to suffer more as the disease progresses.

The attitude of the physician, often stemming from his frustration in not being able to cure the disease, may be keenly sensed by the patient as apparent lack of concern, and contribute to the patient's fear of death, abandonment, and hopelessness. The ability to listen, discuss, and gain the confidence of the patient are necessary aspects of the management of pain. Failure to produce a pain-free state may often be due to ignoring the psychologic dimensions and may lead to unneccessary narcotic use or lead the patient to seek costly and ineffective methods to control pain.

MECHANISMS OF CANCER-RELATED PAIN

The pain in cancer patients is not physiologically unique. It is usually caused by one of the following mechanisms [25]:

1. Compression of nerves by tumor or pathologic fractures adjacent to nerve structures. This pain is localized, sharp, and projecting, typical of neuralgia.
2. Infiltration of the nerves and blood vessels by tumor, producing perivascular and perineural lymphangitis. This pain is commonly diffuse and burning (sympathetic).
3. Obstruction of a viscus, which produces true visceral pain described as dull, diffuse, and poorly localized.
4. Partial or complete obstruction of blood vessels, which causes venous engorgement or arterial ischemia.
5. Infiltration or tumefaction of tissues invested by fascia, periosteum, or other pain-sensitive structures.
6. Necrosis, infection, and inflammation of pain sensitive structures produced by tumors. This pain is usually refractory and excruciating.

PRINCIPLES OF PAIN CONTROL

The management of cancer pain may be aimed at control of the specific pathologic events causing pain, i.e., primary control, or symptomatic control aimed at altering the perception of pain, i.e., secondary control (Table 4).

Primary control
In malignant disease, primary control involves attack against the pain-causing tumor. Even when the cancer is incurable, specific disease-oriented

Table 4. Existing methods of alleviating cancer-related pain [7].

1. *Primary control methods*
   A. Therapy directed toward control of the disease process itself
      1. Surgery
      2. Radiation therapy
      3. Chemotherapy
         Cytotoxic drugs
         Hormonal agents
   B. Therapy directed toward a specific disease-related (reversible) pathophysiologic event, e.g. treatment of
      1. Infection with antibiotics
      2. Inflammation with anti-inflammatory agents
      3. Gout with antihyperuricemic agents
2. *Symptomatic control methods*
   A. Systematic analgesics
      1. Interference with specific chemical substances involved in pain reception peripherally. Anti-inflammatory/antipyretic agents
      2. Interference with conduction of pain away from affected site
         Local anesthetics
      3. Interference with central nervous system perception of pain and affective responses
         Narcotic analgesics
      4. Interference with anxiety, tension, or depression
         Sedatives/hypnotics
         Phenothiazines
         Tricyclic antidepressants
      5. Interference with consciousness
         General anesthetics
   B. Surgical procedures on the spinal cord and brain

therapy may be the most productive of pain relief [7]. In general, such pain control should be attempted at an intensity proportionate to the expected benefit. Symptomatic control is usually necessary during all or part of this process.

Surgery has a role in pain control. Examples of indications for surgery include bypass operations to reconnect obstructed visci or large blood vessels. Surgical ablation of the endocrine glands has produced dramatic relief in endocrine-responsive tumors even when there has not been obvious regression of tumor [26–29]. Surgery is of course used in ablation of neurologic pathways and nuclei, although this is not technically primary control.

Radiation therapy has for a large part of its practice the palliative care of cancer patients. When the pain is focal and due to a tumor, radiation may be very useful. Pain relief from radiotherapy is most likely in bony metastases from tumors of glandular origin [30–31]. A study by the Radiation

Therapy Oncology Group showed that 90% of patients with bony metastases profit somewhat from radiotherapy, while 54% had complete pain relief[32]. Interestingly, low dose, short course schedules were as effective as high dose longer schedules. Patients with breast and prostate cancer metastatic to bone had more relief than those with other primary tumors such as lung. Patients with less pain initially had more proportionate relief than those with more pain.

In the management of pain due to metastatic disease to the brain, concomitant high doses of steroids with palliative radiotherapy can improve or completely control tumor cephalgia in greater than 85% of patients[33–35].

With chemotherapy, control of pain is a consequence of shrinkage of tumor or cessation of tumor growth. Thus, effectiveness depends on the drug sensitivity of the tumor. Regional chemotherapy may be of particular use when the tumor causing pain is in the supply of a single artery. For example, control of hepatic pain from tumor may be accomplished by hepatic artery infusion of chemotherapy, resulting in high local drug concentration with lower systemic toxicity[36–38]. Symptomatic relief has been achieved in as high as 70% of patients so treated[37].

Symptomatic control

Symptomatic control of pain is achieved by either elevating the pain threshold in the central nervous system or by affecting the pathways conducting pain sensation[23]. Either involves analgesia, which implies decreasing pain without loss of consciousness. The specific agent employed must correspond to the specific needs of the patient. Individualization of dosing, constant monitoring, and titration for effect are extremely important.

Considerable variation exists in patient response to analgesics. One drug at one schedule will obviously not suffice. The analgesic regimen of choice is that which achieves as pain free a state as possible while allowing as normal a life as possible.

Analgesics are classified based on their clinical use in relation to pain. Some are suitable for mild pain (non-narcotics), some for moderate pain (combinations of non-narcotics and mild narcotics or narcotic antagonists), and some for severe pain (usually narcotics of higher potency)[39, 40]. Table 5 lists a partial classification.

Basically, one begins with the mildest agents that achieve pain control and progresses to stronger agents when lesser measures are insufficient. Each drug should be given to its maximum dose based on therapeutic effect and toxicity before going on to a more potent agent. Individualization is always important, and attention must be paid to those factors in the patient that

Table 5. Recommended analgesic therapy based on severity of pain.

Degree of pain symptom	Suggested agent for control
Mild pain	Aspirin or acetaminophen
Moderate pain	Add codeine or oxycodone to above Rx (?) zomepirac plus mild narcotic
Severe pain	Morphine, hydromorphone
Very severe pain	Levorphanol, methadone
Overwhelming pain	As above plus adjunctive pharmacologic agents and non-pharmacologic maneuvers

Table 6. Choice of adjuvant therapy [23].

Type of pain	Co-analgesic	Non-drug measures
Bone pain	Aspirin 600 mg 4 hourly or Ibuprofen 400 mg qid	Irradiation
Raised intracranial pressure	Dexamethasone 2–4 mg tid; diuretic (?)	Elevate head of bed, avoid lying flat
Post-herpetic neuralgia, super-ficial dysaethetic pain	Amitriptyline 25–100 mg; HS L-DOPA (?)	
Nerve pressure pain	Prednisolone 5–10 mg tid	Nerve block; irradiation
Intermittent stabbing pain	Valproate 200 mg B-tid or carbamazepine 200 mg T-qid	
Gastric tenesmoid pain/bladder tenesmoid pain	Chlorpromazine 10–25 mg 8–4 hourly	
Gastric distension pain	Metoclopramide 10 mg 4 hourly	
Muscle spasm pain	Diazepam 5 mg bid or baclofen 10 mg tid	Massage
Lymphoedema	Diuretic and corticosteroid (?)	Elevate foot of bed, elastic stocking, compression cuff
Infected malignant ulcer	Metronidazole 400 mg tid or alternate antibiotic	
Activity precipitated pain		Modify way of life (if possible)

have to do with drug pharmacokinetics (e.g., liver and kidney function) and those which predispose to certain toxicities (e.g., a history of duodenal ulceration, a history of sensitivity to aspirin) [40].

PHARMACOLOGIC PAIN CONTROL – GENERAL PRINCIPLES

Successful pain management begins with matching the analgesic to the characteristics of the specific pain. Table 6 lists several situations together with recommendations for analgesic selection. There are many agents within each class of analgesics, and it is prudent for each physician to select a few agents and learn their characteristics with respect to site and mechanism of action, pharmacokinetics, and side effects [41]. Table 7 is an example of this concept of analgesic practice.

Perception of pain involves several levels [42] (Figure 1). Receptors in the injured tissue are activated; stimulation of central nervous system via pathways in the spinal cord and brain stem follows. Central recognition of pain results in avoidance behavior through descending (efferent) mechanisms.

These interactions have been studied intensively. The discovery and isolation of opiate receptors in the mid-70s led to the finding of naturally occurring opiate-like substances (endorphins, enkephalins) which are located in the synapses between nerve fibers [43–49]. These probably function to modify noxious stimuli. Their action seems to be the inhibition of release of another peptide, substance 'p', which transmits such stimuli. Endorphins allay pain centrally and may block both afferent transmission or efferent impulse conductance in the spinal cord and periphery. These substances

Table 7. Guidelines for appropriate use of systemic analgesics in chronic cancer pain [41].

1. Establish a simple, practical analgesic schema (stepladder) to include a representative agent of each class
   a. Non-narcotic – aspirin or acetaminophen
   b. Weak narcotic – codeine
   c. Strong narcotic – morphine

2. Avoid pentazocine, and in patients with renal failure, merperidine

3. If methadone is used, be familiar with its precautions for dosing and dose escalation

4. The proper dose and schedule of a narcotic analgesic is dictated by the intensity of pain and not by the brevity of the prognosis. 'Morphine exists to be given not merely to be withheld.'

5. Diversional therapy is of great value

6. Properly used and monitored – addiction does not occur with narcotic analgesics

7. Physical dependence (not to be confused with addiction) does not prevent a downward adjustment of dose should pain ameliorate

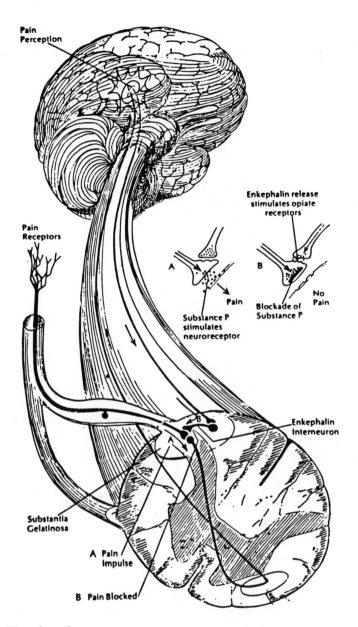

Figure 1. The pain pathway.

have a short half-life, and their tissue levels are increased in both acute and chronic pain.

Noxious stimuli in skin and body tissue can initiate events that result in inflammation and resultant enhancement of pain (Figure 2). An enzyme system exists in all microsome-containing cells [52] (Figure 3). Arachidonic

210

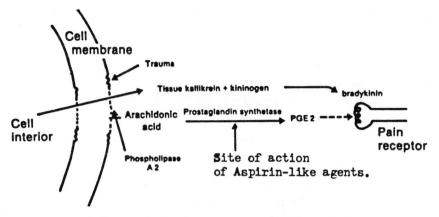

Figure 2. The anti-inflammatory/analgesic action of the aspirin-like agents results from blocking formation of the peripheral nerve stimulator (PGE₂) by inhibiting the needed converting enzyme (prostaglandin synthetase) [52].

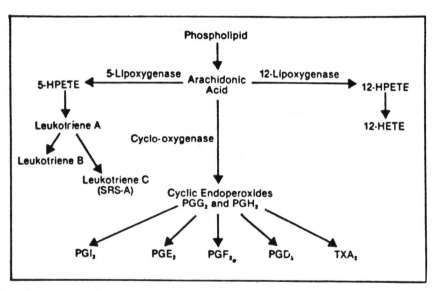

Figure 3. Cyclo-oxygenase and lipoxygenase pathways of arachidonic acid. 12-hydroxyeicosatrienoic acid is 12-HETE; 12-hydroperoxyeicosatrienoic acid, 12-HPETE; slow reacting substance of anaphylaxis, SRS-A; prostaglandin, PG; and thromboxane, TXA₂.

acid, an essential fatty acid, exists as an inactive precursor or prostaglandin in the cell wall until reacted with molecular oxygen by cyclo-oxygenases [50, 51]. This results in the formation of unstable peroxides (cyclic endoperoxides) that in turn form the biologically active prostaglandins. The status of prostaglandins as true primary mediators of inflammation has not been fully demonstrated, but blocking their production has been shown to alleviate inflammation and specific pain perception [50].

Non-narcotic analgesics

Non-narcotic analgesics are non-addictive and include salicylates, acetominophen, and the ever-enlarging class of non-steroidal anti-inflammatory agents. The clinically useful doses of these are generally without psychotropic activity.

Except for zomepirac sodium (Zomax®), newer non-narcotic analgesics have not shown superiority in pain relief to plain aspirin [53–56]. As a drug, aspirin calls for superlatives. It is probably the most widely used medication [67]; it is one of the oldest and least expensive of all drugs; and it is most certainly the most underestimated. If discovered today, it would be heralded as a wonder drug because of its effectiveness in a variety of situations, and would probably be available by prescription only, assuming that the Food and Drug Administration could be convinced to approve it. No doubt it would be extremely expensive to the patient.

Moertel compared the relative effectiveness of nine oral analgesics in pain due to cancer. The first study (Table 8) involved 57 patients and used a double-blind crossover design. Aspirin 650 mg was superior to all agents tested; mefenamic acid (Pontsel®) 250 mg, mentazocine (Talwin®) 50 mg, acetominophen 650 mg, phenacetin 650 mg, and codeine 65 mg, and also showed significant advantage over placebo. Propoxyphene (Darvon®) 65 mg, ethoheptazine 75 mg, and promazine (Sparine®) showed no significant activity. Interestingly, costs of agents other than aspirin were several hundred percent higher [55].

Table 8. Relative therapeutic effect of oral analgesics according to mean percentage of relief of pain achieved in 57 patients (from Moertel [55]).

Analgesic agent	Dose (mg)	Relief of pain (%)	
Aspirin	650	62	Significantly superior to placebo ($p < 0.05$)
Pentazocine	50	54	
Acetaminophan	650	50	
Phenacetin	650	48	
Mefenamic acid	250	47	
Codeine	65	46	
Propoxyphene	65	43	Significantly inferior to aspirin ($p < 0.05$)
Ethoheptazine	75	38	
Promazine	25	37	
Placebo	–	32	

A second study by Moertel on 100 patients with cancer pain, demonstrated that aspirin 650 mg, plus either codeine 65 mg, oxycodone 9.76 mg, or pentazocine 25 mg, produced significantly greater pain relief than aspirin alone. Aspirin plus caffeine 65 mg, pentobarbital 32 mg, promazine 25 mg, ethoheptazine 75 mg, or propoxyphene napsylate 100 mg, did not show significant advantage in analgesic effectiveness over aspirin alone [56].

It has never been demonstrated that formulations of aspirin, phenacetin, and caffeine (APC) are superior to aspirin alone in providing pain relief [57, 60]. Furthermore, these readily available combinations can be abused, and there is a risk of developing analgesic nephropathy, characterized by papillary necrosis and interstitial nephritis [58–60].

There are conditions that preclude the use of aspirin. These include a history of previous gastrointestinal ulceration or hemorrhage, hypersensitivity reactions, and thrombocytopenia. Aspirin is increasingly recognized as a major cause of gastrointestinal bleeding requiring hospitalization. 50 to 94% of patients admitted with that diagnosis have a recent history of salicylate ingestion. Perry stated that almost 100% of patients admitted to hospital with acute gastric erosions and no radiologically demonstrable lesion have a history of recent aspirin consumption [61].

Aspirin allergy is an underrecognized problem [62]. It is usually seen in the third to fourth decade of life, and characterized initially by watery nasal discharge and development of nasal polyps. Bronchial asthma may develop after a time, and attacks may be precipitated by ingestion of aspirin or after nasal polypectomy. Avoiding aspirin does not wholly reverse the asthmatic state, but in its absence, the condition can usually be controlled with the ordinary means. Alcohol, indomethacin, antipyrine, and other drugs and chemicals may precipitate asthmatic attacks in such patients [63].

In one study, five patients with clearly documented aspirin-induced asthma were challenged with acetaminophen, 500 mg, mefenamic acid, 250 mg, indomethacin 25 mg, dextropropoxyphene, 65 mg, phenylbutazone, 100 mg, or lactose tablets. The forced expiratory volume at one second (FEV 1) was measured every thirty minutes after the challenge. Marked decreases in FEV 1 were observed after most of these agents. Acetaminophen, indomethacin, and mefenamic acid caused the most severe reactions. Dextropropoxyphene caused a reaction in one case. Phenylbutazone did not cause any reactions [63].

Thus, there is reason for great caution in prescribing any analgesic or non-narcotic anti-inflammatory agent to patients with a history of aspirin allergy.

Aspirin also inhibits collagen-induced release of adenine diphosphate (ADP) from platelets resulting in impaired aggregation [64–66]. Although this effect may be therapeutically beneficial in ischemic disease of the heart or brain [69], it may be detrimental if used in patients with compromised coagulation systems.

Over 500 products are available without prescription which contain a salicylate as one of the ingredients [68].

Aspirin acts by interruption of prostaglandin synthesis through a blockade of the enzyme prostaglandin synthetase [70] (Figure 2). Prostaglandin E_2 is thought to sensitize local chemoreceptor sites to stimulation. Such pain is dull and throbbing. (Sharp stabbing pain of direct stimulation of nerves is not sensitized by prostaglandin, and is thus not usually ameliorated by aspirin.) Thus, the action of aspirin is peripheral and it does not change the perception of pain as such [71].

Acetominophen, while devoid of substantial anti-inflammatory activity at normal doses, is a suitable alternative to aspirin as an analgesic and antipyretic [72–72]. It does not produce gastritis [76] nor inhibit platelet function significantly [75] at normal doses. Abuse may be associated with hepatotoxicity [77] and analgesic nephropathy [78].

Ibuprophen (Motrin®) was the first of the class of non-steroidal anti-inflammatory agents [79]. These agents, like aspirin, inhibit prostaglandin synthesis at the cyclo-oxygenase level [80]. The half-life, chemistry, and other individual characteristics of these agents are described in Tables 9, 10.

Table 9. Differential profile of the non-narcotic analgesics.

Generic (trade)	Starting dose	Max. rec. daily dose	Milligram tablets price per 100 [a]	Comments
Acetaminophen	650 mg Q 4 hrs	4000 mg	325 mg tab. $1.90/100 tab.	a. Therapeutically equivalent to aspirin except where anti-inflammatory action needed
Aspirin	650 mg Q 4 hrs	3900 mg	325 mg tab. $0.60/100 tab.	a. Agent of choice if not contraindicated
Fenoprofen (Nalfon)	600 mg QID	3200 mg	300 mg tab. $16.68/100 tab.	a. $t_{\frac{1}{2}} = 2-3$ hr b. If gastrointestinal complaints occur, administer with meals or milk
Ibuprofen (Motrin, Rufen)	400 mg QID	2400 mg	400 mg tab. $21.06/100 tab.	a. $t_{\frac{1}{2}} = 3-4$ hr b. FDA-authorized as analgesic and anti-inflammatory
Indomethacin (Indocin)	25 mg BID or TID	200 mg	25 mg tab. $20.50/100 tab.	a. $t_{\frac{1}{2}} = 4-5$ hr b. FDA-approved for rheumatoid arthritis, degenerative joint disease, acute gout, acute painful shoulder

Table 9. Continued.

Generic (trade)	Starting dose	Max. rec. daily dose	Milligram tablets price per 100 [a]	Comments
				c. Not indicated for simple analgesia
				d. Most adverse effects are dose dependent, so use the lowest effective dose possible
Mefenamic acid (Pontsel)	500 mg initially	250 mg q 6 hr	250 mg tab. $22.82/100 tab.	a. $t\frac{1}{2}$ = 4–6 hr b. Not recommended for use longer than 1 week due to possible serious side effects
Naproxen (Naprosyn)	250 mg BID	750 mg	250 mg tab. $31.32/100 tab.	a. $t\frac{1}{2}$ = 13 hr b. Urinary clearance increases with increasing doses
Phenylbutazone (Butazolidin, Azolid)	300–600 mg daily	600 mg	100 mg tab. $16.73/100 tab.	a. $t\frac{1}{2}$ = (phenylbutazone = 84 hr, oxyphenbutazone = 72 hr) b. Indicated for short-term acute use c. Not indicated as simple analgesics
Oxyphenbutazone (Tandearil, Oxalid)	300–600 mg daily	600 mg	100 mg tab. $17.72/100 tab.	d. Serious side effects preclude chronic use in pts over 60 e. Careful patient selection and close supervision are essential f. Serious blood dyscrasias are possible
Sulindac (Clinoril)	150 mg BID	400 mg	150 mg tab. $35.78/100 tab.	a. $t\frac{1}{2}$ of sulfide metabolite = 18 hr b. Parent drug is inactive; activity is due to active sulfide metabolite
Tolmetin (Tolectin)	400 mg TID	2000 mg	200 mg tab. $17.05/100 tab.	a. $t\frac{1}{2}$ = about 1 hr b. Chemically related to indomethacin, but action and toxicity are similar to propionic acid derivatives
Zomepirac sodium (Zomax)	50–100 mg q 4–6 hr	600 mg	100 mg tab. $22.34/100 tab.	a. $t\frac{1}{2}$ = 4–5 hr b. Currently FDA-approved only for relief of mild to moderately severe pain c. Safety and efficacy of zomepirac for chronic use remains to be determined

[a] Average wholesale price – October, 1982.

Several of these agents have been reported to cause acute renal failure [81–83]. Patients with congestive heart failure, lupus, cirrhosis, or chronic renal failure are more at risk for this complication. These patients may have increased renal prostaglandin synthesis as a compensatory mechanism. Because all non-steroidal anti-inflammatory agents are excreted through the kidney, patients on chronic therapy should have renal function monitored [84].

One new agent, zomepirac sodium (Zomax®), has been developed strictly for analgesic potential and warrants separate discussion [85]. Cooper demonstrated that this agent provides greater analgesia in post-operative dental pain than aspirin and equivalent analgesia to codeine [86]. The efficacy of zomepirac sodium was confirmed by Wallenstein who reported in cancer patients with moderate to severe post-operative pain that oral zomepirac produced analgesia equivalent to intramuscular morphine [87].

Stambaugh found that repeated doses of zomepirac were judged less effective by patients who had previous received narcotics, but not by patients who had not received the latter [88]. However, this preference may have been due to non-analgesic effects of the narcotics rather than actual superior analgesia. Reduction of the analgesic effect of zomepirac does not seem to occur over the long term, and overall toxicities are not great [89, 90].

In summary, aspirin and acetaminophen remain the agents of choice when pain is not great. If pain is not controlled with these agents, zomepirac seems to be an appropriate alternative. Due to its peripheral site of action, it may be used in conjunction with an oral narcotic, since the combination

Table 10. General characteristics of non-steroidal anti-inflammatory agents.

All non-steroidal anti-inflammatory agents:

    are as effective as aspirin as analgesic, anti-inflammatory and antipyretic agents

    act by inhibiting prostaglandin biosynthesis

    can cause gastrointestinal toxicity (irritation, nausea, vomiting, bleeding), although usually less than does aspirin

    are more expensive than aspirin

    share many of the side effects of aspirin

    inhibit collagen-induced platelet aggregation; platelet effects are less significant clinically than aspirin's effects on platelets (more bleeding with aspirin)

    can cause significant sodium retention

    have the propensity for cross-sensitization in patients with aspirin tolerance

    are excreted via the kidney

    can cause central nervous system side effects

    can cause rashes

may be synergistic. Zomepirac should not be substituted for narcotics, but may be added to the regimen of patients taking narcotics, with gradual reduction of the narcotic dose when feasible.

Narcotic antagonists

The propoxyphene series of drugs (Darvon®, Dolene®) continue to be frequently prescribed despite eight controlled prospective studies disputing their effectiveness [55, 56, 91–96]. The claim that they have less adverse effects than codeine is the reason for this.

Adverse effects of propoxyphene compounds include nausea, vomiting, constipation, dizziness, and drowsiness. The addiction potential is low compared with codeine, but is real. Young reported nine deaths due to propoxyphene overdosage [97]. Naloxone (Narcan®) is an effective antidote.

Pentazocine (Talwin®) is a benzomorphan derivative which has a weak narcotic antagonist action. Pentazocine 30 mg was found to have analgesic equivalency to 75–100 mg meperidine or 10 mg morphine [98–99]. After intramuscular injection, the effect is noticeable in 20 minutes. Pentazocine causes irritation at the site of injection and has a short duration of action (3 hours). The analgesia produced by oral administration is not dependable because of variable absorption. The most common side effects include sedation, drowsiness, nausea, vomiting, and blurred vision. Other side effects resemble those of the narcotics (see below) [101, 102]. Pentazocine has a dependence potential substantially less than morphine or meperidine, but similar to that of codeine [100]. Prolonged parenteral treatment in moderately high doses can lead to morphine-like dependence.

Other agents of the narcotic antagonist class have little use in the overall management of chronic pain.

Narcotic analgesics

Narcotic analgesics (opiates) are naturally occurring, semi-synthetic, or synthetic drugs which effectively relieve pain without producing loss of consciousness, and which have the potential to produce physical dependence. Although they vary one with another in terms of quantitative and even some qualitative effects, they are sufficiently similar to discuss together. The relative differences are summarized in Table 11.

Chemically, they are classified as phenanthrenes, phenylpiperidines, or diphenylheptanes (Table 12). Modification of the parent structure produces changes in the pharmacologic activity which may alter or eliminate the analgesic potential but increase antitussive, antidiarrheal, or narcotic antagonist properties.

Table 11. Pharmacologic activity of analgesics [7].

Drugs	Analgesic[a]	Antitussive	Sedation	Emesis	Respiratory depressant	Constipation	Addictive	Equianalgesic mg dose[b]	Average adult mg dose[c]
Morphine	V++	++	++	++	++	++	++	10	10–15
Diecetylmorphine (Heroine)	V++	++	++	+	++	+	+++	4	illegal
Ethylmorphine (Dionin)	V+	+++			++		?		15–60
Nalorphine (Nalline)	V++	+	+ or 0	+	++	+		8	15–10[d]
Codeine	V+	+++	+	+	+	+	+	120	15–60 (8–20)
Hydromorphone (Dilaudid)	V++	++	+	+	++	+	++	1	1–2
Methyldihydromorphinone (Metopon)	V+++	++	++	++	+++	+	+	3	3–9
Hydrocodone (Dicodid, etc.)	V++	+++			?	++			(5–10)
Dihydrocodeine (Paracodin, etc.)	V++	+++		+	+		+	60	30–60
Dihydrodesoxymorphine-D (Desomorphine)	V+++					+	+++	1	
Oxymorphone (Numorphan)	V++	+		+++	+++	+++	+++	1	½–1
Oxycodone (Percodan)	V++	+++	++	++	++	++	++	10	10–15 (3–5)
Nalmexone (EN-1620A)	V++		++	+			?	70–90	
Leivorphanol (Levo-Dromoran)	V++	++	++	+	++	?	++	2	2–4
Racemorphan (Dromoran)	V++	++	+	+	++	+	++	2½	1–5
Dextromethorphan (Romilar)		+++	?	?					(10–20)
Levallorphan (Lorfan)	V++	+	+	+	++			2	1[d]
Pentazocine (Talwin)	V++		++ or 0	++	++	+	+	30	20–30
Naloxone (Narcan)									½–1[d]
Naltrexone (EN-1639A)									½[d]
Methadone (Dolophine, etc.)	V++	++	+	+	++	+	+	8	5–15
Propoxyphene (Darvon)	V+		+	+	+	?	+	130	32–65

Table 11. Continued.

Drugs	Analgesic [a]	Antitussive	Sedation	Emesis	Respiratory depressant	Constipation	Addictive	Equianalgesic mg dose [b]	Average adult mg dose [c]
Levopropoxyphene (Novrad)		+++	+	+					(50–100)
Noracymethadol	V++		++	++	++		+	10	8–30
Dextromoramide (Palfium, etc.)	V++	++	+	++	++	+	+	5	5–10
Meperidine (Demerol, etc.)	V++		+	?	++	+	++	100	30–75
Alphaprodine (Nisentil)	V++		++	+	++	+	++	40	25–60
Anileridine (Leritine)	V++	+	++	?	++	+	++	30	25–50
Piminodine (Alvodine)	V++		+	+	++	+	++	7½	10–20
Ethoheptazine (Zectane)	V+				++		+	200	100

[a] V = visceral and deep traumatic pain in contrast to somatic and joint pains.
+ = degree of activity from the least (+) to the greatest (+++) activity.
0 = produces the opposite effect.
? questionable activity.
Blank space indicates that no such activity has been reported for this compound.
[b] Equianalgesic to morphine sulfate, 10 mg SC.
[c] Oral antitussive dose in parentheses.
[d] Used solely as narcotic antagonist and not as analgesic.

Table 12. Chemical classification of narcotic analgesics [10].

Phenanthrene derivatives
    Codeine
    Hydromorphone (Dilaudid)
    Levorphanol tartrate (Levo-Dromoran)
    Morphine sulfate
    Opium alkaloids, concentrated (Pantopon)
    Oxycodone
    Oxymorphone (Numorphan)

Phenylpiperidine derivatives
    Alphaprodine (Nisentil)
    Anileridine (Leritine)
    Fentanyl (Sublimaze)
    Meperidine (Demerol)

Diphenylheptane derivatives
    Methadone (Dolophine)

Table 13. Side effects of narcotic analgesics as manifested in terms of end-organ function [7].

A. *Central nervous system*
euphoria (dysphoria)
sedation
lowering of seizure threshold
central depression of respiration, cough reflex, nausea, vomiting

B. *GI tract*
decreased secretions
constipation
increased smooth muscle tone in biliary tract

C. *Genitourinary tract*
urinary retention

D. *Circulatory system*
postural hypotension

E. *Miscellaneous*
anaphylactoid reaction
autonomic reactions (diaphoresis, hyperglycemia, miosis, dry mouth)
antidiuresis
adverse interaction with monoamineoxidase inhibitors (especially meperidine)

Pharmacologic effects (Table 13)

1. Central nervous system. Narcotic analgesics exert their effect by directly interacting with central and spinal chord opiate receptors. They may act centrally to cause modification of the response to pain and may also affect the emotional response to pain [103]. They produce a broad spectrum of effects which are dependent in part on the circumstances under which they are administered [106]. Narcotic analgesia is accompanied often by sedation and euphoria. (Sedation and euphoria may also be secondary to the relief of pain rather than a direct effect.) In the absence of pain, dysphoria, apprehension, apathy, mental confusion, hallucinations, and delirium have been seen. Narcotics may lower the seizure threshold, and thus must be administered cautiously in patients with seizure disorders.

2. Respiratory effects. Opiates produce respiratory depression by a direct effect on chemoreceptors in the respiratory centers of the brain stem. This results in a decreased sensitivity to increases in serum carbon dioxide tension. The narcotic analgesics also depress the pontine medullary centers responsible for regulation of the rate of respiration. Initially there is a reduction of tidal volume followed by a decreased respiratory rate. The heavily narcotized patient has slow, irregular periodic respiration. Patients with respiratory insufficiency who lose their response to carbon dioxide retention may suffer hypoxic coma as a result of opiate administration. Such patients may continue to breathe through the hypoxic drive mechanism regulated by the carotid and aortic chemoreceptors. Administration of oxygen may reduce this drive and precipitate apnea unless mechanical ventilation is provided.

Patients with intracranial malignancies may develop arteriolar dilatation as a result of increased carbon dioxide retention following opiate use, and paradoxically develop more severe pain as a result of a rise in cerebral blood flow and cerebrospinal fluid pressure.

Opiates may also affect the respiratory system by depressing the cough reflex through an action on the cough centers in the medulla. This may occur with subanalgesic doses. This action could be adverse in patients with pneumonia or those whose condition predisposes them to pneumonitis.

3. Gastrointestinal effects. Narcotics produce gastrointestinal effects directly and through centrally mediated mechanisms. Gastric, biliary, and pancreatic secretions are decreased by opiates. Smooth muscle tone of the bowel is decreased, resulting in gastric retention and constipation. The morphine congeners, meperidine and methadone, are less constipating than morphine. In contrast, the smooth muscle tone of the biliary tract and the sphincter of Oddi is increased, and bile duct pressure may rise from 20 ml to as high as 300 ml of water, precipitating biliary colic.

Similar effects on pancreatic ducts can occur, and plasma amylase and lipase levels may rise.

Nausea and vomiting are common with initial administration of narcotics, as a probable consequence of direct stimulation of the chemoreceptor trigger zone in the medulla. However, with continued administration there is depression of the vomiting center and subsequent administration of the drugs is less associated with this side effect. Narcotics may sensitize the auditory vestibule, and this may explain why nausea and vomiting are more common in ambulatory patients than those who are bedfast.

4. Urinary tract effects. Narcotics increase smooth muscle tone in the urinary tract, and spasm may result. Tone and amplitude of contraction, especially in the lower third of the ureter, may be increased, resulting in urgency. Because of increased tone in the vesicle sphincter, however, urination may be difficult. Patients who are somnolent and those with prostatic hypertrophy or urinary stricture may be prone to develop urinary retention with narcotic use.

Urinary excretion initially decreases with narcotic administration. This may be due to a central action causing increased secretion of antidiuretic hormone (ADH). However, one study suggested that decreased urinary output can occur without apparent release of ADH and may be attributed solely to decreased renal plasma flow and increased tubular reabsorption [104].

5. *Cardiovascular effects.* Narcotics depress the vasomotor center and stimulate medullary vagal nuclei; circulatory effects may also be due to stimulation of histamine release and a direct effect on peripheral receptors. When therapeutic doses are given, bedfast patients rarely demonstrate a significant cardiovascular effect. Ambulatory patients, however, may have orthostatic hypotension as a result of peripheral vasodilatation. The adverse circulatory effects are increased in the presence of reduced blood volume and with concomitant use of drugs which have alpha-adrenergic blocking activity.

Narcotics usually decrease heart rate. This effect can be ablated by atropine. Meperidine, which has anticholinergic effects, is an exception. Myocardial tone and contractility is increased by small doses and decreased by large doses of narcotics.

6. *Endocrine effects.* Opiates produce endocrine effects due in part to central nervous system effects. In addition to inappropriate ADH secretion, narcotics have been reported to inhibit release of adrenocorticotropic (ACTH) and gonadotropic hormones. In patients with narcotic induced hypoadrenalism, the effect can be ablated by administering ACTH.

Narcotics can inhibit thyroid stimulating hormone leading to a clinically detectable suppression of thyroid hormone production.

Hyperglycemia may occur as a result of a direct action on paraventricular receptor sites near the foramen of Monro or as a result of the stimulation of epinephrine release.

Choice of narcotic analgesics

Most narcotic analgesics produce equal effects in equianalgesic doses. Factors such as oral effectiveness, duration of action, degree of action on smooth muscle, route of metabolism, and individual variation in patient response should be considered in the selection of an agent.

The most effective agents are the morphine surrogates, but even though the range of relative potency may be several hundred-fold that of morphine, there are not appreciable differences in 'ceiling' effects. A more potent drug is not necessarily a more effective drug.

Differences in degree of side effects at equianalgesics doses tend to be insignificant. However, the spectra of side effects among drugs of different classes may be quite different. Higher degrees of pain relief can be encountered before limiting toxicity with drugs of the morphine type than is possible with the narcotic antagonist types or with salicylates or non-steroidal anti-inflammatory agents (Table 14).

Table 14. An equianalgesic comparison of the most common analgesics [21].

Generic and (trade) name	Dose	Equivalent to [a]	Peak effect	Duration	Plasma half-life	Comments	Precautions
Non-narcotics							
Acetaminophen (Tylenol, Tempra, etc.)	600 mg po 600 mg rectal suppos.	Aspirin 600 mg po	2 hrs Slower than oral	3–4 hrs	1–4 hrs	Antipyretic and anti-inflammatory action is weak	In large doses, may cause liver toxicity
Acetylsalicylic acid (aspirin)	600 mg po 600 mg rectal suppos.	Morphine 2 mg IM	2 hrs Slower than oral	3–4 hrs	15 min	Has antipyretic and anti-inflammatory activity	Used with steroids, it may increase gastric bleeding
Methotrimeprazine (Levoprome)	20 mg IM	Morphine 10 mg IM	1 hr	4–6 hrs	Unknown	A phenothiazine; recommend starting with 5 mg dose	May cause over-sedation, orthostatic hypotension, liver toxicity
Zomepirac (Zomax)	100 mg po	Morphine 16 mg IM	1–2 hrs	4–6 hrs	1–4 hrs	Has anti-inflammatory and antipyretic activity	Use with caution in patients with urinary tract infection, elevated BUN, crea-tinine, and in patients with aspirin sensitivity
Narcotic antagonists							
Butorphanol tartrate (Stadol)	2 mg IM 2 mg IV	Morphine 10 mg IM	1 hr 30 min	3–4 hrs 3–4 hrs	2.7 hrs	Mixed agonist–antagonist, may produce psychoto-mimetic effect	May cause abstinence reaction in patients physically dependent on narcotics

Table 14. Continued.

Nalbuphine HCl (Nubain)	10 mg IM / 10 mg IV	Morphine 10 mg IM / Pentazocine 60 mg IM	1 hr / 30 min	4–5 hrs / 3–4 hrs	5 hrs	Mixed agonist–antagonist, but less psychotomimetic effect than pentazocine	Same precautions as with butorphanol
Pentazocine HCl (Talwin)	60 mg IM / 30 mg po / 180 mg po	Morphine 10 mg IM / Aspirin 600 mg / Morphine 10 mg IM / Pentazocine 60 mg IM	1 hr / 2 hrs	3–4 hrs / 3–4 hrs	2–3 hrs / 2–3 hrs	Mixed agonist–antagonist, may cause psychotomimetic side effects	Same precautions as with butorphanol; use with caution in patients with cardiac abnormalities
Narcotics							
Codeine sulfate	30–60 mg po / 200 mg po	Aspirin 600 mg / Morphine 10 mg IM / Codeine 120 mg IM	2 hrs	3–4 hrs	$2\frac{1}{2}$–3 hrs	Same as morphine, but weaker	Not for IV use
Hydromorphone HCl (Dilaudid)	7.5 mg po / 3 mg rectal suppos.	Morphine 10 mg IM / Hydromorphone 1.5 mg IM	1 hr	3–4 hrs	2–3 hrs	Quick onset of action	Same precautions as with morphine
	1.5 mg IM / 1 mg IV	Morphine 10 mg IM	30 min / 15 min	3 hrs / 2–3 hrs	2–3 hrs	Has similar time effect as heroin; highly soluble	Same precautions as with morphine

Table 14. Continued.

Levorphanol tartrate (Levo-Dromoran)	4 mg po	Morphine 10 mg IM Levorphanol 2 mg IM	2 hrs	4–5 hrs	15 hrs	Same as morphine	Same precautions as with morphine
	2 mg IM	Morphine 10 mg IM	1 hr	4–5 hrs			
	1 mg IV		15–30 min	3–4 hrs			
Meperidine HCl (Demerol, Pethadol)	50 mg po	Aspirin 600 mg po	2 hrs	3–4 hrs	3 hrs	Causes CNS excitation ranging from irritability to seizures	Not for chronic administration in patients with renal dysfunction
	300 mg po	Morphine 10 mg IM Meperidine 75 mg po					
	75 mg IM	Morphine 10 mg IM	1 hr	2–4 hrs			
	50 mg IV		5–15 min	2–3 hrs			
Methadone HCl	20 mg po	Morphine 10 mg IM Methadone 10 mg IM	2 hrs	4–5 hrs	15–22 hrs	Same as morphine	Same precautions as with morphine
	10 mg IM	Morphine 10 mg IM	1 hr	4–5 hrs			
	5 mg IV		15–30 min	3–4 hrs			

225

Drug	Dose	Equivalent				Comments	Contraindications
Morphine sulfate	60 mg po	Morphine 10 mg IM	2 hrs	4–5 hrs	2½–3 hrs	May cause oversedation, confusion, visual disturbances, urinary retention	Contraindicated in patients with: impaired ventilation, asthma, elevated intracranial pressure, liver failure
	10 mg IM		1 hr	4–5 hrs			
	5 mg IV		15–30 min	2–4 hrs			
Oxycodone (with aspirin-Percodan; with acetaminophen-Percocet)	5 mg po	Codeine 60 mg po	1 hr	3–4 hrs	2–3 hrs	Not available in IM or IV form	
	30 mg po	Morphine 10 mg po					
Oxymorphone HCl (Numorphan)	1 mg IM	Morphine 10 mg IM	1 hr	4–5 hrs	Unknown	Highly soluble; not available orally	Same precautions as with morphine
	5 mg IV	Morphine 10 mg IV	15–30 min	3–4 hrs			
	10 mg rectal suppos.	Morphine 10 mg IM Oxymorphone 1 mg IM	2 hrs	6 hrs			
Propoxyphene HCl (Darvon, Dolene)	65 mg po	Aspirin 600 mg po	2 hrs	3–4 hrs	12 hrs	A 'weak' narcotic; structurally related to methadone	Overdose can be complicated by convulsions
Propoxyphene napsylate (Darvon N) (with acetaminophen-Darvocet N)	100 mg po	Aspirin 600 mg po	2 hrs	3–4 hrs	12 hrs		

[a] The oral/parenteral efficacy ratio refers to the ratio of doses given by the two routes of administration necessary to produce equivalent 'total' analgesic effect when both intensity and duration of effect are taken into account. If only maximal intensity or 'peak' effect is considered, however, oral administration yields even less effective analgesia than parenteral administration. These studies were done on cancer patients. In other types of pain, equivalencies may not be the same.

The determination of equivalent analgesic doses is made on comparison of a drug to a standard such as morphine or aspirin. Equianalgesic doses are expressed either in terms of peak effect (peak of the time-effect curve) or duration of effect (area under the time-effect curve). Thus, when time-effect curves are not equivalent, these measurements do not adequately express the differences.

Virtually all drugs are less effective orally than parenterally in terms of peak effect. Morphine and oxymorphone have relative low oral to parenteral potency ratios, whereas codeine, oxycodone, and methadone have higher ratios.

Tolerance due to narcotics is associated with a shift in time-effect curve to the right. Narcotics have cross-tolerance, but this is not complete [105]. Tolerance to other than analgesic effects develops at the same rate as analgesic tolerance, so increasing a dose of a narcotic to keep pace with pain control needs carries little risk of increased toxicity. Physical dependence also develops at the same rate as tolerance; however, patients who have received morphine for one to two weeks show only mild withdrawal symptoms if the drug is stopped abruptly.

Withdrawal symptoms differ quantitatively from drug to drug. Those with a long duration of action are associated with milder withdrawal symptoms than those with a short duration of action. Administration of narcotic antagonists, of course, produces severe withdrawal symptoms in any patient using narcotics.

Studies have shown that fear of producing drug addiction is the major reason for underprescribing narcotics [4]. Other reasons include a misunderstanding of the optimal effective doses and duration of action, and inordinate concern over side effects.

Table 15. Guidelines for choosing the proper dose, schedule, and route of administration of analgesics.

---

1. Use the oral route of administration whenever and for as long as possible when giving systemic analgesics.

2. Chronic (persistent) pain requires chronic (preventative) therapy. To use an administration schedule that is dependent on pain to be present before the analgesic may be administered (i.e. prn) is both irrational and inhumane.

3. Each patient will require close monitoring of doses initially to establish the true pain-free interval achieved with each dose – ultimately, the right dose is that which achieves a pain-free state for at least 3–4 hours duration.

4. Attention should be given to the expected side effects which accompany use of analgesics.

   A. Use adjuvant therapy to prevent or minimize the expected sequelae, e.g. constipation, nausea/vomiting, dysphoria/anxiety, CNS depression.

The chance of a hospitalized patient becoming psychologically addicted to narcotics given for pain is very slight. Undertreatment may in fact produce a craving for the drug, which may be interpreted as addiction, rather than a desire for pain relief. Addiction and tolerance may in fact be delayed by adequate dosing. Principles of operant conditioning would suggest that dosing on demand (prn), making reception of the drug conditioned on the patient's complaint of pain, would be more likely to lead to addictive behavior than when the drug is given at regular intervals so that non-pain behavior is encouraged [106] (Figure 4) (Table 15).

Combining narcotics with psychotropic agents may be useful in some situations to reduce the fear of pain, which is also a factor in addictive behavior.

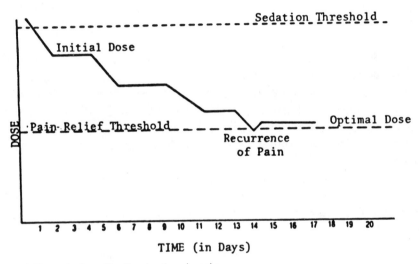

Figure 4. Narcotic dose titration in chronic pain.

NEW METHODS OF MORPHINE ADMINISTRATION

Intravenous infusion

Recent studies have shown that intravenous infusions of morphine may be very useful in management of intractable pain of cancer [107–112]. There are obvious dangers associated with this, and proper guidelines should be established in each institution regarding the conditions and means by which this is done [113].

1. Indications. Morphine infusions are reserved for hospitalized patients with intractable pain who are not sufficiently controlled by intermittent injections or for whom there is a contraindication for oral or intramuscular dosing. At least one study suggested that a smaller daily dose of morphine was required than with intermittent administration.

2. Dosage and administration. Doses most commonly used range from 40 to 95 mg/day, although dosage ranges from 0.5 to 200 mg/day have been used. The usual dose is 0.04 to 0.07 mg/kg per hour. A safe starting dose is one fourth the previously used intermittent dose per hour. If a patient has been without narcotics for four hours or more, the initial calculated dose is given as an i.v. push prior to beginning the infusion. Dose increases by one to three mg/hour, not more often than every twelve hours, may be performed until pain control is achieved. A cautious, gradual approach is man-

Table 16. Intravenous morphine infusion for chronic pain.

Investigator	Patient population	Medications	Comments
Holmes [107]	3 patients with terminal cancer	Morphine sulfate 40–95 mg/hr for 30–70 days	Patients were coherent and alert. No escalation of dose needed once a steady state achieved
Ensworth [108]	2 patients with terminal cancer	Morphine drip at 30 mg/hr; increased to 144 mg/hr over 5 days	Patient was pain-free. Alert but agitation noted
		Morphine drip at 5–10 mg/hr; increased to 20 mg/hr over 6 days	Patient not completely pain-controlled at 20 mg/hr, infusion D/c' ed due to phlebitis. Significant CNS toxicity noted
Miser et al. [110]	8 children with terminal cancer	Morphine infusion. Initial dose based on pain meds in previous 24 hours. Adjustments made to provide pain relief. Duration of therapy = 1–16 days	Complete pain control at 0.025 to 2.6 mg/kg/hr (0.8–80 mg/hr). Median dose = 0.04–0.07 mg/kg/hr. Toxicity: constipation, drowsiness. Respiratory depression to 10/min
Kowolenko [109]	12 patients with terminal cancer	No information provided	Patients became less lethargic and more coherent; less anxious regarding pain med dose

datory. The drug is mixed with dextrose 5% in water at a 1 mg to 1 ml ratio and prepared in 500 cc lots.

3. Precautions. a) Respiratory depression with narcotic infusions should not be treated with narcotic antagonists for fear of precipitating a sympathetic crisis [109]. Rather, ventilatory support should be used while the narcotic is discontinued; b) narcotic infusions should only be administered using an infusion pump or a volume controlled i.v.; c) drug infusion rates should be accomplished by changing rate of flow rather than concentration of drug.

Morphine infusion avoids the peaks and troughs of blood levels which occur with intermittent dosing and anxiety is reduced [111]. Doses are easily adjustable; nursing time and effort are actually reduced.

Intraspinal administration of morphine

Since opiate receptors exist in the spinal chord [120, 121], administration of morphine by the epidural or subarachnoid route for the control of pain

Table 17. Intraspinal administration of analgesics.

Investigator	Patient population	Medications	Comments
Oyama et al. [114]	14 patients with advanced cancer	B-endorphin (synthetic)	100% relief in all patients with 3 mg IT dose; mean duration = 33 hrs; toxicity = mild disorientation ± euphoria in 3 patients
Leavens et al. [115]	6 patients with advanced cancer	Lumbar intrathecal morphine (2 pts.); intraventricular morphine (4 pts.)	1 mg IT produced relief for 10–14 hrs; 2.5–4.0 mg intraventricularly produced relief for 12–24 hours; treated for 3–7 months with gradual increase dose, but no complication
Poletti et al. [116]	2 patients with advanced cancer	Epidural morphine via indwelling Broviac catheter	2 mg dose = 8–12 hours pain relief for 6 months without tolerance developing
Onofrio et al. [117]	1 patient with advanced cancer	Intrathecal morphine via continuous infusion using Infusaid (implanted pump)	Pain free on 1.8 mg/24 hours by continuous infusion

230

seems reasonable to produce analgesia at the level of spinal sensory integration [114–118]. An excellent review of this subject by Yaksh should be consulted [119]. Table 17 summarizes published reports of successful intraspinal analgesia.

Two recent reports have described intraspinal analgesia with new surgically implanted delivery systems. Poletti implanted indwelling Broviac catheters into the spinal epidural space, and later, used a morphine reservoir connected to a shunt pump and a valve system which permitted patients to administer epidural morphine themselves (Figure 5). Leavens described the use of an Ommaya reservoir with its catheter tip in the lumbar space or the lateral ventricle. This permitted percutaneous injection of morphine, and also could be used in the out-patient setting, but required the training of a family member [116].

Onofrio in a recent review concluded that chronic intrathecal morphine was superior to standard neurosurgical procedures for pain relief, in that there was preservation of motor and sensory modalities while achieving a pain-free state [117].

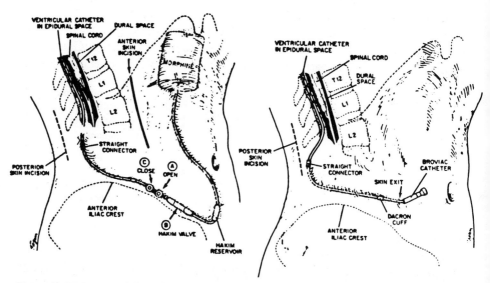

Figure 5. Diagram on left: diagram of a completely indwelling catheter system, consisting of morphine reservoir, shunt pump, and on-off valve, for long-term administration of morphine into the epidural space. For the placement operation, the on-off valve is opened (A), the Hakim valve is pumped 20 times (B) delivering 2 ml of morphine, and the on-off valve is then closed (C).
Diagram on right: diagram of a partially indwelling Broviac catheter system for long-term administration of morphine into the epidural space. After healing, the skin exit wound requires clean rather than sterile dressing.

Intrathecal morphine achieves a clinically significant effect on pain, but unlike parenteral morphine, does not result in a suppression of supraspinal centers. The use of morphine in this way, however, does have some problems: a) there is the necessity for multiple punctures; b) respiratory depression can occur with redistribution of bolus morphine to supraspinal centers; c) with bolus morphine, tolerance develops fairly rapidly.

Onofrio recently reported a successful case of pain control with the use of a continuous infusion of morphine into the intrathecal space using a subcutaneously implanted pump (Infusaid® drug delivery system). This has the advantage of not requiring as many injections and assuring that the absolute level of morphine in the spinal fluid at any moment is low.

The continuous infusion of a low dose of morphine may slow the development of tolerance in as much as the initial peaks of receptor activation seen with bolus injection do not occur.

Intrathecal morphine has one great advantage over neurosurgical pain ablation in that it does not depend on the creation of a sensory deficit. Neurosurgical procedures also are associated with occassional motor system deficits and sometimes fail to produce long-standing analgesia because of partial recovery. Furthermore, the higher the locus of pain being treated, the more risky and less successful the neurosurgical procedure used to treat it. Since supraspinal centers are not affected to the same degree as when parenteral morphine is given, voluntary motor function is in fact enhanced by virtue of the relief of pain. No effects on autonomic function have been observed with this modality.

As systems are developed which are safer and easier to apply, intrathecal morphine administration should have a significant impact on chronic pain control in cancer.

CONTROVERSIES IN ANALGESIA

1. Brompton's cocktail

In the 1890s a solution of morphine and cocaine in a gin and honey base was given to patients to be taken by mouth ad libitum to control pain [122]. In the 1930s a similar approach was popularized at the Brompton Chest Hospital to manage post-operative pain in thoracotomy patients. The Brompton Hospital compendium published the formula in 1952 and the British Pharmaceutical Codex officially recognized this in 1973. Recently, this approach has gained popularity in the United States.

As no commercial formulations are available, there are many variations of 'Brompton's cocktail', but the official formula consists of morphine,

10 mg; cocaine, 10 mg; 95% ethyl alcohol, 5 ml; and cherry syrup, 5 ml, in a chloroform water base to 20 ml.

The beneficial effects of the solution regarding analgesia are primarily attributable to morphine, despite the implication that the cocaine and alcohol are synergistic.

Cocaine was originally added to the mixture for its stimulant and euphoric properties. Cocaine is absorbed through the gastrointestinal tract (60% of an equal intravenous dose is bioavailable) [124–125], and in large doses causes side effects such as confusion, restlessness, hallucinations, hypertension, and arrhythmias. For these reasons, modifications have been made. Forrest [126] studied a dextroamphetamine–morphine combination in 450 post-operative patients. He reported that dextroamphetamine significantly augmented the analgesic effect of morphine, and counteracted the sedation and loss of alertness in these patients. He proposed that the added analgesia was by selective stimulation of inhibitory pain neurons. The study, however, only evaluated the effect of a single dose of the combination.

Researchers at the Fox Chase Cancer Center developed a modification of Brompton's cocktail consisting of morphine 30 mg and dextroamphetamine 5 mg in an aromatic elixir base, total volume, 10 ml [127]. Ten ml of the solution is given every six hours and at bedtime; dextroamphetamine is withheld. This preparation has been quite effective in rendering patients pain-free without undue sedation.

In a double-blind crossover trial, plain morphine in syrup was compared to Brompton's mixture in 30 patients with intractable cancer pain [128]. All received the preparation for two weeks. Pain relief was evaluated by an independent observer using a pain rating scale. No statistically significant difference was noted in the two formulations.

Another study, also double-blind crossover in design, was conducted in 61 patients with chronic cancer pain [129]. When cocaine 10 mg was added to each dose of morphine, there was a significant initial increase in alertness, but tolerance to this stimulant effect occurred rapidly and deletion of the cocaine at that point produced minimal consequences.

Based on these trials, a simple morphine solution, such as the one which has recently become commercially available [123], is probably sufficient for oral control of severe pain in the majority of patients.

2. Heroin

Controversy continues regarding the use of heroin in the treatment of chronic cancer pain. Some studies have suggested that heroin may produce greater euphoria and fewer side effects than morphine in equal analgesic doses. Karko prospectively compared the analgesic and mood altering effects of heroin to morphine in chronic cancer pain [130]. Heroin reached its peak effectiveness in about one hour, whereas morphine did so in about 90 minutes. Patients' moods improved about equally, the effect being seen sooner with heroin, but lasting longer with morphine. The side effects of either preparation were similar.

The greater solubility of heroin has been advanced as a reason for its use in patients where high doses of narcotics have been required. However, there are commercially available preparations such as hydromorphone hydrochloride (Dilaudid®) which is both more soluble and more potent than morphine [131].

Due to the wide variety of morphine congeners, the difficulty in safeguarding against theft, and the lack of demonstrated important differences between heroin and morphine, the legalization of heroin for medical use seems unreasonable.

SUMMARY

There are a wide variety of pharmacologic agents useful in the management of pain. New methods of delivery hold forth the promise of better ability to manage pain in patients with cancer. If an attack against the tumor is possible, this is desirable as palliation; but in most patients with incurable cancer, analgesic use will be necessary. The physician who treats patients with cancer pain can serve them best when pain is approached like any other symptom – when it is treated specifically and when it is treated with sympathy, care, and full attention to the uniqueness of the patient. It is only the rare patient who will need psychiatric consultation or referral for neurosurgical procedures.

Further research regarding optimum use of presently available agents is promising. Patient-controlled analgesic systems using modern technologic advancements hold hope for maintaining patients in a functional pain-free state [132].

ACKNOWLEDGMENT

The author wishes to thank Mrs Dorothy Rossi and Mrs Donna Marinucci for their expert assistance in the preparation of this manuscript.

REFERENCES

1. Bonica JJ: Cancer pain: the importance of the problem. In: Advances in Pain Research and Therapy, Vol. 2, Bonica JJ, Ventofridden V (eds). New York, Raven Press, 1979, pp 1–11.

2. Houcle RW: Pain and the patient with cancer. In: The Medical Clinics of North America – Symposium on the Medical Aspects of Cancer, Karnofsky DA, Rowson RW (eds). Philadelphia and London, WB Saunders Co, 1956, pp 687–703.

3. Shimm DS, Logue GL, Maltbie AA, Dugan S: Medical management of chronic cancer pain. JAMA 241:2408–2412, 1979.

4. Marks RM, Sachar EJ: Undertreatment of medical in-patients with narcotic analgesics. Ann Intern Med 78:173–181, 1973.

5. Saunders CM: Care of the terminal stages of cancer. Ann Royal Coll Surg (England), Volume 41.

6. Houde R, Fink BR: Management of pain of advanced cancer: systemic analgesics and related drugs. In: Advances in Pain Research and Therapy, Vol 2, Bonica JJ, Ventofridde V (eds). New York, Raven Press, 1979, pp 301–302.

7. Catalano RB: Supportive care of the seriously ill cancer patient: control of pain. In: Oncologic Emergencies, Yarbro JW, Bornstein RS (eds). New York, Grune & Stratton, 1981, pp 365–393.

8. Dant RL, Cleeland CS: The prevalence and severity of pain in cancer. Cancer 50: 1913–1918, 1982.

9. Oster MW, Vizel M, Turgeon MS: Pain of terminal cancer patients. Arch Intern Med 138:1801–1802, 1978.

10. Catalano RB: Medical management of pain caused by cancer. Semin Oncol 2:379–392, 1975.

11. DuBe' SE: Hospice care and the pharmacist. US Pharmacist 2:25–38, 1981.

12. Wilkes E: Some problems in cancer management. Proc R Soc Med 67:23–27, 1974.

13. Twycross RG: Clinical management with dramorphine in advanced malignant disease. Int J Clin Pharmacol 93:184–198, 1974.

14. Bonica JJ: Cancer pain: a major national health problem. Cancer Nurs J 4:313–316, 1978.

15. Pannuti F, Martoni A, Rossi AP, Prana E: The role of endocrine therapy for relief of pain due to advanced cancer. In: Advances in Pain Research and Therapy, Vol 2, Bonica JJ, Ventofridden V (eds). New York, Raven Press, 1979, pp 00–00.

16. Parker CM: Home or hospital? Terminal care as seen by surviving spouse. J R Coll Gen Proct 28:19–30, 1978.

17. Twycross RG: Choice of strong analgesic in terminal cancer: diamorphine or morphine? Pain 7: 93–104, 1977.

18. Silverberg E: Cancer statistics, 1982. Cancer – A Cancer Journal for Clinicians 32:15–31, 1982.

19. Bonica JJ: Fundamental considerations of chronic pain therapy. Postgrad Med 53: 187–194, 1973.

20. Murphy TM: Cancer pain. Postgrad Med 53:187–194, 1973.

21. Roger DG: 21 problems in pain control and ways to solve them. Your Patient and Cancer: 65–69, 1981.

22. Black PM: Management of cancer pain: An overview. Neurosurg 5:507–518, 1979.

23. Twycross RG: Overview of analgesia. In: Advances in Pain Research and Therapy, Vol 2, Bonica JJ, Ventofridden V (eds). New York, Raven Press, 1979, pp 617–633.

24. Foley KM: Pain syndrome in patients with cancer. In: Advances in Pain Research and Therapy, Vol 2, Bonica JJ, Ventofridden V (eds). New York, Raven Press, 1979, pp 59–75.

25. Bonica JJ: The management of pain. Philadelphia, Lea & Febeger, 1953.

26. Kennedy BJ, Fortuny IE: Therapeutic castration in the treatment of advanced breast cancer. Cancer 17:1197–1202, 1964.

27. Scott WW: Rationale and results of primary endocrine therapy in patients with prostatic cancer. Cancer 32:1119–1125, 1973.
28. Fracchia AA, Farrow JH, Miller TR: Hypophysectomy as compared to adenolectomy in treatment of advanced breast cancer. Surg Gynecol Obstet 133:241, 1971.
29. Murphy GP et al.: Hypophysectomy and adrenalectomy for disseminated prostatic carcinoma. J Urol 105:817–825, 1971.
30. Parker RG: Pain relief for the cancer patients through selective radiation therapy. Northwest Med 69:1022–1025, 1968.
31. Rubin P: Current concept in cancer: metastases and disseminated cancer. V. Bone. Int J Rad Oncol Brol Phys 1:1199–1200, 1976.
32. Tong D, Gillick L, Hendrickson FR: The palliation of symptomatic osseous metastases. Cancer 50:839–899, 1982.
33. Horton J, Barter OH, Olsen KB: The management of metastases to brain by irradiation and corticosteroids. Am J Roentgenol Rad Ther Nucl Med 111:334–336, 1971.
34. Weinstein EA: The effects of dexamethasone on brain edema in patients with metastatic brain tumours. Neurology 23:121–129, 1973.
35. Black P: Brain metastases: current status and recommended guidelines for management. Neurosurg 5:617–631, 1979.
36. Cady B, Oberfield RA: Regional infusion chemotherapy of hepatic metastases from carcinoma of the colon. Am J Surg 127:220–226, 1974.
37. Mawsey WH, Fletcher WS, Judkins MP et al.: Hepatic artery infusion for metastastic malignancy using percutaneous-placed catheters. Am J Surg 121:160–164, 1971.
38. Ensminger W, Niederhuber J, Dakhel S, Thrall J, Wheeler R: Totally implanted drug delivery system for hepatic arterial chemotherapy. Cancer Treat Rep 65:401–411, 1981.
39. Halpern LH: Analgesic drugs in the management of pain. Arch Drug 112:861–869, 1977.
40. Houde RW: Systemic analgesics and related drugs: narcotic analgesics. In: Advances in Pain Research and Therapy, Vol 2, Bonica JJ, Ventofridden V (eds). New York, Raven Press, 1979, pp 263–273.
41. Twycross RG: The Brompton cocktail. In: Advances in Pain Research and Therapy, Vol 2, Bonica JJ, Ventofridden V (eds). New York, Raven Press, 1979, pp 291–300.
42. Dawson DM, Fischer EG: Host effects of cancer: pain. In: Cancer Medicine, 2nd ed, Holland JF, Frei E (eds). Philadelphia, Lea & Febeger, 1982, pp 1205–1219.
43. Pert CB, Pasternak GW, Snyder SH: Opiate agonists and antagonists discriminated by receptor binding in brain. Science 182:1359–1361, 1975.
44. Snyder SH: Opitate receptors in the brain. New Engl J Med 296:266–271, 1977.
45. Guillemin R: Endorphins, brain peptides that act like opiates. New Engl J Med 296:226–228, 1977.
46. Anon: Encephalins: the search for a functional role. Lancet, October 14:819–820, 1978.
47. Snyder SH, Pert CB, Pasternak GW: The opiate receptor. Ann Intern Med 81:534–540, 1974.
48. Loh YP, Loriaux LL: Adrenocorticotropic hormone, B-lipotropian, and endorphin-related peptides in health and disease. JAMA 247:1033–1034, 1982.
49. West AB: Understanding endorphins: our natural pain relief system. Nursing 81:50–53, 1981.
50. Higgs GA: Arachidonic acid metabolism. pain, and hyperalgesia: the mode of action of non-steroid mild analgesics. Br J Clin Pharmacol 10 (suppl 2):2335–2353, 1980.
51. Ramwell PW: Biologic importance of arachidonic acid. Arch Intern Med 141:275–279, 1981.
52. Pruss AG: Evaluation of zomepirac. J Clin Pharmacol 20:215–222, 1980.

236

53. Vandam LD: Analgetic drugs – the mild analgetics. New Engl J Med 286:249–252, 1972.
54. Richlin DM, Brand L: The use of oral analgesics for chronic pain. Hosp Formulary: 32–41, 1982.
55. Moertel CG, Ohmann DL, Taylor WF et al.: A comparative evaluation of marketed analgesic drugs. New Engl J Med 286:813–815, 1972.
56. Moertel CG, Ohmann DL, Taylor WF et al.: Relief of pain by oral medications. JAMA 229:55–59, 1974.
57. Beaver WT: Mild analgesics: a review of their clinical pharmacology. Part II. Am J Med Sci 251:576–599, 1966.
58. Abels: Analgesic nephropathy. Clin Pharmacol Ther 12:583–587, 1971.
59. Goldberg M, Murray TG: Analgesic-associated nephropathy: an important cause of renal disease in the United States? New Engl J Med 299:716–717, 1978.
60. McLeod DC: Analgesic nephropathy. New Engl J Med 300:319, 1979.
61. Perry DJ, Wood PHN: Relationship between aspirin taking and gastrointestinal hemorrhage. Gut 8:301–308, 1967.
62. Chafee FH: Aspirin intolerance. I. Frequency in an allergic population. J Allergy Clin Immunol 53:193–199, 1974.
63. Smith AP: Response of aspirin-allergic patients to challenge by some analgesics in common use. Br Med J 2:494–496, 1971.
64. Weiss HJ, Aledorf LM: Impaired platelet/connective tissue reaction in man after aspirin ingestion. Lancet 2:499, 1967.
65. Harris WH et al.: Aspirin prophylaxis of venous thromboembolism after total hip replacement. New Engl J Med 297:1246, 1977.
66. Horter HR et al.: Prevention of thrombosis in patients on hemodialysis by low-dose heparin. New Engl J Med 301:577, 1979.
67. Taylor F: Aspirin: America's favorite drug. FDA Consumer 14(10):12, 1980.
68. Anon: Aspirin products. Medical Letter 23:65, 1981.
69. Anon: Aspirin after myocardial infarction. Lancet 1:1172, 1980.
70. Flower RJ, Moncada S, Vane JR: Analgesic-antipyretic and anti-inflammatory drugs. In: The Pharmacological Basis of Therapeutics, 6th ed, Gilman AG, Goodman LS, Gilman A (eds). New York, MacMillan Publishing Co, 1980, pp 682–728.
71. Ferreira SH: Inflammatory pain, prostaglandin hyperalgesia and the development of peripheral analgesics. Trends Pharmacol Sci 2:183, 1981.
72. Ameer B, Greenblatt DJ: Acetaminophen. Ann Intern Med 87:202–209, 1977.
73. Koch-Weser J: Acetaminophen. New Engl J Med 295:1297–13101, 1976.
74. Cooper SH: Comparative analgesic efficacies of aspirin and acetaminophen. Arch Intern Med 141:282–285, 1981.
75. Mielke CH: Comparative effects of aspirin and acetaminophen on hemostasis. Arch Intern Med 141:305–310, 1981.
76. Jick H: Effects of aspirin and acetaminophen in gastrointestinal hemorrhage. Arch Intern Med 141:316–320, 1981.
77. Zimmerman HJ: Effects of aspirin or acetaminophen on the liver. Arch Intern Med 141:333–341, 1981.
78. Schreiner GE, MacNally JF, Winchester JE: Clinical analgesic nephropathy. Arch Intern Med 141:349–357, 1981.
79. Anon: Ibuprofen (Motrin) – a new drug for arthritis. Medical Letter 16:109–110, 1974.
80. Kantor KG: Ibuprofen. Ann Intern Med 91:877–882, 1979.
81. Katz SM, Capaldo R, Everts EA, DiGregorio JG: Tolmetin, association with reversible renal failure and acute interstitial nephritis. JAMA 246:243–245, 1981.

82. Smith VT: Anaphylactic shock, acute renal failure and disseminated intravascular coagulation, suspected complication of zomepirac. JAMA 247:1172–1173, 1982.
83. Robertson CE, Ford KJ, Someran V: mefenamic acid nephropathy. Lancet 2:232–233, 1980.
84. Plotz PH, Kimberly RP: Acute effects of aspirin and acetaminophen on renal function. Arch Intern Med 141:343–348, 1981.
85. Lewis JR: Zomepirac sodium, A new non-addicting analgesic. JAMA 246:377–379, 1981.
86. Cooper SA: Efficacy of zomepirac in oral surgical pain. J Clin Pharmacol 20:230–242, 1980.
87. Wallenstein SL, Rogers A, Karko RF et al.: Relative analgesic potency of oral zomepirac and intramuscular morphine on cancer patients with postoperative pain. J Clin Pharmacol 20:250–258, 1980.
88. Stambaugh JE, Tejada F, Trudnowski RJ: Double-blind comparison of zomepirac and oxycodone with APC in cancer pain. J Clin Pharmacol 20:261–270, 1980.
89. Honig S: Preliminary report: long-term safety of zomepirac. J Clin Pharmacol 20: 392–396, 1980.
90. Rouoff GE, Andelman SY, Cannella JJ: Long-term safety of zomepirac: a double-blind comparison with aspirin in patients with osteoarthritis. J Clin Pharmacol 20:377–384, 1980.
91. Cass LJ, Fredrich WS: Clinical comparison of the analgesic effects of dextropropoxyphene and other analgesics. Antibiot Med Clin Ther 6:363–370, 1959.
92. Graber CM: The post-partum patients in evaluating analgesic drugs. Clin Pharmacol Ther 2:429–440, 1961.
93. Procko LD: Evaluation of D-propoxyphene, codeine and aspirin. Obstet Gynecol 16: 113–118, 1960.
94. Berdon JK: The effectiveness of D-propoxyphene in the control of pain after peridontal surgery. J Periodont 39:106–111, 1964.
95. Chilton NW: Double-blind evaluation of a new analgesic agent in post extraction pain. Am J Med Sci 242:702–706, 1961.
96. Hopkinson JH: Acetaminophen vs. propoxyphene for relief of pain in episiotomy patients. J Clin Pharmacol 7:251–263, 1973.
97. Young DJ: Propoxyphene suicides. Arch Intern Med 129:62–66, 1972.
98. Beaver WT, Wallenstein SL, Houde RW: A clinical comparison of the effects of oral and intramuscular administration of analgesics: Pentazocine and phenazocine. Clin Pharmacol Ther 9:582–597, 1968.
99. Beaver WT, Wallenstein SL, Houde RW: A comparison of the analgesic effects of pentazocine and morphine in patients with cancer. Clin Pharmacol Ther 7:740–751, 1966.
100. Lewis JR: Misprescribing analgesics. JAMA 228:1155–1156, 1974.
101. Bellville JW, Green J: The respiratory and subjective efforts of pentazocine. Clin Pharmacol Ther 7:740–751, 1966.
102. Reichenberg S, Pobers F: Severe respiratory depression following Talwin. Am Rev Resp Dis 107:280–282, 1973.
103. Vandam LD: Analgetic drugs – the potent analgetics. New Engl J Med 286:249–251, 1972.
104. Papper S, Papper EM: The effects of preanesthetics, anesthetics, and post-operative drugs on renal function. Clin Pharmacol Ther 5:205, 1964.
105. House RW, Wallenstein SL, Beaver WT: Clinical measurement of pain. In: Analgesics, de Stevens G (ed). New York, Academic Press, 1965, pp 75–122.
106. Bonica JJ: The total management of the patient with chronic pain. Drug Therapy 3:33–47, 1973.

238

107. Holmes H: Morphine IV infusion for chronic pain. Drug Intell Clin Pharm 12:556, 1978.
108. Ensworth S: Morphine IV infusion for chronic pain. Drug Intell Clin Pharm 13:297, 1979.
109. Kowolenko M: Morphine IV infusion. Drug Intell Clin Pharm 14:296–297, 1980.
110. Miser AW, Miser JS, Clark BS: Continuous IV infusion of morphine sulfate for control of severe pain in children with terminal malignancy. J Pediat 96:930–932, 1980.
111. Ruller PC, Murphy F, Dudley HAF: Morphine: controlled trial of different methods of administration for postoperative pain relief. Br Med J 1:12–13, 1980.
112. Fraser DG: Intravenous morphine infusion for chronic pain. Ann Intern Med 93:781–782, 1980.
113. Menard PJ: Use of continuous narcotic infusions. Am J Hosp Pharm 39:1459–1460, 1982.
114. Oyama T, Jin T, Yamaya R et al.: Profound analgesic effects of B-endorphin in man. Lancet 1:122–124, 1980.
115. Leavens ME, Hill CS, Cech DA, Weyland JB, Weston JS: Intrathecal and intraventricular morphine for pain in cancer patients: initial study. J Neurosurg 56:241–245, 1982.
116. Poletti CE, Cohen AM, Todd DP, Ojemann RG, Sweet WH, Zervos NT: Cancer pain relieved by long-term epidural morphine with permanent indwelling systems for self-administration. J Neurosurg 55:581–584, 1981.
117. Onofrio BM, Yahsh TL, Arnold PG: Continuous low dose intrathecal morphine administration in the treatment of chronic pain of malignant origin. Mayo Clin Proc 56:516–520, 1981.
118. Richelsen E: Spinal opiate administration for chronic pain: a major advance in therapy. Mayo Clin Proc 56:523, 1981.
119. Yaksh TL: Spinal opiate analgesia: characteristics and principles of action. Pain 11:293–346, 1981.
120. Goldstein A: Opioid peptides (endorphins) in pituitary and brain. Science 193:1081–1086, 1976.
121. Snyder SH: Opiate receptors in the brain. New Engl J Med 296:266–271, 1977.
122. Anon: The Brompton cocktail. Lancet 1:1220, 1979.
123. Glover DD, Lowry TF, Jacknowitz AI: Brompton's mixture in alleviating pain of terminal neoplastic disease: preliminary results. South Med J 138:278, 1980.
124. VanDyke C et al.: Oral cocaine: plasma concentrations and central effects. Science 200:211, 1979.
125. Wilkinson P et al.: Intranasal and oral cocaine kinetics. Clin Pharmacol Ther 27:386, 1980.
126. Forrest WH et al.: Dextroamphetamine with morphine for the treatment of post-operative pain. New Engl J Med 296:712–715, 1977.
127. Catalano RB: Personal communication, 1982.
128. Melzack R, Mount BM, Gorden JM: The Brompton mixture versus morphine solution given orally. Effects on pain. Canad Med Assoc J 2:1348, 1977.
129. Twycross RG: Value of cocaine in opiate-containing elixirs. Br Med J 2:1348, 1977.
130. Karko RF, Wallenstein SL, Rogers AG, Grabinski PY, Houde RW: Analgesic and mood effects of heroin and morphine in cancer patients with postoperative pain. New Engl J Med 304:1501–1505, 1981.
131. Lasagna L: Heroin: a medical 'me too'. New Engl J Med 304:1539–1540, 1981.
132. Bennett R: Results are better when patients control their own analgesia. JAMA 247:945–947, 1982.

11. Psychological Adjustment in the Mastectomy Patient

GERALD J. MARGOLIS and ROBERT L. GOODMAN

Similar to many problems for which he is consulted, the physician's role in helping in the psychological adjustment of mastectomy patients depends upon his recognition and understanding of the factors involved and his ability to intervene. This discussion will focus on the psychological impact that the diagnosis and treatment of breast cancer has upon women, with particular emphasis on the feelings which the patient is likely to be struggling with when seen by her physicians, as well as some suggestions about how best to handle these problems. This problem will be approached from the point of view of prevention, as well as the handling of those problems which may occur in the post mastectomy patient.

Since breast cancer is the leading cause of cancer mortality in American women and since the standard treatment, modified radical mastectomy, is known to be effective in improving the survival rates of women diagnosed as having early breast cancer, medical and public service organizations have, in recent years, heavily promoted the advantages of early detection and treatment. Frequent self examination, regular physician physical examinations, mammography, etc. have been promoted by mass media campaigns. Women have by and large responded to these campaigns with more awareness of the problem, and there has probably been relative success in apprehending the disease more often in its earliest stages, thereby increasing chances of therapeutic success. Heightening the awareness of the importance of early detection has, however, had the consequence of heightening anxiety about the disease in the general population. This phenomenon is unavoidable, but one must nevertheless be aware both of its existence and of its consequences. Women who have discovered a lump by self examination come to the physician with a sense of anxiety whether it is overtly expressed or not. That many patients do express it directly, even dramatically, is evident to any physician who has dealt with these patients. Those who hold their feelings in may be more easy to manage initially in the office, but will

Higby, DJ (ed), Supportive Care in Cancer Therapy. ISBN 0-89838-569-5.
© *1983, Martinus Nijhoff Publishers, Boston. Printed in The Netherlands.*

not necessarily have a smoother course of adjusting to disease and treatment at a later time. It is the physician's responsibility to understand that anxiety under such a circumstance is normal and to face it with his patient by giving her an opportunity to talk with him and share with him her feelings about what may lie ahead for her. The potential psychological problems of the mastectomy patient begin at this point, and the prophylactic treatment of the problems should also begin here. Why are women so anxious about the initial visit and how do we know that they are?

A number of studies indicate that 'emotional suffering appears to far outweigh the physical pain in women who have undergone mastectomy' [1, 2], as well as the importance in these patients of a 'sense of mutilation, loss of feelings of femininity and fear of death [3]. Our own ongoing study of the psychological aspects of breast cancer and its treatments confirms these observations. Feelings of disfigurement and mutilation are compounded by feelings of an insult to the integrity of the body image (vide infra) and to the sense of femininity. This difficulty is further worsened by feelings of loss of sexual desirability as well as loss of an important organ of erotic arousal with consequent difficulties with sexual enjoyment. Most patients anticipate and fear these problems preoperatively and following mastectomy experience them for varying periods of time. Most patients eventually make at least some degree of psychological adjustment after a few years (some more quickly than this, others more slowly). However, the adjustment is usually incomplete to a degree and some measure of difficulty with body image and sexuality persists even for years. The majority of women eventually find ways to carry on their lives without dwelling on these problems excessively but are reminded of them and bothered about them frequently. For some patients an adequate psychological adjustment is not possible.

The breast is a highly invested body part for the vast majority of adult women. This observation is as true of the normal women we interviewed as it is of those with breast cancer. The breast is an integral part of body image, a symbol of femininity in a physical sense, important to feelings of attractiveness and sexual desirability and an important erotic organ as well. The body image is, as this term implies, the way in which a person views the physical aspects of his or her self. It is a part of the overall self image which includes many other non-physical aspects of one's views of oneself as well (e.g. intelligent or dull, loveable or irascible, happy or unhappy, etc.). For women the body image is a more important aspect of self image than is the case for most men, due to a combination of interacting factors including biological (especially endocrinological), intrapsychic (within the mind) and societal (including interpersonal) factors.

As far as women are concerned, the biological changes at puberty and adolescence, particularly the onset of menstruation and the development of breasts, are much more dramatic than that which occurs in the male. The newly developed female breast is a brand-new organ that only a short time before was entirely absent. From this time until menopause a women undergoes bodily changes during each menstrual cycle. Pregnancy, post-partum changes in the function of the breast, and menopause also cause more dramatic bodily changes than the man experiences during comparable periods of his life and focus the woman's attention on her own body to a greater extent.

Intrapsychic aspects are complicated and can only be discussed briefly. They derive principally from the fact that the very young (i.e. pre-school age) girl notices that she has nothing visible in the erotically arousable place where a little boy has a penis. Since 'more equals better' to the very young child, the young girl erroneously concludes that she is physically genitally inferior. This envy of the penis has profound effects on the child's psychology. In this discussion, only one aspect of this psychology will be examined, namely that one of the ways in which the child handles this insult to her self esteem, is to begin to hope for and to look forward to the development on her chest of appendages like those which her mother has in order to make up for her supposed genital lack. This uniquely feminine organ is something that she can have that males do not. This 'upwards displacement' [4] of psychological investment from penis to breast is an extremely important factor in the high investment women place in their breast as an essential part of body image. It is not understood by most men and probably not by most male physicians since they do not go through the same psychological developmental stages in the same way. For most men a chest is a chest. It is either male of female; a genital is a genital and is either male or female. For the woman, the breasts are experienced as much more because they are invested with the additional significance given the male to his penis [5]. The breasts become, for the adolescent and adult woman, the most visible physical personal symbol of her feminity as well as an integral part of her physique. Since her genitalia are for the most part hidden, her breasts are what differentiates her the most from men. It is important to her personal feelings of sexual desirability. The breast's significance as an important source of erotic stimulation also becomes functional during adolescence and continues throughout adulthood.

The societal (or environmental) factor makes its contributions via the role models, social role expectations and peer interactions of the girl. This aspect is subject to more change than the first two aspects discussed, since society frequently changes. In the environment of the majority of the breast cancer population (>40 years of age), social roles are determined and limited by biology to a much greater extent than is the case with men. Central in their lives as women is marriage and motherhood and primary gratification from work outside the home was considered to be aberrant when they were younger. Being physically attractive is, therefore, much more important than it is to men of this generation. This observation reinforces the emphasis on the importance of the body image aspect of self image already heightened in the female because of biological and intrapsychic differences. All three factors interact within the mind of the woman, the more basic (i.e. biological and intrapsychic) limiting the possible scope of operation of the least basic (i.e. societal). This discussion is brief and is presented as background to enable us to grasp the experience of the woman anticipating and finally experiencing life without a breast.

With this understanding of the psychological meaning of the breast to women, it is easier to grasp the feelings of anxiety and sense of dread which accompanies the patient to the physician's office with a newly discovered breast lump. Utilizing this knowledge for the proper handling of patients can provide for a prophylactic approach to potential psychological problems in a large percentage of women. The initial physical exam in any particular case may: 1) lead the physician to feel certain that there is no malignancy; or 2) to believe that further diagnostic tests are warranted; or 3) that the mass is so likely to be malignant that a biopsy is indicated regardless of what other tests may show. In any event, it is incumbent upon the physician to present to the patient his opinion in a manner that reflects his understanding of how she is going to hear and comprehend it. Handling the fortunate first group of women (certain benignity) is the easiest. It is the physician's role, in such a case, to reassure his patient that he has good news for her, that she has no physical problem even though he can understand her anxiety about the disease and to suggest that she return if any other problems occur. To scold or chastise a patient who has mistaken normal breast tissue or a medically insignificant 'lump' for breast disease is never helpful to a patient and may, with some women, make it very difficult for them to return if they become suspicious in the future. This suggestion would almost seem to be too basic to mention if it were not for the fact that a number of the women we have interviewed who finally did develop breast cancer, report just such experiences in their previous history. This experience played a role in a few patients, in causing them to delay examination when a new mass appeared. In some cases it interfered with the ability to form a rapport with the physician, a rapport that is necessary in the successful management of the patient.

Naturally, the more serious the mass appears to be, the more kindness, gentleness and understanding are required. How the physician handles the future mastectomy patient at this point will have a major effect on her ability to adjust later on. In one recent retrospective study of mastectomy patients [6], the greatest fear immediately after discovery of a lump in the breast was, for about half the patients, a fear of cancer. The second greatest number of women expressed a fear of losing their breast as the greatest fear that occurred to them at this point (13%), and about the same number, that is 12%, expressed a fear of death as their greatest fear. In addition, 73% of the women indicated that they were aware at this point of some degree of fear about losing a breast. It is not difficult to understand why this fear would be so. These women, in most cases, are healthy in every other respect and yet are faced with a possible deprivation in the near future of an essential aspect of body image, a symbol of femininity, an important aspect of sexual desirability and an important source of erotic arousal in sexual love.

It is at this juncture that the physician can prepare for the future psychological adjustment of the patient. If he can make an ally of his patient, enlist her cooperation in the prospective work and encourage in her a sense of active participation in this important aspect of her health care, he can prevent many common post mastectomy psychological problems. Anxiety, a sense of dread, and feelings of helplessness are the natural accompaniments of a patient faced with breast cancer, but they can be lessened by directing the patient's attention to what she can do for herself in cooperation with her physician. The first step in this process is to inform the patient about the findings in an empathic manner that is cognizant of the psychological implications to her of the possibility that a mastectomy may be necessary. Honesty without undue alarm is the proper approach. The patient about whom the initial exam is questionable, and for whom further studies will determine the necessity of a biopsy, should be made aware of this uncertainty and have explained to her what a mammogram, needle biopsy, etc. may reveal. In those cases in which the physician is certain that a biopsy is indicated (whether upon initial examination or following further studies), a frank discussion in a relaxed atmosphere is imperative. The discussion should take place in the doctor's consulting room rather than the examining room, in an unhurried manner. The patient should be encouraged to ask questions and the doctor should answer them fully. What the patient is told must be done so with compassion. We have interviewed patients who were allegedly told abruptly, 'You have cancer! Off with the breast!' or 'Stop crying! You're going to have the breast removed whether you like it or not.' or 'Don't ask so many questions. It is not going to change anything.' It is frequently not easy for the busy physician to find time to sit down and discuss such matters with a patient, but it is nevertheless essential. It may, also, frequently not be easy for the physician to have to face such unpleasant feelings with the patient, but it is an integral part of the treatment and will set the stage for how the patient will likely view her illness following mastectomy: hopefully as something she worked on with her doctor to overcome rather than as a victim of something that has already ruined her life and will sooner or later kill her.

It is with these principles in mind that the controversy over the 'so-called' one stage or two stage treatment must be viewed. Our goal is, as much as possible, to make the patient a partner in the treatment procedure with the view of enlisting her cooperation in her post mastectomy health care. The most reasonable approach is to recommend to the patient a two stage procedure so that upon being informed of the findings she can participate in the decision to undergo a treatment that is going to have such profound effects on her life. To anesthetize a patient under conditions where she does not know whether she is going to wake up with or without a breast, sets the stage not only for an acute depressive reaction but for chronic feelings of helplessness, dependency, victimization and emotional invalidism as well. Hostile feelings towards the doctor in such circumstances can be expected. There are occasional patients who may express a preference for a one stage procedure and say, in effect, 'I don't want to know about it, I'll be too upset to decide anyway!' Because of considerations of future adjustment to the disease and the mastectomy itself, we recommend that such patients be gently encouraged to opt for the two stage procedure. It should be explained to them that women generally adjust better to mastectomy if they have had an opportunity to participate more fully in the decision making process about the treatment following the biopsy and that the treatment does not need to be accomplished the next day. The patient may take a few days to think about things. Naturally, for those few woman who insist upon a one stage procedure even after such an explanation, wishes must be respected. However, there is a greater likelihood of later psychological morbidity from this choice. The patient may, at this point, ask about what the treatment recommendations will be if the biopsy is positive; if she does ask in such a fashion, the treatment should be discussed fully. Other patients may not ask about treatment until they have learned that the biopsy is positive.

From this point on, the manner in which patient–physician interaction occurs becomes critical in regard to providing the best chances for avoiding future problems. The finding of a positive biopsy must be discussed with the patient with delicacy and tact. The most prominent fears of the patient are likely to be associated with death and cancer, but fears of becoming disfigured, no longer whole, unfeminine, deformed, mutilated, unattractive, and asexual will plague her as well [6, 7]. In one study of 41 mastectomy patients [2], the 'pre-mastectomy period' was considered to be the worst time emotionally for almost half of the patients. Delivering the patient the 'bad news' on the telephone or on the run after sticking one's head in the door, or via a nurse or relative, actually increases chances for psychiatric problems in the future. It is the obligation of the physician to engage his patient in a frank and open discussion of the problems which face her.

Which physician should be involved in this aspect of her care depends on the patient and on the circumstances. If the general surgeon or gynecologist has a previous relationship with the patient then, ideally, he is the one to interact with the patient. He is likely to be viewed with a sense of awe by the patient: 'knowledgeable, skilled and god-like' by a patient 'eager to believe in his power to cure both the body and the psyche' [3]. Unfortunately, some physicians are unable to deal with the patient because of busy schedules or personalities which may include an inability to tolerate the emotional accompaniments of the patient's illness. The physician should recognize if either one or both of these potential problems exist so that the most suitable physician substitute can be found to handle the psychological aspects of care. If the patient already has an ongoing relationship with an interested family physician, internist, or gynecologist, then this individual should become involved in the medical and support care. In situations where no such prior physician is available (or where this physician can not or is not suited to assume such a role) or particularly where post-operative chemotherapy is likely, a medical oncologist may become the most suitable substitute. Such an interested physician (e.g. the medical oncologist) must become involved with the problem prior to the biopsy to facilitate the patient's experiencing him as a full participant in the treatment. It is the responsibility of the surgeon to determine whether or not he will be able to talk with his patient and, if not, to arrange for the early involvement of this team approach with the medical oncologist or other physician. Such an alternative will offer the patient a maximum opportunity to invest her faith in this physician rather than entirely in the surgeon. The emphasis must be on the physician, as expert about breast disease and its treatment, discussing with his patient what she expects to anticipate in the way of psychological distress post-operatively. For this reason, turning this aspect of the job over to a nurse, social worker, or even a psychiatrist is not as good an option for most patients. It is the physician who is treating her, the physician she hopes to cure her, the physician who will be 'disfiguring' her in order to save her life, and for these reasons, the physician on whom she will feel most in need of working with.

It is at this point that the patient with early (clinical Stage I or II) breast cancer should receive information about alternative treatments (if any) to further the patient's sense of participating as a partner in her treatment. A discussion of the efficacy of primary radiation therapy [8] in controlling early breast cancer as measured against the standard treatment, modified radical mastectomy, is not pertinent to our present topic. However, it is a viable alternative which offers the patient the possibility of control of her cancer without the disfigurement, and without the insult to her body image, feelings of femininity, sexual desirability and sexual enjoyment that she will be anticipating from mastectomy. Suicidal ideation occurs in about 20% of breast cancer patients [2, 5, 6]. In an ongoing study, the suicidal ideation in approximately one half of these patients, that is 8%, was directly related to concerns about having to have a mastectomy and disappeared completely upon learning about and choosing the radiation therapy alternative [5]. If the physician explains the choice to the patient, including, of course, his own opinion about which treatment offers the best chances for recovery and/or control of disease and other aspects about the pros and cons for each, then those patients who do choose mastectomy can be expected to have a smoother post-operative course. Not only will much psychological morbidity attendent upon feelings of helplessness and being victimized be avoided, but the therapeutic partnership thus fostered will prove useful in gaining the mastectomy patient's participation in post-surgical care (exercise, self examination, chemotherapy, etc.) as well. For similar reasons, a frank discussion of whether or not post-mastectomy breast reconstruction is desirable should be initiated at this point with the patient.

In addition to stressing the team work aspects with the patient, the physician should emphasize whatever other positive factors exist for the individual patient, e.g. size of tumor, presence or absence of involved lymph nodes, supportive family, etc. [3]. This emphasis may foster optimism, may increase the ability to make healthy use of the mental mechanism 'denial' and help to prepare for life changed by breast loss. An unhealthy use of denial is not a good sign, however, and certainly should not be encouraged by the physician. Most common examples of this extreme denial occur in patients who do not want to talk about disease at all, just want to 'get it over and done with', will not talk to people close to them, etc. Physicians do not like to see people suffer and some may welcome this kind of withdrawal in a patient. Some physicians even encourage it, rationalizing that if the patient does not think about it, it will not bother her or it will not be as real to her. Their actual motive may often have more to do with their own desire to avoid having to deal with their patient's emotions. However, mastectomy is real and it has real and significant psychological effects on a patient. An overuse of denial at this point usually leads to crashing at some later point: post-operative depression and chronic smoldering depressions later on.

Most of these psychological problems can be adequately dealt with by the interested surgeon or medical oncologist utilizing the treatment partnership in the manner previously described. Occasionally, patients present clues that the impending mastectomy may be precipitating a more serious psychiatric problem for which psychiatric consultation is indicated. A too grossly escap- ist attitude (overuse of denial), uncontrollable anxiety and/or depression, hints about bizarre fantasies concerning the outcome of treatment, frank expressions of delusions or hallucinations, serious suicidal ideation, etc. warrant psychiatric consultation. The temporary pre-operative use of small doses of a minor tranquilizer may prove effective in calming an excessively anxious patient (e.g. Diazepam 5 mg up to four times a day) and obviate the need for a psychiatrist. This kind of medication, however, should never be used in the normally anxious patient as a way to silence her in order to avoid dealing with her questions about mastectomy. Nor should they be used in large doses to make a patient groggy until the operation is over. Such uses would only serve to avoid the difficult but important tasks with the important goal of dealing with the patient now in order to avoid more serious psychological problems later. Shutting off the working through (i.e. the psychological work necessary in giving something up) of anticipated loss in the mastectomy period enhances the likelihood of chronic psychological problems later on. If small doses of the minor tranquilizer do not work well enough, psychiatric consultation is indicated.

It is usually preferable to discuss with the patient the availability of Reach for Recovery Volunteers and self help groups prior to surgery. These groups should never be forced on a patient, but are a resource which many find useful in the post-operative period. Knowing about their availability pre- operatively is reassuring to many patients.

Following mastectomy, the patient is likely to experience feelings of depression, crying spells, insomnia and nightmares [3]. About 70% of pa- tients experience some degree of depressive affect and almost half have some feelings of reactive elation (with an overlapping of the two groups) [6]. (Our ongoing study appears to confirm this.) The elation is best understood as a result of denial of depression, i.e. a fragile and transient defense against depression. If the treatment alliance (therapeutic partnership) has been well established, the physician is in a position to lend a friendly and understand- ing ear to his patient partner in this temporary period of distress. The reac- tions are natural and not difficult to understand, namely, the psychological significance of the new disfigurement. The physician must be available to listen sympathetically to the patient's cries of distress or even horror when she first confronts her mastectomy scar. This period is often one of intense feeling for a woman, and it is helpful for her to know that her physician can share this feeling with her and that she can rely on him and will continue to be able to rely on him for support. We can now see the value of the treat- ment alliance we were at such pains to set up. The better the stage has been set for the patient to be a true partner in the treatment, the better will be her chances of avoiding prolonged psychological distress and psychiatric sequelae. In a calm and non-pressured manner the physician can now begin to enlist his partner's aide in her own recovery. The emphasis in the discussions should be on what 'we' can do and on what the patient can do rather than on what the physician alone can do. The emphasis on 'we' fosters the 'physician–patient' partnership and helps the patient to identify an active role for herself in her own care. Discussions of wound care, proper exercise, etc. should be approached in a positive but non-pressured manner. Emphasis on what the patient can do and is expected to do should gradually lead to discussions of what can be expected in terms of resumption of normal activities of work and of love. Patience and non-pressure are emphasized because the patient should never be required to do more than she is ready to. One must avoid making the patient feel guilty or feel that she is not measuring up to the physician's expectations. Such feelings would only worsen whatever tendencies this patient may have to post-operative depressive feelings. The goal instead is to encourage the patient's active participation and a sense of being able to do something to further her own health care. One is attempting to minimize feelings of victimization, passive acquiescence to tragedy, and depression. The physician must gauge how active a role the patient is able to take, praise her for what she does, perhaps encourage her to do a little more if he senses that she is ready to, but never insist on more than she is able to do.

The emphasis of this discussion has purposely been on dealing with the patient and her problems rather than with her husband and family. The breast loss is experienced as her loss, a very personal loss. Contrary to the expectations of many, the majority of women in our study, both pre- and post-mastectomy, were much more concerned about the injury to their own personal body image than with concerns about what husbands or others would think of them. Concerns about how they appear to others (especially husbands) are often present and are often important, but in most cases not nearly as important as feelings of no longer being physically the same to themselves [5]. Nevertheless, husbands (and, less often, other family members and intimate friends) can often be enlisted to assist in the patient's psychological recovery. The fact that the patient has suffered a significant insult to her body image does not mean that she can not adjust to this loss and make the best of a changed body image. Most women can and do adjust. They do not dwell obsessively on the disfigurement and are able to resume normal lives even though they are frequently bothered by thoughts of breast loss. The physician should, early on, sound out the patient and her husband and make a clinical estimate about whether or not, in this particular marriage, the husband can assume a useful post-mastectomy role. If it is judged that he can, he should be enlisted and a frank discussion with him about the likely psychological effects on his wife pursued. He should be advised that his wife will suffer increased doubts about her personal feelings of femininity, sexual desirability, ability to enjoy and participate in sexual relations, and attractiveness. Verbal and physical reassurances of love and affection and, once she is able, the resumption of sexual relations will be helpful to her in making the necessary readjustment. Since she is going to consider the change in her body to be of much more significance than he will (and probably much more than he can even imagine she will), he is in a position to be supportive and reassuring about the additional concerns she may have about the mastectomy affecting his feelings for her. Reassurance by the husband that he does not consider her to be significantly disfigured and that she is still attractive and sexually desirable to him, can help her to modify her own personal feelings of disfigurement and to make readjustments in her sexual life. The husband, if able, may be helpful from the painful moment when the patient first sees and feels her mastectomy scar through the weeks and months required for full psychological adjustment to her breast loss in her personal life. However, the physician must first sound out the husband to see how capable and willing he is to participate. The minority of spouses who do not feel willing and able to be helpful should not be coerced in any way by the physician; under such circumstances more harm than good may ensue.

One of the factors in a woman's fears about losing a breast often relates to concerns about its effect on the sexual relationship with her husband. Numerous studies (over 200 in the past 25 years beginning with Bard and Sutherland in 1955 [9]) on this subject have been reported. In our study, such concerns do play an important role, though usually not the most important role in the fear of losing a breast. In our patients, this concern was not as great as were those about disfigurement and change in personal body image; the majority felt that they could eventually make adjustments, with some degree of difficulty, in their sexual relations with the help of their husbands, but that adjusting to a changed and deformed self image (body image) would be much more difficult and might never be accomplished. Here is an opportunity at this point to make use of the patients' temporary sexual problem. This change is associated with obvious potential psychiatric difficulties, yet the patient usually feels optimistic about overcoming this problem. As she makes her sexual adjustment and finds her husband more accepting of her and less affected by her disfigurement than she had imagined, her own ability to accept her changed body image is often enhanced. The greatest difficulty encountered is with women whose relationships with their husbands (or male friends) are ambivalent and tenuous so that this source of 'testing herself' with a likelihood of positive feedback is absent.

Since the physician will continue to see the patient, follow-up visits should also serve the purpose of reassessing her psychological adjustment to mastectomy. It should be made clear at the time of discharge from the hospital that the patient can call for an earlier appointment if psychological problems arise, just as she can for physical problems. Since a close rapport should now exist, the most common adjustment problems can usually be handled by the physician. These problems will often include revulsion upon looking at herself in the mirror, touching herself bathing, feeling less feminine than and, therefore, inferior to other women at a gathering, concerns that others can tell she is wearing a prosthesis and look down at her for it, shame at her husband seeing her nude, difficulty engaging in sexual relations, inability to enjoy sex once engaged because of thoughts about breast loss disfigurement, inability to resume friendships, work and leisure activities, etc. A sympathetic ear accompanied by a brief explanation of what the physician thinks is bothering her in terms of her personal body image concerns can be helpful in helping her over this difficult period. These explanations should be aimed at utilizing what the physician knows about the difficulty she is having with her changed body image and the attendent effects on her present psychological complaints. Every attempt should be made to aide the patient in speaking frankly about her problem and to utilize the physician's understanding of what is causing it in order to reinforce her sense of intellectual mastery over it. Attempts to reinforce denial by trying to have the patient stop talking about her problem will not work. This type of response is an automatic tendency of many people including physicians, especially with someone who is dwelling fruitlessly upon something about which she can do nothing. However, scolding or kidding a patient into not talking is more likely to make her feel lonely, isolated and not understood. A better approach is a combination of a frank facing of this problem which the patient has already pre-operatively indicated that she can adjust to (since she has chosen this form of treatment over other alternatives) and emphasis on positive aspects that do exist to facilitate her own automatic devices for calling forth defense mechanisms of denial and rationalization. The patient is then allowed to integrate the new and painful experience into what is a newly changed self image utilizing defense mechanisms with the help of her treatment partner, the physician.

The physician should repeatedly emphasize the mutual involvement of the physician–patient partnership in her continuing care and expect that the patient may need to continue to see him for support and reassurance from time to time. In most cases, frequent contact will be very brief and will diminish greatly with time but for some women it may continue indefinitely. It is for this latter patient that it is important for the physician who does enter into this type of relationship with the patient to be one who can take a sincere interest in her as a person attempting to become physically healthy and to resume a normal life. At any time that problems seem to become overwhelming, it is wise to have the patient return again in a week or two for a brief talk to see how she is progressing. Such an approach is usually sufficient and can turn a potentially chronic problem into a temporary one. Naturally, if these problems worsen over the course of several months and if other psychiatric symptoms (such as those mentioned earlier) appear, referral to a psychiatrist may be warranted.

SUMMARY

The main emphasis of this chapter has been to describe the emotional problems experienced by patients prior and subsequent to mastectomy, the developmental background of these problems, and the manner in which the physician should attempt to prevent, recognize, and treat these problems. The most important aspect in dealing with these problems is the development of a patient–physician relationship pre-diagnosis in which the patient is made to feel a full participant in the therapeutic plan.

REFERENCES

1. Ervin CV: Psychological adjustment to mastectomy. Medical Aspects of Human Sexuality 7:42–65, 1973.
2. Jamison KR, Wallisch DK, Pasnair RO: Psychological aspects of mastectomy: I. The woman's perspective. Am J Psychiatry 135:432–436, 1978.
3. Asken MJ: Psychoemotional aspects of mastectomy: a review of recent literature. Am J Psychiatry 132:56–59, 1975.
4. Sperling M: Conversion hysteria and conversion symptoms: a revision of classification and concepts. J Am Psychoanalytic Association 21:4, 1973.
5. Margolis GJ, Goodman RL: Changing the psychological morbidity of mastectomy. Presented at Annual Meeting of the American Psychiatric Association, Toronto, Canada, May 19, 1982.
6. Grandstaff HW: Behavior changes related to mastectomy. Presented at the 14th Annual San Francisco Cancer Symposium, March 1979.
7. Schwartz MD: An information and discussion program for women after a mastectomy. Arch Surg 112:276–281, 1977.
8. Hellman S, Harris JR, Levene MB: Radiation therapy of early carcinoma of the breast without mastectomy. Cancer 46:988–994, 1980.
9. Bard M, Sutherland AM: Psychological impact of cancer and its treatment. Cancer 8: 656–672, 1955.

12. Enterostomal Therapy: Supportive Care for the Cancer Patient

MARILYN A. WILLIS, JERILYN A. LOGEMANN, JACQUELINE B. BANGERT, MARY POWERS and SANDRA SHILLER GELBER

INTRODUCTION

The ostomy patient has undergone a prescribed treatment which impacts on every significant aspect of living [1]. The goal of rehabilitation with these patients is to restore them to optimal levels of functioning within their appropriate environment (home, work and social arena) given the limits imposed by their medical status [2].

To implement successful rehabilitation for this population, the attending physician must: 1) be accepting of the patient's altered state (the ostomy); 2) be committed to managing those problems that can be anticipated, and to preventing or reducing the occurrence of unnecessary complications; 3) be actively and consistently assessing patient needs; and 4) be able to use available resources successfully. This is an awesome responsibility because of the variety and complexity of problems encountered by the ostomy patient [1, 3].

There are a number of health care specialists available to assist the physician in identifying and addressing the ostomy patient's needs: the enterostomal therapist, the social worker, the psychologist, and the oncology nurse as well as lay self-help groups. This chapter focuses on the role of the enterostomal therapist, a professional speciality in nursing which provides direct patient care, patient and family teaching and rehabilitation for patients with colostomies, urinary diversions, ileostomies, or fistulas and draining wounds [4].

THE DEVELOPMENT OF ENTEROSTOMAL THERAPY AS A NURSING SPECIALITY

Colostomies have been performed since the early eighteenth century, when they were solely emergency, life-saving procedures. Today, over a

Higby, DJ (ed), Supportive Care in Cancer Therapy. ISBN 0-89838-569-5.
© 1983, Martinus Nijhoff Publishers, Boston. Printed in The Netherlands.

million people in the United States are living with some kind of permanent stoma-colostomy, ileostomy, ileal conduit or ureterostomy [5]. During the past two decades increasing emphasis has been placed on the pre-operative and post-operative teaching and care required by the ostomy patient. The medical focus is no longer limited to the successful completion of the surgical procedure and the healing process. It has been expanded to include rehabilitation activities often initiated prior to surgery to ensure that the patient's potential for resumption of pre-disease functioning is maximized [6].

Among the developments that have fostered and supported the expansion of ostomy patient rehabilitation has been the introduction of a new specialty area, enterostomal therapy, to address more effectively the complex needs of this patient population. In October 1958, when Norma Gill started working with ostomates at Cleveland Clinic, Dr Rupert Turnbull coined the title 'Enterostomal Therapist' to describe her position [7]. In 1971, therapist was changed to therapy to indicate an area of specialization for the R.N., L.P.N., E.T. or paramedic. By 1961, a training program was organized at Cleveland Clinic to fill the need for additional therapists.

By 1968, the North American Association for Enterostomal Therapy (NAAET) was founded in Phoenix, and held its first meeting in Cleveland, Ohio in January of 1969 for the purpose of communication and standardization. As the specialty grew, interest in enterostomal therapy became international and during the third conference of the NAAET the name of the Association was changed to The International Association of Enterostomal Therapy (IAET). In 1972 at the Fourth Annual Conference, the first set of by-laws was drafted and educational standards for Enterostomal Therapy schools were established including length of training and requirements for certification. At this time five schools were accredited.

At the Fifth Annual Conference (Chicago, 1973) the articles of the association were ratified and the membership file included 227 certified enterostomal therapists. A code of ethics, job description, and objectives of the organization were written in 1975, and the American Cancer Society invited the IAET to serve on the Service and Rehabilitation Committee of its National Board. In 1976, it was decided that only RNs would be admitted to enterostomal therapy educational programs for certification. Since that time the IAET has continued to grow until the profession now has over 1,500 enterostomal therapist members and 13 accredited training programs (Appendix A). Its annual conventions promote communication and continuing education activities and conduct the association's business. Seminars are presented by various regional groups throughout the year.

The educational programs offered by the 13 IAET approved schools vary in length from six to eight weeks and include intensive, individual classroom and clinical experiences (Appendix A). The curriculum focuses on: 1) a specific knowledge base related to the patient population, anatomy and physiology of the alimentary, genitourinary and integumentary systems, human sexuality, psychosocial, emotional, nutritional and pharmacological considerations, diagnostic techniques and treatment approaches, and basic nursing care of patients with stomas, pelvic exenteration, internal reservoir and perineal wounds; 2) *specific principles* to guide the delivery of care, including principles of rehabilitation, teaching, communication; and 3) *specific technical skills*, e.g., marking of stoma sites, use of prosthetic ostomy equipment and communication techniques.

OVERVIEW OF E.T. INTERVENTIONS WITH OSTOMY PATIENTS

Enterostomal therapists have the unique education to: 1) initiate and carry out pre- and post-operative ostomy management; 2) develop and implement effective teaching strategies which facilitate patient learning and self care; 3) evaluate psychosocial/emotional and sexual adjustment and implement interventions as appropriate; and 4) serve as a resource to both the patient and other professionals for the management of ongoing patient problems. Enterostomal therapists function, with some autonomy, in a variety of settings including acute care and chronic hospitals, clinics, visiting nurse associations and independent practice. It is important to stress that the care provided is not limited to the site of the ostomy, or only to ostomates, but can include other patient problems for which similar principles and knowledge apply. These services may include, for example, management of leaking gastrostomy tubes, decubitus care, and control of fecal and urinary incontinence. As nursing specialists, they have assumed the roles of care providers, educators, patient advocates, consultants and researchers.

The discussion that follows outlines the potential pre- and post-surgical involvement of the E.T. with the newly diagnosed and hospitalized cancer patient. Numerous examples are provided to illustrate the scope of services that are available and the focus of interventions by the E.T. Details of care, which may vary with the differences in therapy approach or individualized patient care plans, are omitted.

Pre-surgical intervention

E.T.'s are usually involved pre-operatively in patient care and teaching as a result of referral by the physician or nursing staff. Responsibilities of the E.T. include: a) examining the available medical data; b) interpreting contemplated surgical procedures to patient and family; c) assessing the physical and emotional status of the patient in order to establish priorities for post-operative care and management; d) teaching the patient and family; and e) pre-operative marking of the optimal stomal site.

Patient medical records are reviewed with focus on radiology and biopsy pathology reports. Discussion with the surgeon to elucidate anticipated surgical procedures is sometimes needed. Since patients and their families are not usually medically oriented, previous explanations about the surgery need to be repeated and clarified as appropriate. As an aid to patient understanding, the E.T. uses diagrams and pictures to explain the anatomy of the G.I. system and the possible effects of surgery.

The therapist uses this opportunity to identify physical disabilities and other factors which may hinder the patient's ability to manage ostomy care post-operatively. Observations are also made of interactions between patient and family members, if they are present. Particular emphasis is given to decreasing fears of the family by providing information and answering questions as appropriate. Educating the significant others is imperative pre-operatively since they will be providing much of the emotional support needed by the patient post-operatively. Reservations and concerns that family and friends might have regarding the stoma and anticipated recovery may keep them at a distance or restrict their involvement. These actions are often interpreted by the patient as signs of rejection.

Pre-operative marking of the optimal stoma site, at a time when the abdomen can be observed in many positions, is vital. Delay until the patient is in the operating room increases the chances of poor site selection, e.g. drapes may cover the bony prominences; a large breast may fall laterally; and it is difficult to be sure where a flaccid panniculus will hang. To quote Dr D'Orazio 'All our efforts to supply psychologic support are seriously jeopardized if there is not a decent stoma on which to build ... every patient needs a well-placed, well-constructed stoma that can be seen easily' [8]. Dr Turnbull showed that bringing the stoma through the rectus muscle and separating rather than cutting the rectus and fascia will prevent peristomal hernia [9].

In addition to teaching and stoma site marking, some E.T.'s set up a contract with their patients regarding post-operative expectations. Much anxiety is allayed if patients know they will not be required to take responsibility for their stoma until they regain the strength to do so, and if they know they will not be discharged until they are proficient in care of the stoma and appliance. Reassurance that help is available after hospital discharge, through local ostomy groups and ostomy out-patient clinics, also assists in sending well-prepared patients to surgery and simplifies post-operative care. These discussions pre-operatively provide evidence to patients that the therapist is accepting of the anticipated post-operation physical change.

Post-surgical interventions

Stomas can be designated by location, type and output:

Location — ileum
          — ascending, transverse, descending and sigmoid colon
          — colon or ileum (for urinary diversion)

Type   — end, with or without mucus fistula loop
          — double barrelled
          — ileal loop (for urinary diversion)

Output — fecal
          — urinary

Unfortunately, cancer may be diagnosed too late for definitive surgery and cure. For those persons with advanced cancer, a diverting loop ostomy is often indicated to alleviate obstruction.

Regardless of the type of ostomy, the goal after surgery and prior to hospital discharge is to have a patient who is confident in his/her ability to care for himself (with or without the help of family or friends). This goal can be achieved in a predictable and orderly sequence of interventions, although individual patient skills and recovery from the surgical experience dictate the speed and ease with which it occurs. The therapist supports and maintains open communication between patient, family, physician and nursing staff as a vital element in reaching the desired patient outcomes.

Focus of interventions (days one–three post-surgery)

The first task, particularly if no pre-operative teaching has been possible, is to create the trust that is necessary for learning to occur. During this period the enterostomal therapist assumes responsibility for ostomy care and utilizes this opportunity to demonstrate his/her acceptance of the patient's altered state as well as to observe the patient's reaction. Critical tasks to be accomplished include:

1. Identification and application of the appropriate equipment and materials (appliances, skin barriers, adhesives and deodorants).
2. Assessment of the patient's progress in recovering from the surgical experience.
3. Identification and recording of the stoma appearance, skin condition and the nature of the effluent.
4. Establishment (through negotiation with patient and staff) of a target date for self-sufficiency in ostomy care.
5. Creation of an open environment in which the patient and family can express feelings without fear of rejection or retaliation.

Focus of interventions (days four–six post-surgery)

As the patient regains strength and begins to actively interact with the environment, the therapist gradually introduces the knowledge and teaches the skills needed for ostomy care. As the E.T. begins to shift the responsibility for care to the patients, their ability to do their own care is assessed. A family member or friend is asked to assist if needed. Criteria for assistance include severe arthritis or other physical disability in hands and arms, senility, cataracts or blindness, or severe emotional problems. Children under age seven generally also require assistance. In addition, consideration may be given to future referral to a home health care agency or the visiting nurse association.

Discussions are instituted with all patients on topics such as diet, methods of coping with odor and elimination, and peristomal skin care. Specific areas of concern for particular types of ostomies are also reviewed. If the patient has a descending or sigmoid colostomy, a premorbid bowel history is obtained. Using this information, the physician's recommendations and the patient's personal preferences, the pros and cons of irrigation are discussed. Irrigation may or may not be started at this time. With urostomates, the need to prevent ascending tract infections through adequate fluid intake, maintenance of urine acidity and the use of night gravity drainage is emphasized. Discussions with the ileostomate center on the importance of preventing electrolyte imbalance, protecting peristomal skin and preventing intestinal blockage. Written instructions on self-care are given and discussed for each type of ostomy. The provision of emotional support through the use of an ostomy visitor is instituted at this time also, if earlier contacts have not been arranged.

Focus of interventions (days seven–ten post-surgery)

The responsibility for stoma care now rests for the most part on the patient with or without the assistance of a family member or friend as previously discussed. The enterostomal therapist assists by providing verbal reinforcement as the patient changes his appliance independently, at least twice. The significant other observes or assists, if warranted, at one of those times.

FOCUS OF DISCHARGE PLANNING

The enterostomal therapist's duties immediately prior to hospital discharge include:
1. Securing sufficient equipment and supplies for three to four weeks' care after discharge.
2. Providing an out-patient stoma clinic appointment in three to four weeks to re-evaluate stoma changes.

3. Instructing the patient to call sooner if a stoma problem develops.
4. Providing addresses of ostomy supply dealers near the patient's home.
5. Discussing methods to make the appliance less obtrusive during sexual intimacy.

If patient problems are anticipated, the E.T. will initiate referral to an appropriate community agency for follow-up assistance in the home setting.

Interventions post-hospital discharge

During the hospital stay, enterostomal therapists interact with patients who are in the process of adjusting to a series of major physical and emotional changes. Efforts are directed towards providing support and at the same time teaching the necessary management skills and measures to reduce or minimize potential problems. However, the professional staff recognize that transfer to the home environment, with its attending differences in structure, routines, roles, and resources can be problematic for even the well-prepared, new ostomate. In addition, once home, changes in patient needs, expectations, physical state and performance abilities can create difficulties that warrant continued professional intervention.

Currently, there are varying practices for ostomy patient follow-up by the E.T. post-hospital discharge. Some institutions have established out-patient stoma clinics which offer comprehensive services (including enterostomal therapy) on a routine basis. Other therapists have established various arrangements to see patients periodically on an out-patient basis, with more intensive scheduled follow-up based on the specific presenting problem. In other instances, for a variety of reasons, enterostomal therapists are primarily available to patients by telephone or through contacts at local ostomy club meetings.

In addition to variability in ostomy patient access to the E.T., there is also variability in intervention plans utilized by therapists during the post-hospitalization period. In an attempt to provide uniformity in approach during out-patient handling of ostomy problems, a multi-disciplinary, multi-institutional advisory committee to the Illinois Cancer Council developed a series of E.T. protocols to serve as a guide for patient problem identification and management [10]. The protocols were specifically planned for use with patients who received care from the E.T. during hospitalization, and who were being followed on a regularly scheduled basis for out-patient care.

The protocols are designed as decision trees for patient problem resolution in 10 potential areas of concern, including: abnormal bowel elimination (diarrhea and constipation); equipment management (appliance and irrigation); gas and odor; skin irritation and breakdown; inadequate nutritional intake, inadequate sexual adjustment; and patient anxiety. These problems are believed to represent difficulties for this target population during the post-discharge period [1, 3, 11].

The guidelines are based on standard care practices currently utilized by enterostomal therapists in the hospital setting, which are now being extended to the post-discharge period. The major components of each set of guidelines include: a) *specification* of major problem areas to be explored; b) *identification of consistent E.T. interventions*; and c) recommendation of *referral* resources. The protocols focus on process, with details provided for clarification.

The protocols for each problem area follow. In addition, one protocol, management of equipment, is discussed in detail to illustrate the potential usefulness of these decision trees. Only highlights or points of emphasis are reviewed from the other guidelines.

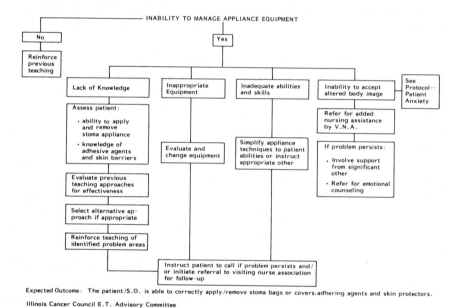

Expected Outcome: The patient/S.O. is able to correctly apply/remove stoma bags or covers, adhering agents and skin protectors.

Illinois Cancer Council E.T. Advisory Committee

Figure 1. Protocol: Management of appliances.

This protocol identifies some of the more common causes of patient problems with equipment management. One reason for patient difficulties may be the lack of knowledge regarding appliances. In teaching patients about equipment selection and management, the primary care provider must first assess the type of ostomy, the patient's dexterity and learning ability, as these factors will affect the application and removal of an appliance. Instruction covers the various types of adhesive products and the skin barrier to protect skin integrity. The nurse/E.T. continually evaluates previous teaching strategies for their effectiveness and selects alternate methods when necessary. It is important to reinforce teaching, especially in those areas identified as patient care problems.

If the equipment is inappropriate (i.e., it is not providing an adequate seal or adequate containment for effluent, is too large or too small, or is not odor-proof) then the care provider needs to evaluate the available equipment on the market. Once an assessment has been made of the patient's physical condition, a recommendation for change can be initiated to provide the appliance appropriate for this patient's individual needs.

Sometimes the patient has a difficult time with complex instructions or with poor hand coordination. If this situation occurs, the patient is fitted with disposable equipment, whenever possible. After the patient is discharged from the hospital, problems are managed by a referral to the Visiting Nurses Association or to an E.T. out-patient clinic. The IAET is developing a directory of existing clinics across the country. A current membership list of E.T.'s is available from the IAET and is helpful in determining the closest specialized E.T. in your area.

After surgery, patients may have problems accepting their altered body image. Many refuse to look at their stoma. Especially after temporary colostomies, patients have a tendency toward denial and often refer their care to another family member, friend or aid. If there is refusal to be independent and take charge of self-care, referral to the visiting nurse as well as other professionals for support and problem resolution is needed.

Most patients experience anxiety immediately after surgery, especially because of the change in body image. With time, support and teaching this anxiety is alleviated and the individual progresses again to a state of independence. If patients are having continued problems with self-acceptance, they may need a psychological consultant. The ultimate goal is for patients to be able to apply and remove their own stoma pouch, adhering agents, and skin protectors correctly with enough frequency to prevent leakage, odor and skin problems [11, 12].

Figures 2 and 3 outline the potential problems of patients with abnormal elimination. For the patient with constipation, the nurse will assess whether there is reduced physical activity, inadequate or poor fluid and fiber intake, abuse of medication such as laxatives, and the presence of disease or an obstructive process. The patient is referred to the physician for evaluation of bloating, abdominal cramping, pain, bleeding, diarrhea, stoma adhesions and swelling. Chronic constipation is reduced by drinking four to six glasses of water along with adding raw bran as bulk daily.

It is important to note that diarrhea may be a result of chemotherapy or radiation. During these treatments a patient who is wearing a security or closed-ended pouch should change to an open-end pouch. Continuing colostomy irrigations at this time may cause frustration since the patient cannot

262

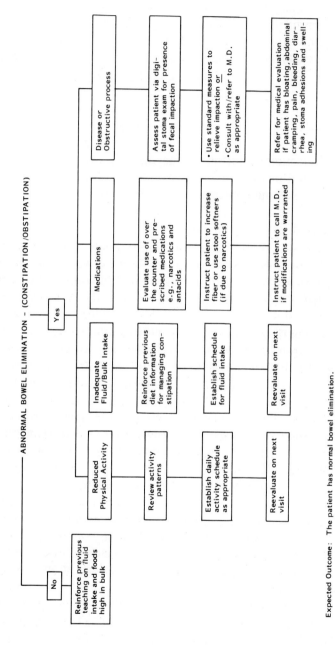

ABNORMAL BOWEL ELIMINATION – (CONSTIPATION/OBSTIPATION)

No

Reinforce previous teaching on fluid intake and foods high in bulk

Yes

Reduced Physical Activity

Review activity patterns

Establish daily activity schedule as appropriate

Reevaluate on next visit

Inadequate Fluid/Bulk Intake

Reinforce previous diet information for managing constipation

Establish schedule for fluid intake

Reevaluate on next visit

Medications

Evaluate use of over the counter and prescribed medications e.g., narcotics and antacids

Instruct patient to increase fiber or use stool softners (if due to narcotics)

Instruct patient to call M.D. if modifications are warranted

Disease or Obstructive process

Assess patient via digital stoma exam for presence of fecal impaction

• Use standard measures to relieve impaction or
• Consult with/refer to M.D. as appropriate

Refer for medical evaluation if patient has bloating, abdominal cramping, pain, bleeding, diarrhea, stoma adhesions and swelling

Expected Outcome: The patient has normal bowel elimination.

Illinois Cancer Council E.T. Advisory Committee

Figure 2. **Protocol: Management of constipation/obstipation.**

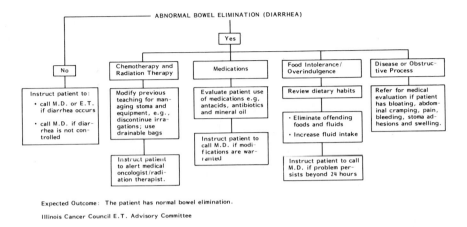

Figure 3. Protocol: management of diarrhea.

control diarrhea with irrigations. Diarrhea may also occur from a food intolerance or an overindulgence, and the individual's dietary habits need to be reviewed to find the offending food or fluid. The patient is instructed to contact the physician if the problem persists beyond 24 hours. Immediate follow-up is warranted because in addition to potential electrolyte imbalance, skin irritation is a real possibility. This latter problem may occur because of the increased volume and enzymes in liquid stools and the frequent appliance changes needed, due to poor adherence. If skin problems do arise, the patient has limited means to contain the effluent [13, 14].

A patient who has an ileostomy, ascending and temporary colostomy, ileal conduit, fistula and/or a wound is subject to skin irritation and breakdown from the discharging effluent. The epidermal skin layer is of primary concern to every patient. Variables that influence peristomal skin integrity are the composition, consistency, and quantity of effluent along with the underlying disease and treatment. Other variables are the patient's individual medication, surgical construction and location of the stoma, the skills of those caring for the patient, interest of the patient in self-care, and lastly the availability of proper supplies. When a fungal infection is present it is necessary for the physician to support rehabilitative patient care by prescribing an antifungal, non-greasy, topical medication to facilitate early and speedy recovery. In some cases, results are seen within 24 to 48 hours [15, 16] (see Figure 4).

In the cancer patient, adequate in take is difficult to manage since anorexia along with nausea may be present. It is important to have the physician and dietitian assess individual metabolic needs and instruct the patient and family in implementing a set regime to maintain the patient's usual or appropriate weight level [14, 17].

264

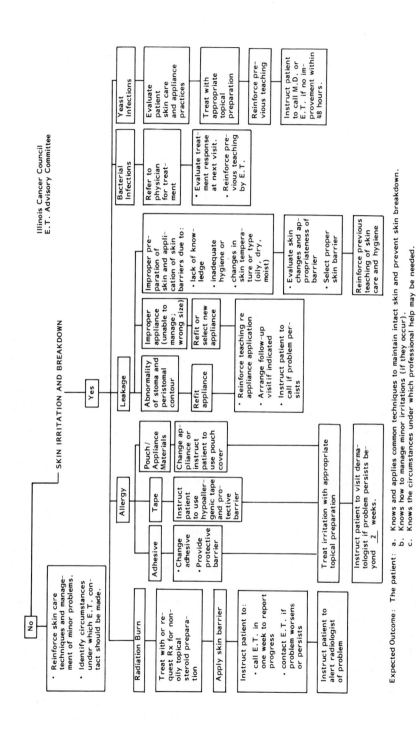

Figure 4. Protocol: care of skin.

Illinois Cancer Council
E.T. Advisory Committee

SKIN IRRITATION AND BREAKDOWN

No

• Reinforce skin care techniques and management of minor problems.
• Identify circumstances under which E.T. contact should be made.

Yes

Radiation Burn
Treat with or request Rx for non-oily topical steroid preparation

Apply skin barrier

Instruct patient to:
• call E.T. in one week to report progress
• contact E.T. if problem worsens or persists

Instruct patient to alert radiologist of problem

Allergy

Adhesive
• Change adhesive
• Provide protective barrier

Tape
Instruct patient to use hypoallergenic tape and protective barrier

Pouch/Appliance Materials
Change appliance or instruct patient to use pouch cover

Treat irritation with appropriate topical preparation

Instruct patient to visit dermatologist if problem persists beyond 2 weeks.

Leakage

Abnormality of stoma and peristomal contour
Refit appliance

Improper appliance (unable to manage: wrong size)
Refit or select new appliance

• Reinforce teaching re appliance application
• Arrange follow-up visit if indicated
• Instruct patient to call if problem persists

Improper preparation of skin and application of skin barriers due to:
• lack of knowledge
• inadequate hygiene or
• changes in skin temperature or type (oily, dry, moist)

• Evaluate skin changes and appropriateness of barrier
• Select proper skin barrier

Reinforce previous teaching of skin care and hygiene

Bacterial Infections
Refer to physician for treatment

• Evaluate treatment response at next visit.
• Reinforce previous teaching by E.T.

Yeast Infections
Evaluate patient skin care and appliance practices

Treat with appropriate topical preparation

Reinforce previous teaching

Instruct patient to call M.D. or E.T. if no improvement within 48 hours.

Expected Outcome: The patient: a. Knows and applies common techniques to maintain intact skin and prevent skin breakdown.
b. Knows how to manage minor irritations (if they occur).
c. Knows the circumstances under which professional help may be needed.

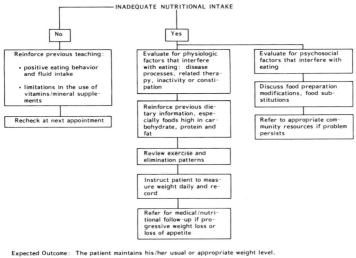

Expected Outcome: The patient maintains his/her usual or appropriate weight level.

Illinois Cancer Council E.T. Advisory Committee

Figure 5. Protocol: management of nutritional intake.

After a sigmoid colostomy, care of the stoma may include irrigation or the wearing of an odor-proof pouch [18, 19]. Initially the physician usually orders irrigation based on the individual's prior bowel history, dexterity, learning ability, and daily activity schedule. Irrigation is a practical technique only if there is reason to expect the patient to remain continent for approximately 24 hours. Within the framework of this expectation, the protocol (Figure 6) lists other problems which may arise.

Currently there is controversy surrounding the need for irrigations for sigmoid colostomy management. In addition, there are differences in practice regarding when these techniques are taught and implemented. Some E.T.'s instruct patients to irrigate while they are in the hospital. Others are reluctant to initiate the activity during this period because of possible patient discomfort and limitations. For example, distention of the bowel with a liter of irrigating fluid may cause incisional discomfort and soreness of the perineal area, or low energy level may preclude the patient from sitting for the protracted period needed to accomplish an irrigation. In addition, if chemotherapy or radiation therapy is initiated, the diarrhea which may result will frustrate the patient's attempts to stay continent for 24 hours after irrigating. Under these circumstances, and after consultation with the physician, therapists will discuss the procedure as a later possibility and let the patient go home wearing a drainable bag.

If the option exists, it is often helpful to have patients keep a bowel diary for four to six weeks after discharge before deciding on irrigation. Many

266

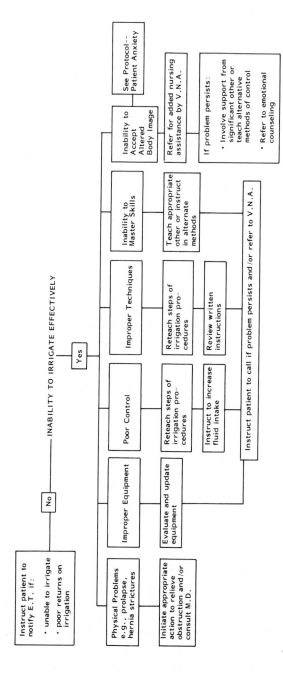

Instruct patient to notify E.T. if:
• unable to irrigate
• poor returns on irrigation

— INABILITY TO IRRIGATE EFFECTIVELY

No

Yes

Physical Problems e.g., prolapse, hernia strictures
Initiate appropriate action to relieve obstruction and/or consult M.D.

Improper Equipment
Evaluate and update equipment

Poor Control
Reteach steps of irrigation procedures
Instruct to increase fluid intake
Instruct patient to call if problem persists and/or refer to V.N.A.

Improper Techniques
Reteach steps of irrigation procedures
Review written instructions

Inability to Master Skills
Teach appropriate other or instruct in alternate methods

Inability to Accept Altered Body Image
Refer for added nursing assistance by V.N.A.
If problem persists:
• Involve support from significant other or teach alternative methods of control
• Refer to emotional counseling

See Protocol— Patient Anxiety

Expected Outcome: The patient is able to correctly perform the irrigating procedures and to maintain adequate control.

Illinois Cancer Council E.T. Advisory Committee

Figure 6. Protocol: management of irrigation equipment.

patients with sigmoid or descending colostomies who are not receiving oncological therapy settle down to one, or sometimes two, bowel movements a day. Obviously, they can gain little from an hour in the bathroom irrigating. Also, delaying the implementation of irrigation practices gives the E.T. time to see what, if any, oncological therapy will be instituted and what its effect will be. A colostomate who becomes accustomed to wearing a drainable appliance is not nearly as upset by diarrhea as one who has the impossible goal of continence during these trying periods.

Referring the patient to an out-patient stoma/ostomy clinic to learn irrigation at four to six weeks post-discharge, with a physician's order to have irrigation techniques taught if the bowel diary so indicates, solves many of these problems.

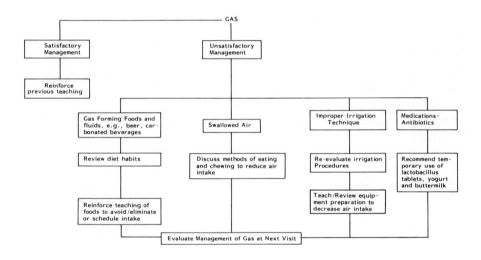

Expected Outcome: The patient knows and applies techniques to decrease gas.

Illinois Cancer Council E.T. Advisory Committee

Figure 7. Protocol: management of gas.

With the ileostomate, colostomate, and fistula patient gas may be a problem. Gas distends the pouch. Thus, an excessive amount of gas or ignoring gas as it fills the appliance leads to breaking the seal or dislodgement of the collecting pouch. Some foods causing gas are beans, beer, carbonated drinks, cucumbers, onions, peas, cabbage, broccoli, cauliflower, yeast and dairy products [20].

268

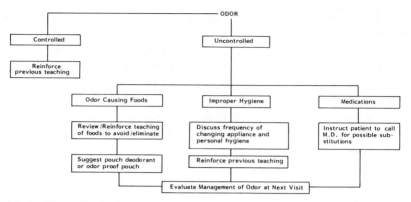

Expected Outcome: The patient knows and applies techniques to minimize odor.

Illinois Cancer Council E.T. Advisory Committee

Figure 8. Protocol: management of odor.

A problem with odor is frequently alleviated by eliminating foods such as onions, cabbage, broccoli, asparagus, peas, beans, turnips, eggs, fish, garlic and some spices from the diet. Odor perception is individualized and patients may be concerned when changing or draining the appliance. They need to be reassured that odor is normal and no different than that experienced with the usual methods of elimination. The goal is proper hygiene along with dietary discretion to reduce or prevent potential problems [20].

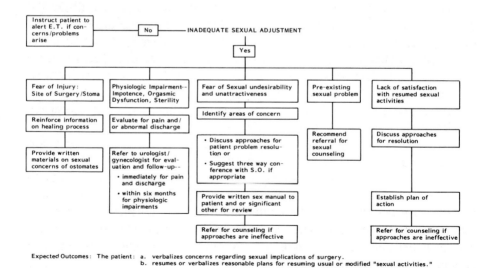

Expected Outcomes: The patient: a. verbalizes concerns regarding sexual implications of surgery.
b. resumes or verbalizes reasonable plans for resuming usual or modified "sexual activities."

Illinois Cancer Council E.T. Advisory Committee

Figure 9. Protocol: management of sexual adjustments.

During the course of their hospitalization or after discharge, patients must confront issues of sexual adjustment. An ostomy can assault a patient's self-concept through altered body functions, self-esteem and sexuality [21]. The etiology of potential sexual problems generally results from: 1) physical impairment; 2) psychological adjustment disorders; and 3) pre-existing sexual problems.

Physical impairment from cancer and its therapies can result in impotence, orgasmic dysfunction and sterility. For the male, the ability to have an erection and to ejaculate is affected by the amount of tissue removed and the resulting temporary or permanent damage to the parasympathetic nerves. Intercourse for some females may be painful while the perineal wound is healing. In those with resections, including the vaginal wall and other genital organs, sexual union may be unsatisfying or even impossible [22]. Chemotherapy and radiation can dry vaginal secretions, render males impotent and lead to infertility. More subtle, but equally important, is the decreased libido that accompanies fatigue and dysphoria induced by the disease and medical interventions [23].

The E.T. and other members of the health care team can help prepare patients and their partners pre-surgically by providing them with information regarding the potential effects of medical intervention on their sexuality. In situations that require expert intervention, the E.T. assesses the problem and refers patients and partners for extensive physical work-up by the urologist/gynecologist and/or to sexual counselors.

Body image is understandably distorted in the ostomate. The sight of the stoma, the time and frequency of discharge, the potential of spillage, the appearance of the appliance and the fear of injury all have a dramatic effect on physical relationships, from holding hands and friendly kisses to intercourse [23]. Patients who feel repulsive and who repulse their partners have little chance of effective sexual contact of any kind. The anxiety and depression that result from patients' concerns regarding the pain of treatment, resulting disability, loss of employment and/or death are other psychological barriers that may impede sexual adjustement.

E.T.'s set the tone that conveys an openness, acceptance and importance of sexual concerns. They must assess the intensity of the problem, then identify and utilize appropriate resources in the hospital or community to provide required intervention. Pre-existing sexual problems will usually resurface during this time. Many patients or their partners will seek to blame the ostomy for all their interpersonal difficulties. Frequently the surgery provides one partner with justification to avoid intimacy. This physical rejection is often evidence of long-standing emotional turmoil and requires recognition by the E.T. The therapist again must identify problems, set the stage for discussion and make referrals to counseling.

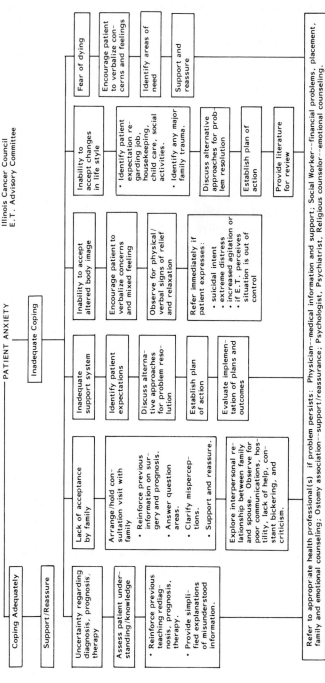

Figure 10. Protocol: management of patient anxiety.

Pre-surgical intervention by the enterostomal therapist including adequate instruction and explanation, facilitates patient acceptance and reduction of anxiety. Anxiety, as a response to a stressful event, is an essential ingredient in coping. It is not the experience of anxiety, but the way the patient handles the anxiety, that constitutes the difference between emotional adjustment and mental disturbance. Protocol 10 identifies potential sources of anxiety and provides direction in helping the ostomate restore adequate coping.

PSYCHOLOGICAL OVERVIEW

Cancer affects a patient's sense of psychological as well as physical well-being. The professional role of E.T.'s frequently places them in the position of being the member of the medical team who becomes most intimately involved with patient and family dynamics. For this reason, it is often the E.T. who first identifies and intervenes in problems of psychological adjustment.

Because individuals are unique, patients will respond in their own style to the diagnosis of cancer and the reality of life with an ostomy. Studies confirm that the majority of patients adjust adequately to their ostomy and only rarely does a severe neurotic or psychotic reaction result [24]. But all patients and their families must be prepared for a tremendous investment of time, energy, money and emotional and physical pain. Having an ostomy will bring stress that can either become a destructive force or serve to reaffirm the strengths and resources patients and families possess. E.T.'s believe the difference lies in early, intensive rehabilitation. In general, patient and family coping depends on: 1) the premorbid personality; 2) the cancer experience; and 3) the reactions of significant others.

The premorbid personality refers to the psychodynamics patients bring into the medical situation. In other words it defines who the person was before the medical crisis. Though crisis provides an opportunity for personal growth as old, non-functional coping mechanisms are discarded for new more functional ones [25], radical personality changes rarely occur. Patients, who before their diagnosis were passive and private, cannot be expected to reach out and readily verbalize their feelings and needs after surgery.

Crisis is also a time when old, unresolved past conflicts resurface. As a procedure which permanently alters bowel function and control, this surgery and its aftermath are likely to rekindle the emotionally charged issues surrounding early life toilet training and self-discipline [26]. Therefore, how a patient responds and adjusts to the ostomy is frequently determined by the conscious or unconscious value of the affected organ and its function [27].

The E.T. must, therefore, make an assessment of patient and family functioning pre-disease in order to anticipate areas of intolerable stress and to plan intervention to minimize potential disequilibrium, disintegration and social isolation. Four critical areas for pre-surgical assessment of patient and family include: 1) premorbid functioning – coping mechanisms, life styles, roles, communication patterns and social networks; 2) religious and cultural philosophies and attitudes; 3) adaptation to past crises; and 4) real or imagined value of rectum, anus and bowel control.

The ultimate goal is not to force patients or families into a preconceived format for adaptation, but to assist them in attaining *their* maximum level of adjustment. Recognizing patients' unique traits allows the medical team to anticipate and plan for potential problems and special needs. For example, if a patient is from a subculture which dictates that men take care of women, problems may arise when the male patient is forced to be dependent on a female nurse. Knowing this the E.T. can plan to institute early self-care and assign the patient to male staff when feasible.

Combining this awareness of patient and family functioning and cultural attitudes with an understanding of how the patient and family faced past crises and the value of sphincter control leads to an assessment and treatment plan which identifies and utilizes strengths as well as recognizing and compensating for limitations. The presurgical period is thus a critical time. It marks the beginning of the 'cancer experience'. To be effective, intensive psycho-social and rehabilitation intervention must begin during this phase.

After surgery patients must deal with the physical and psychological stress and pain of recovery. Days are absorbed by illness. Time becomes a measured segment between skin care and dressing changes [28]. Faced with adjustment to altered body function, disfigurement, the need to regress to incorporate new bowel habits and temporary dependency on family, medical staff and appliances, it is not surprising that the ostomy patient views the post-surgical period as an infantilizing, dehumanizing experience. The added problems of odor, spillage, noise and appearance of the stoma can be repugnant to family and staff. If these factors influence people to stay away from the patient, then the patient will feel isolated and withdraw from others at a time when they most need support and acceptance.

Combined with this lack of control over body functioning, patients feel a lack of control over future well-being. To compensate, patients often exert more rigid controls over other areas of their lives. They frequently develop obsessive-compulsive behavior patterns. Some become 'irrigation addicts' spending as long as 24 to 56 hours a week irrigating [29].

During the post-surgical phase there is an understandable preoccupation with one's body and grief for loss of self-intactness. Druss describes the fantasies patients develop as a result of changes in body image [26]. Many patients experience a period of depression and irrational grieving for real or presumed loss of bowel control, loss of sphincter control, and loss of sexual attractiveness and potency. Others develop phantom rectum sensation or equate the stoma with a sexual organ and 'derive erotic gratification from stimulation of their stoma' [24].

The E.T.'s role during the post-surgical period involves enhancing patient/family adaptation by providing them with adequate information, encouraging autonomy and focusing on maintaining internal equilibrium [29]. To accomplish this, E.T.'s consult with and refer to the mental health professionals available to them.

At the time of discharge from the hospital, patient and family anxiety frequently peaks. Now concerns that previously took a backseat to physical pain and survival needs can no longer be ignored. Patients must confront issues of altered body image, sexuality and intimacy as previously described. Hospital discharge often disrupts family equilibrium further as patients attempt to resume or redefine their roles and responsibilities in the home. Weaning from the security of the hospital floor and dependency on the medical staff can produce fear in many patients as well as overwhelm family members. It is also at this point when financial pressures begin to take a toll. The cost of continued medical treatment, dwindling insurance coverage and employment concerns are a reality for most families. In order to prevent or minimize the trauma that surrounds discharge, E.T.'s begin helping patients and families prepare for this event from the day they are first admitted to the hospital.

In making the transition from hospital to home and community, patients will have to deal with the reactions of the significant people in their lives – grandchildren, employers, neighbors. The results of Dyk and Sutherland's study [30] on adaptation of colostomy patients echoed the conclusions of Prudden who found that 'those who did best were those whose period of adjustment had been strongly supported by those persons who were most important to them' [24]. Family and friends are therefore often the key to a patient's success or failure in adjusting to life with an ostomy.

Unfortunately the climate in most communities interferes with positive of adaptation. Our society has a health, youth, beauty focus that is rejecting cancer patients. Fairy tales condition us to it at an early age. The hero/heroine is depicted as young, strong and vital which equals good. But the witch is old, disfigured and unclear; this symbolizes something bad. Our T.V. commercials proclaim that 'when you have your health, you have everything', falsely implying that without health you have nothing. As one cancer patient put it 'to have Cancer is to be Cancer. People treat you as the disease itself and are afraid to get physically and emotionally close'. The social isolation, either real or imagined, is often the cruelest side effect from surgery.

The medical team cannot ignore their impact on patient and family coping. Staff sets the tone for how patients view themselves and staff–patient interaction represents a model for families in interpersonal interactions. Because patients are exquisitely sensitive to non-verbal communications, staff members must realize that patients will always uncover staff's true feelings and attitudes. People working with ostomates must investigate their feelings about and experiences with cancer, disfigurement and loss, and understand their motivation in working with this patient population. Staff must also be prepared to accept the limitations of their professional skills and expertise. Many patients will fail to respond to medical treatment; others will fail to adapt.

Patients who do survive go through a process of shedding their cancer. This means reaching the dates and anniversaries which symbolize leaving their illness behind. This is an interesting phenomenon in which patients experience both a wish for cure and a fear that they will not be able to continue to adapt. The joy of living is marred by the threat of recurrence and the fear of the quality of their new life. When a patient has come to a full acceptance that he/she will live, he/she begins to realize that he/she is not the only person whose future involves medical uncertainty [28]. Many patients are then able to incorporate painful, frustrating experiences into their personalities and grow towards a new maturity. This is when they get in touch with inner strengths and courage and learn that they do have the capacity to cope and adjust – a capacity they may never have realized they possessed. This can lead both patients and family members to an emergence of new self-worth and a feeling of heroism as they appreciate that they were able to endure an extremely theatening experience. The role for the E.T. and medical team at this stage is ... to let go.

RELATED RESEARCH AND ISSUES IN THE FIELD

There have been extensive reports in the literature on: 1) optimal surgical interventions; 2) specific management tcchniques for identified problems; 3) psycho-social issues; and 4) experiences of patients living with ostomies. However, because of the newness of the field, there is limited information on the impact of the enterostomal therapist on patient outcomes or of specific ostomy rehabilitation programs.

Review of research on the problems of ostomy cancer patients
Studies on ostomy patient problems conducted during the early 1950s and

1960s reveal a myriad of difficulties involving both the physical and psycho-social domain. A classic study of the day-to-day problems created by the establishment of a colostomy and the methods by which the cancer patient solves these problems was reported by Sutherland and others in 1952 [27]. The investigators attempted to identify systematically the major change in, or curtailment of functioning and to relate these areas to the adaptive mechanisms and previous experiences of the patient. Fifty-seven men and women were interviewed in the areas of surgical experiences, colostomy management, adaptation patterns and social participation. Although the detailed findings are too lengthy to include, the following select patient problems serve to highlight issues that in many instances are still of prime importance. Almost all of the patients reported a change in their social life and problems with irrigations and spillage; one third reported serious handicaps to business and personal life due to the frequency of the latter. Forced reduction in work or household activities, particularly strenuous tasks, were related by the majority of the study group. Approximately one third of the patients were depressed during hospitalization or during convalescence. In addition, of the men who were totally impotent (50% of the male sample) all but three were considerably distressed by their state. Females on the other hand were reluctant to discuss sexual performance. The suggestion was made that women who were frigid prior to surgery used the presence of the colostomy to justify termination of future sexual activity.

The authors concluded that on the average, when serious curtailment of function or activity occurs, with the exception of sexual impairment in men, it represents a failure in management. Their recommendations were directed towards the health professional and include suggestions for: 1) a heightened awareness by the surgeon of potential patient problems and involvement of the surgeon during the pre- and post-operative period; 2) increased attention to family reactions, the ability of members to understand patient needs and the capacity to provide appropriate support; 3) an appreciation of the personal and situational components of the teacher–learner relationship (when specific management techniques are being taught); 4) an awareness of the potential for psychological distress and the need for timely interventions; and 5) close collaboration between health team members.

Dyk and Sutherland also interviewed the same patients to determine their perception of the response of their spouse and other family members during the pre-operative, hospital, convalescent and post-convalescent period [30]. Family reactions were varied. They differed according to the period examined and were intimately tied to the nature of the pre-existing relationship. The most consistent pattern across patients was noted during hospitalization when positive accounts of visiting were frequently recalled. This phenomenon may be due to attempts by both patient and family to conform to expected behaviors as well as to the fact that the responsibility of day-to-day care requirements in the constraints of the home setting were not yet a reality. The authors suggest that the nature of the family's response after surgery is consistent with their attitudes observed earlier, for example, when symptoms first manifest themselves, at the time of visits to the physician or during the surgical experience. Dyk and Sutherland affirm that the spouse is often the key to the patient's success or failure in making the necessary life-style adjustments after surgery.

Patient problems have been further delineated in subsequent studies, and some efforts made to identify health care delivery and related issues. Rowbotham identified the reasons why 134 persons with transverse and sigmoid colostomies visited the Stoma Rehabilitation Clinic in Boston in 1971 [6]. Odor, a correctable problem, was the number one stated purpose for the visit across both groups. Other difficulties included skin irritation, a leaking appliance, prolapse, hernia and stenosis. He suggested that it often takes time and several visits for staff to understand some of the complexities of patients living with an ostomy. The voicing of a small complaint may be an excuse for a follow-up visit. In truth, an underlying depression which does not readily manifest itself, may be present. Rowbotham recommends a comprehensive clinic setting rather than a doctor's office as the ideal place for addressing the needs of the out-patient ostomy population.

Lenneberg likewise advocates the need for both stoma clinics and enterostomal therapists as resources supportive of quality care and teaching for ostomates [31]. In addition to characterizing the types of assistance sought by ostomy patients when returning for follow-up visits, her study pinpointed time frames in which patients sought help. Fifty-six percent of the 300 patients studied were seeking assistance after the first post-operative year. Given that problems may be reasonably anticipated, she raises the question as to why systematic provisions for care have not been more widely instituted.

Other investigators have raised similar concerns as a result of their posthospital discharge surveys of ostomy patients through interview or questionnaire. In England, Eardley et al. interviewed 76 patients who had a permanent colostomy for six months or more; 95% had a diagnosis of cancer [32]. The interview covered the topics of the hospital experience, early adjustment and current adjustment. More than 25% of the patients felt that they had received insufficient information about the colostomy during hospitalization. Thirty-three percent of the patients were not satisfied with after-care facilities and 63% were still having problems with management post-surgery. In general, although Eardley concluded that patients had coped well, 39% were currently restricted in some aspect of social life, leisure or employment. The total percentage of patients experiencing residual problems increased to 53% when depression and sexual problems were included. The authors strongly recommended that patients should not be discharged until they are able to manage their stomas and that efforts should be made to minimize discomforts and limitations through the provision of effective post-discharge services. The possible design of those post-discharge services was not addressed.

Follick and Turk designed a survey to assess problems common to all forms of ostomies as well as to identify problems specific to particular types of ostomy patients [3]. A list of potential problems was generated from discussions with select health professionals, ostomy patients and family, and review of the literature. The questionnaire was administered to 131 patients with colostomies, ileostomies and urostomies ranging from several months to 30 years post-surgery. Six categories of problems were assessed: technical management, occupational adjustment, social adjustment, marital/sexual adjustment, family adjustment and emotional adjustment. Data from this unpublished report indicates that 1) 84% of the patients studied identified problems with one or more aspects of technical management; 2) a large percentage felt that their needs for information were unfulfilled; 3) 41% of the patients reported problems with sexual relationships while 51% reported a change in sexual activity (three quarters of whom identified a decrease); 4) 70% of the patients reported a change in social activities (39% indicated an increase, 31% reported a decrease) and 31% felt that their concerns over leakage and odor directly influenced their social activities; 5) 33% indicated more frequent depressions since ostomy surgery; and 6) 36% experienced unusual amounts of anxiety in social situations.

The research studies cited above, while identifying problems and difficulties that patients encounter at various points in time relative to their surgery, do not correlate or interrelate these experiences with the specific management interventions provided or utilized by the patient population. Professionals intimately involved with the care of the ostomy patient report techniques for successful management of a variety of the patient difficulties identified. Ostomates themselves have outlined the positive benefits received from such resources as family members, enterostomal therapists, local ostomy clubs, visiting nurse and home health care agencies, medical staff and other professionals. Yet, there are no definitive studies evaluating various interventions designed to eliminate specific problems experienced.

Care options currently available to ostomy patients

Without this definitive information identifying optimal interventions, providers of health services have responded to perceived patient needs by initiating a variety of systems of care delivery. Subjective judgment would indicate that the most ideal approach is one that provides multi-disciplinary follow-up during hospitalization and a planned, accessible out-patient program with established linkages to community resources. This plan may be best examplified by various Stoma Clinics which have been instituted in several areas of the country. These programs however, are few in number and are usually most readily available in urban settings and larger metropolitan hospitals.

SUMMARY

This chapter has provided an overview of the practice of enterostomal therapy as it relates to the cancer patient who has undergone surgery resulting in an ostomy. Typical roles that the therapist may assume with the patient and family during the pre- and post-surgery period are outlined. Sample protocols for care after discharge from the hospital are presented and briefly discussed. Other roles and training of the E.T. are also reviewed.

Psycho-social considerations for this population are highlighted since these factors are intimately intertwined with the overall achievement of rehabilitation goals. It is hoped that the data presented not only provide evidence of the diversity and complexity of the issues involved in caring for cancer ostomy patients, but also pinpoint the vital need for appropriate and timely utilization of various health care personnel, and for collaboration among members of the health team, including the enterostomal therapist.

APPENDIX A. IAET-APPROVED PROFESSIONAL EDUCATION PROGRAMS

State/City	Institution
Arizona, Tucson	Tucson Medical Center
California, Los Angeles	USC Coslar
San Diego	University of California
Canada, Vancouver, BC	St. Paul's Hospital
Georgia, Atlanta	Emory University
Kansas, Kansas City	University of Kansas School of Nursing
Minnesota, Minneapolis	Abbott-Northwestern Hospital, Inc.
Missouri, St. Louis	The Jewish Hospital
New York, Buffalo	Roswell Park Memorial Institute
New York	Memorial Sloan-Kettering Cancer Center
Ohio, Cleveland	Cleveland Clinic Foundation
Pennsylvania, Harrisburg	Harrisburg Hospital
Texas, Houston	M. D. Anderson Hospital and Tumor Institute

REFERENCES

1. Kirkpatrick JR: The stoma patient and his return to society. Front Radiat Ther Onc 14: 20–25, 1980.
2. Mayer NH: Concepts in cancer rehabilitation. In: Oncologic Medicine, Sutnick AI, Enstrom PF (eds). Baltimore, University Park Press, 1976, pp 333–344.
3. Follick MJ, Turk D: Problem specification by ostomy patients (Phase I). Paper presented at the 12th annual meeting of the Association for the Advancement of Behavior Therapy, Chicago, 1978.
4. Rodriguez DB: Enterostomal therapy: an editorial. The Cancer Bulletin 33(1):3, 1981.
5. Lenneberg E et al.: When a patient has or needs an ostomy. Patient Care 2(13):112–151, 1977.
6. Rowbotham JL: Advances in rehabilitation of stoma patients. Cancer 36(2):702–704, 1975.
7. Rizzo M: Here's to progress: the IAET comes of age. E.T. Journal: Winter, 1977.
8. D'Orazio ML: Rehabilitation of ostomy patients. In: The Cancer Patient: Social and Medical Aspects of Care, Cassileth BR (ed). Philadelphia, Lea and Febiger, 1979, pp 185–199.
9. Turbull RB, Weakley FL: Atlas of Intestinal Stomas. St. Louis, The CV Mosby Company, 1967.
10. The Illinois Cancer Council E.T. Advisory Committee: Bangert J, Bozinovitch D, Eatough D, Keithley J, Kemp M, LaGesse J, Logemann J, Nicosia J, Powers M, Willis M.
11. Donovan MI, Pierce SG: Cancer Care Nursing. New York, Appleton-Century-Crofts, 1977, pp 165–168.
12. Broadwell DC, Appleby CH, Bates MA, Jackson BS: Principles and techniques of pouching. In: Principles of Ostomy Care, Broadwell DC, Jackson BS (eds). St. Louis, CV Mosby Company, 1982, pp 565–643.
13. Click C: Special considerations for the ostomy patient. The Cancer Bulletin 33(1):24–26, 1981.
14. Thawley C, Stadnik L: Nutrition Information for Ostomates. Delaware, The Wilmington Medical Center Cancer Program, 1980.
15. Reardon M: Care of the patient with an ileostomy. The Cancer Bulletin 33(1):12–14, 1981.
16. Lazar P, Sarbacker JD, Kowalski M: Recognizing, Treating, and Preventing Ostomy-Related Skin Problems. Illinois, Hollister Inc, 1978.
17. Hunter E: Nutritional therapy for the cancer patient. In: Nursing Care of the Cancer Patient, Bouchard-Kurtz R, Speese-Owens N(Aut). St. Louis, The CV Mosby Company, 1978, pp 68–85.
18. Hampton B: Colostomy care. The Cancer Bulletin 33(1):8–11, 1981.
19. Goode PS: Postoperative considerations. In: Principles of Ostomy Care, Broadwell DC, Jackson BS (eds). St. Louis, The CV Mosby Company, 1982, pp 369–380.
20. Rowbotham JL: Managing colostomies. CA-A Cancer Journal for Clinicians 31(6):336–345, Nov/Dec 1981.
21. Schain WS: Sexual functioning, self-esteem and cancer care. In: Frontiers of Radiation Therapy and Oncology, Vaith JM, Beomberg RC, Adler L (eds). 14th Annual San Francisco Cancer Symposium, S Karger, 1980, pp 12–19.
22. Dericks VC: The psychological hurdles of new ostomates: helping them up ... and over. Nursing '74, October, 1974.
23. Derogates L, Kourlesis S: An approach to evaluation of sexual problems in the cancer patient. CA-A Cancer Journal for Clinicians 31(1):46–50, Jan/Feb 1981.

24. Prudden JF: Psychological problems following ileostomy and colostomy. In: Rehabilitation of the Patient with a Colostomy. The American Cancer Society Reprint, 1971.
25. Lindemann E: Coping with long-term disability. In: Coping and adaptation, Caelhoe GV et al. (eds). New York, Basic Books, pp 127–139.
26. Druss RG et al.: Psychologic response to colectomy. Archives of General Psychiatry 18:53, 1968.
27. Sutherland AM et al.: The psychological impact of cancer and cancer surgery: adaptation to the dry colostomy; preliminary report. Cancer 5:857–872, 1952.
28. Zubrod GC: Success in cancer treatment. Cancer 36(1):250–269, 1975.
29. White RW: Strategies of adaptations: an attempt at systematic description. In: Coping and Adaptation, Caelhoe GV et al. (eds). New York, Basic Books, pp 55–58.
30. Dyk RB, Sutherland AM: Adaptation of the spouse and other family members to the colostomy patient. Cancer 9:123–138, 1956.
31. Lenneberg E: Role of enterostomal therapists and stoma rehabilitation clinics. Cancer 28:225–228, 1971.
32. Eardley A, George WD, Davis F, Schofield PF, Wilson MC, Wakefield J, Sellwood RA: Colostomy: the consequences of surgery. Clinical Oncology 2:277–283, 1976.

13. Care for Adolescent Oncology Patients

CAMERON K. TEBBI

INTRODUCTION

The past two decades have seen a marked improvement in the treatment and survival of adolescents and young adults with malignant disorders. For the physician who treats adolescents, this success has introduced a new challenge: to extend the treatment considerations to address the concerns of the individual who is at an age involving emancipation and entrance into an independent life [1]. In recent years, it has become increasingly evident that the needs of the adolescent are sufficiently unique to warrant special care facilities when medical intervention becomes necessary. Nowhere are these needs more prominent than in the treatment of adolescent oncology patients. Extensive chemotherapy and other medical interventions presently used in the treatment of cancer intertwine with difficulties inherent in the process of adolescence and emancipation, and introduce a difficult task for patients, their families, and the medical profession. Parallel to improvement in the medical management and prognosis of cancer patients, increasing attention is directed toward the psychological effects of the disease on the host.

The efficacy and success of current therapeutic regimens have significantly altered the philosophy of treatment of malignant disorders. At the present time, therapy is often given with curative rather than palliative intent. This trend is increasingly applied to various types of malignancies. With increased sophistication in the use of current non-specific therapeutic modalities and the better definition and knowledge of prognostic factors, the therapeutic regimens ideally should be individualized and suited for the degree of risk involved.

As the rate of survival for cancer increases, it is recognized that the scars of treatment far exceeds those which are visible. These effects can be lifelong, especially when initially experienced during a critical stage of life.

Higby, DJ (ed), Supportive Care in Cancer Therapy. ISBN 0-89838-569-5.
© *1983, Martinus Nijhoff Publishers, Boston. Printed in The Netherlands.*

Attention must be given to the developmental stage of the patient, for adolescence is probably the most difficult and least understood of all periods of human development. Coping with the stress of cancer added to the already difficult challenges stemming from changes in physical and mental development, is difficult under the best of circumstances even when good health and vigor prevail. Coping with cancer at the time when mechanisms to face the stress are not fully developed and shaped is a difficult task that significantly alters the orderly pattern of development which normally takes place at this time. Furthermore, cancer and its consequences present an emotional crisis of major proportions for every member of the patient's family. Providing various means of assistance to cope with these adverse psychological effects during and after therapy requires major understanding on the part of health care providers of the nature of adolescence. It is increasingly recognized that such a task should be performed by a coordinated multidisciplinary team including physicians, psychologists, nurses, physical and occupational therapists, social workers and others.

Finally, until a more specific mode of prevention and treatment replaces present therapies, the challenge to the oncologist who treats adolescent patients remains to design treatment regimens providing maximal therapeutic benefits with minimal short- and long-term side effects, and to reduce to any extent possible the psychological trauma to the patients [1].

BACKGROUND

To better understand and face the problems magnified by cancer during adolescence, knowledge of normal growth and development in this age group is essential. Adolescence is not merely a transition from childhood to adulthood, but it is a distinct phase of growth and personality development [2-3]. This period of life is characterized by marked emotional and physical changes [4-6]. This is the period in which the rapidly maturing person organizes internal and external realities more in accordance with the adult perceptions. Ego organization at this age is enriched by means of identifications.

Adolescence arbitrarily is divided into early, middle and late stages. Major characteristics of these stages are shown in Table 1. Reviewing the experiences of adolescence reveal that the most important tasks in the early and middle stages are body image and independence, respectively. These issues are superseded by identity development in the later stages of this period.

Characteristics of early adolescence, approximating the years twelve to fifteen, include questioning and rebellious behavior against parental and societal rules. This activity is an effort to sever previous dependent emotional ties [7]. In this regard, the young adolescent's effort is filled with uncertainty and ambivalence, i.e., there is a simultaneous emerging desire for freedom and emancipation from the family while a need persists for security and support of childhood identity [4].

Another integral part of the young adolescent's early attempt to establish independence is an increased concern for and awareness of body image [8]. The hormonally induced physical changes occurring at this time generate new somatic sensations which the adolescent evaluates for their 'normalcy' [9]. At this stage the body image tends to remain idealized and strongly linked to the opinions, perceptions, and evaluations of others [10].

Middle adolescence is applied to the ages fifteen through eighteen. At this stage, physical maturity is nearly complete. This period is characterized by the need to establish a strong peer group alliance as fledging attempts at emancipation from family and establishment of independent identity continues [4, 11]. The peer group rather than the family serves as the basis upon which the adolescent experiments with efforts to become self-reliant [10]. At this point, the emerging sense of identity is focused primarily on meeting gender-role expectations [11]. This developmental task of psycho-sexual differentiation behaviorally is accomplished by establishing a more realistic body image and by developing an interest in, and ability to attract, the opposite sex [10].

Late adolescence comprises the years eighteen to twenty-two. At this time, autonomy and sexual orientation have been fairly well established and the adolescent is concerned primarily with defining and achieving functional roles. During this period, completion of education and formulation of at least preliminary plans for career and marriage are main goals. The major effort to achieve emancipation from family has been accomplished [4] and parental communication is again open. The peer group has less of a binding influence [10], and the adolescent/young adult has achieved a positive, stable identity that is essentially congruent with societal norms [6].

Body image

The concept of body image appears to be a product of real and fantasized experiences. This in part stems from a combination of the adolescent's own physical development, peer emphasis on physical attributes, and the individual's awareness of cultural expectations [12]. Developmental tasks include the confidence which individuals acquire with mastery over the environment and reflects in motor, intellectual, and emotional skills. Achievement of these abilities can change the coping strategy and in turn determine the individual's orientation. To assure 'normality' in early adolescence, com-

Table 1. Major characteristics of stages in adolescence.

Early adolescence (approximately age 12–15)

Rapid physical growth
Freedom from family
Accepting self-responsibility
Questioning and rebellious behavior
Move from influence of home to that of peer group
Minor conflicts at home
Consciousness of body image
New drives (particularly sexual)
Desire to be 'normal'

Middle adolescence (age 15–18)

Increased thinking
Peak of struggle with parents to exercise authority
Reactions of great intensity
Establishment of peer standards of stress behavior, etc.
Establishment of realistic body image
Attempts to be attractive to opposite sex
Sexual fantasies
Interest in outside work
Desire for association with members of the opposite sex

Late adolescence (age 18–22)

Increased stability
Acceptance of self
Establishment of autonomy
Capability to relate to members of the opposite sex
Establishment of standards by dating partners
Replacement of parents or peers as source of greatest influence
Definition and achievement of a functional life role
Increased importance of education, career, marriage, family, community and life-style

---

parisons of body parts with peers of the same sex is not unusual. During this period uncertainty with body parts and their growth can result in clumsiness in arm and leg coordination, producing a degree of concern. The idealized body image can resemble that of an admired individual, composite features from several persons, or totally fantasized shapes based on common stereotypes. By mid-adolescence when the peak rate of physical development is over, idealized body image is replaced by a more realistic view. Acceptance of one's physical features, even if wishing they were different, is established. By late adolescence, reality and certainty in one's attractiveness replace former thoughts. The development of body image and its relation to physical characteristics may affect the individual's psychological adjustment. In this stage of adolescence, the competition for popularity and status in the peer group, relation to the opposite sex, and adult privileges are often affected by body image. An altered or unfavorable image, such as that resulting from various medical interventions and treatments used in cancer care can cause discrimination, ostracism and rejection by the peer group and the opposite sex. Initial formation of body image can have a long-lasting and far-reaching effect on an individuals's future.

Peer membership

Development of close friendship bonds is a characteristic of the adolescent period and an integral part of self-understanding and acceptance. This can serve to bring comfort when necessary, lend courage, and provide reassurance of 'normalcy' of action and thoughts. It can result also in obtaining acceptance, increasing self-esteem and forming of identity. Peer relationships during early adolescence are used for support and mutual understanding. During middle adolescence the influence of peers can conflict with that of parents [10, 12]. Participation in group activities and having the same idols, a characteristic of adolescence, is tantamount to being a part of a family [10]. Ultimately, in late adolescence the reliance on and conformity to the peer group is replaced largely by self-confidence and rational decisions. Friendship at this point is based on mutual need and respect rather than sharing of confidences. Since independence and self-determination are an outgrowth of experiences in the peer environment [13], impact of social isolation arising from cancer and its treatment is substantial.

Autonomy

Another important adolescent task is the achievement of autonomy, with of emotional ties with family, particularly the parents, and establishment of self-dependence. While rapid physical and cognitive growth and the struggle for separation and freedom may cause conflict in the parent/adolescent relationship, the process is important for full emancipation. In late adolescence, when a certain degree of autonomy and stability is achieved, desire for parental guidance and reinforcement to insure high self-esteem and a sense of competence often reemerges. The need for dependence on parents during a catastrophic disease such as cancer interrupts the quest for autonomy and brings a regression in the degree of freedom already achieved by adolescents.

Vocational choice

The adolescent is surrounded by social pressures to select a vocation, more often than not requiring advanced training and education which may induce a certain anxiety and stress. Vocational achievement brings future financial security and acceptance by the society, which generally promotes the philosophy of a duty to work hard and evaluates individuals according to the extent of their success.

Deprivation of proper training and vocational opportunities caused by interruption due to cancer and its therapy potentially can provoke a lack of security and retard social growth.

Sex role identity

By and large, cultural influences and expectations determine a person's eventual sex role identity. In most societies, the traditional roles for males and females are subject to constantly changing sexual values which in turn add to the complexity and confusion of adolescence. During the early stage, a member of the same sex is taken as a love object arising from the influence of the ego ideal. By mid-adolescence, there is a decisive turn toward heterosexuality and a final and irreversible renunciation of earlier love ties. Throughout adolescence, the level of psycho-sexual maturity in girls is generally two to three years ahead of the boys. Regardless of sex, by late adolescence, a well-developed capacity for heterosexual intimacy is expected.

Formation of sexual identity, ordinarily fostered by the freedom to move in and out of brief and less intense friendships with peer groups and the opposite sex, when interrupted due to cancer and its treatment, can result in substantial delay or disorder of sexual development.

Physical growth

The physical process of puberty is heralded by sudden spurts in height and appearance of subtle first signs of sexual maturity, followed by a period of profound physical and emotional growth. These visible developments are preceded by biological changes. The sequence of growth during adolescence generally is the same in all individuals, but the magnitude, rate, time of onset and completion may be extremely variable. Patterns of changes involving skin, skeleton musculature, reproductive systems, facial contours, fat distribution, pelvic proportions and secondary sexual development follow an orderly sequence in males and females [14]. Individual background (including sex, race, nutrition, previous illness, and environment), however, has significant effects on these developments. Physical maturation does not necessarily parallel psychological emancipation.

The process of physical maturation occurs one to two years earlier in girls than boys. The time for pubescence can vary significantly among populations. Marked variability of the timing of pubertal development has importance both in health and disease. The 'normal' adolescent has a tendency to compare him/herself with peers; the timing of pubescence may have a substantial effect on perception of one's body image. Individuals with delayed development are more likely to have difficulty securing a sense of self-esteem and may be unsure of their biological integrity. The timing of pubertal development has significance for coping with cancer. Depending on the stage of growth and development, the individual's response to the physical changes and restrictions imposed by the disease or its treatment can differ significantly.

EFFECTS OF ILLNESS AND HOSPITALIZATION ON DEVELOPMENTAL TASKS OF ADOLESCENCE

During the process of emancipation, the adolescent's concern mainly involves body image, self-concept, and the definition of intellectual, sexual and functional identities. Illness and hospitalization pose a profound threat to the successful completion of these developmental tasks [11]. Physical and psycho-social immobility caused by the disease and its treatment constrains freedom of movement and self-determination, and involvement in the supportive and faciliative peer environment [15]. Any threat by illness to the body image surely will affect the self-concept and sexual role identity [16]. In general, ill teenagers are fearful about what is happening to their bodies [11]. Any insult that disrupts biological integrity automatically is perceived in a heightened and exaggerated manner. Often the disease is conceptualized in terms of alteration in body image and feelings rather than in medical terms.

As previously indicated, confinement and the limitations imposed on freedom of movements as components of illness, affect the adolescent's autonomy. Thus, disability is particularly overwhelming when one is struggling for emancipation and self-determination. Chronic illness can cause adolescents to become overly self-centered and greatly affected by emotional forces that can act as powerful stimulants or depressants. This preoccupation may extend to a point that a significant amount of energy is spent simply in compensating for illness or disability and coping with demands at the expense of everyday living and maturational activities. Sickness can highlight the significance of physical attributes to the detriment of other human values. Under stress and frustration, regression to the earliest learned behavior that is appropriate to the situation is not unusual [17]. This reaction can be in the form of a return to a formerly acquired response (historical regression) [18].

Childhood experiences underlie adolescent coping mechanisms, and under conditions of illness these earlier behaviors may be reasserted. Regression to dependence often results in feelings of apprehension and discouragement, leading to anxiety and depression. Independence is achieved by 'acting' rather than only thinking or wishing, and illness reduces the ability to act and assume responsibility [16]. Meanwhile, parents also develop a regressive identification with their child, as they find in the relative helplessness of the adolescent an opportunity to regain their control and reassert their mastery.

Psychological stress and the impact of cancer on adolescent development

Current data indicates that emotional stress as reaction to the diagnosis of cancer and its treatment follow a pattern similar to that characteristic of severe trauma [19]. A traumatic stress is defined as 'an extreme disturbance of biological and psychological functioning brought on by an unusually threatening, damaging, or demanding life condition' [18]. The reactions of the cancer patient are a result of a number of threats including disabling illness, death, change in appearance, alienation, and pain [19–21]. Emotional responses may include one or more of four classes used to index stress, i.e., disruptions in affects and moods; impairments in cognitive functioning; changes in motor activities and behavior; and physiological changes. Which class or which combination of these areas predominate depends on a multitude of biological and environmental variables such as age, sex, initial psychological stability, socio-economic level, degree of other stress situations, past experiences with stress, and available supportive resources.

Often the initial response to the impact of cancer is one of shock and disbelief, followed by a period of denial [22]. The expression of shock and denial is a psychological attempt on the part of the patient to maintain some semblance of the status quo and to avoid a disruption in psychological equilibrium [23]. At this stage, the integrity of personality is defended by denying the stressful situation. Often no behavioral modification is made, and information concerning the diagnosis is refused [24]. The duration of this level of denial depends on the individual and the circumstances involved, but it is usually short-lived because reality forces cognitive awareness upon the individual [19].

The second response pattern is anxiety. In this stage, cognitive input concerning the diagnosis of cancer is perceived and attempts are made to deal with the situation on an intellectual basis [23]. As the intellectual and emotional aspects of acceptance are separated and distinguished, the behavioral manifestations of anxiety and anger become apparent. This response is followed by cognitive perception of the changes caused by cancer, emotional adjustment to the situation, and a search for relevant, hopeful information to reduce anxiety and return to psychological equilibrium [22, 26].

The third sequence in the emotional response to cancer is anger and/or guilt caused by frustration at the inability to adjust to the situation on a purely cognitive basis [19, 23, 27].

The fourth and final response is depression which can be defined as habituation to repeated frustrations [22]. At this stage, a new psychological equilibrium is established at the emotional level.

The relevance to the adolescent patient of the above generally agreed responses to cancer is not clear. Limited available information indicates that the psychologic problems of adolescents can be defined as alteration of self-concept and body image, difficulty in interpersonal relationships and interference with future plans. The response may vary depending on the stage of development, i.e., in early adolescence body image is threatened; in middle stages, independence and fear of rejection by others are concerns; and by late adolescence, the threat is shifted to career and marriage plans.

The adaptation process

The behavioral manifestations of stress have been referred to as the adaptation process. Coping might be defined as the manner in which an individual deals with stress in order to obtain relief and regain equilibrium [28]. Adaptation, therefore, can be considered a process and not just an isolated set of independent actions [18]. The coping process combines elements of perception, performance, appraisal, and correction [28]. The adaptation process of coping includes external and internal aspects [24]. The external aspect is social and functional, while the internal component of coping refers to the manner in which the individual psychically defends against manifest anxiety. General coping strategies for adult cancer patients are many, ranging from rational inquiry to moral masochism [28]. These coping strategies often interact and seldom remain as distinct entities.

In adolescent patients, mechanisms to adapt to stress are not well formed or functional. Common adolescent coping strategies are denial, intellectualization, regression and compensation [11]. Adolescent cancer patients can suffer from increased dependency on parents, social isolation from siblings, physical and psychological immobility, environmental deprivation, and delayed developmental task achievement. Comparison of normal adolescents with cancer patients reveals that the latter group is more likely to turn against themselves and be concerned with body image and physical health. From the previous information, it is apparent that cancer and its therapy can have a significant effect that, unresolved, can be detrimental to the patient's future.

Hospitalization of the teenager can lead to fear of rejection or even abandonment. The adolescent commonly adapts via denial of his illness. With serious illness, parents also may foster this denial compounding this problem. Adolescents may attempt to cope with hospitalization by intellectualizing their illness and attempting to separate emotion from fact. They also may cope via non-compliance or even rebellion. With the stess of a severe or chronic illness, an occasional adolescent may regress to a younger emotional stage of life. Adolescents often believe that their illness is a punishment for their sins.

Fear of the unknown, inherent in the present management of cancer; confusion; anxiety about the outcome of the illness; stress caused by forced dependency; alteration in the body image configuration; fears of abandonment; isolation from peers; diminished self-esteem; and interrupted educational, vocational, marriage, family, and life plans, separately or simultaneously can overwhelm adolescents with cancer.

The preceding discussion should not imply that adolescents with cancer necessarily represent a psychologically deviant population. Many teenagers and young adults are able to develop coping strategies which enable them to overcome successfully the problems posed by their disease and its treatment. A prime example is our study revealing that patients who have undergone amputation due to cancer, adjust well, in general, to their situation and lead a successful and productive life [29].

Adolescence and cancer care

In contrast to adults, most adolescents have had little experience with health providers and hospitals, are unsure of themselves or how to present their complaints and problems, and are often worried about the normalcy of their bodies [15]. It is established that, unlike children where the physician works with or via the child's parents, the adolescent must become the center of concern and communication, with the parental figure present on the periphery.

Most adolescents feel they are invincible, and the necessity of being in a hospital may bring about severe reactions. They may have great difficulty in coping with a serious illness or surgical procedure because of real or imagined threats to their body images.

The difficulties faced by adolescents in the ordinary hospital setting for acute diseases often are magnified for youths with cancer. Medical advances have enhanced vastly the life expectancy and survival rate for cancer, thus increasing the expectation for individuals to recover and reenter the job market. Longer survival and sophisticated therapeutic options have significantly increased the number of patients and the frequency of their admission to the major medical or cancer centers. In most hospital settings, however, adolescent patients are dispersed according to their age or type of malignancy rather than grouped for their adolescent needs. Often these individuals experience difficulty adjusting to other patients on the same floor. In pediatric wards, adolescents are treated much like children, a matter they resent, and feel demeaned. On adult services they are treated as adults, which they are not and experience conflicts often characterized as the 'generation gap'. 'Every objective study in the past ten years has indicated that the older child is always aware of the seriousness of his predicament, is concerned by a conspiracy of silence, and is anxious to discuss his worries with a sympathetic person' [30]. Fortunately for all concerned, in recent years openness has replaced a 'hush-hush' policy of keeping patients from knowledge of their disease and its consequences. The result is direct communication between the physician and adolescent without going through the parents as intermediaries. This policy decreases distortion of the facts and confusion produced by variation in stories presented to the patient. Confidence in knowing that the medical staff share the truth has replaced suspicion on the part of patients and has resulted in honest, open and clear discussion about the disease and its therapy. In this way, confusion and disappointments are reduced, and patient participation in care, decision making and planning for the future are increased.

A multidisciplinary approach to patient care has enhanced the input of various disciplines and opened new avenues for patients to voice their opinions. The effectiveness of a hospital program which makes use of psychological principles has been previously demonstrated [31]. The fact remains that, due to the complexity and involvement of therapy, most adolescent specialists as a rule avoid caring for cancer patients, leaving a void where the expertise and experience is most needed. The physician who treats adolescents with cancer needs to become familiar with and be sensitive to the

Table 2. Mortality of leading malignancies in adolescents in the United States (1978).

Age	Type of cancer	Deaths	Death rate
		Male/female	Male/female
15–19	Leukemias	237/119	22.3/11.5
	Bone	100/57	9.4/5.5
	Brain and central nervous system	95/77	8.9/7.4
	Non-Hodgkin's lymphomas	74/27	7.0/2.6
	Testicular	46/–	4.3/–
	Hodgkin's disease	–/32	– /3.1
20–24	Leukemias	214/126	21.2/12.4
	Testis	106/–	10.5/–
	Non-Hodgkin's lymphoma	93/41	9.2/4
	Hodgkin's disease	90/47	8.9/4.6
	Brain and central nervous system	88/73	8.7/7.2
	Ovary	–/35	– /3.5
15–34	Leukemias	827	22.1
	Brain and central nervous system	467	12.5
	Non-Hodgkin's lymphoma	380	10.1
	Testicular	329	8.8
	Hodgkin's disease	335	8.9

needs of his/her patients and to capitalize upon the social awareness of the adolescents.

Cancer in adolescents

In the United States, cancer is the leading cause of death from disease in the adolescent and young adult age groups [32]. In 1978 in the United States 7,283 young adults (3,937 males and 3,346 females) ages 15–34 died of cancer [33]. The rate of death from cancer is estimated to be 68.6 per million for ages 10–19 years, or one for each 14,577 persons in this age group [34, 35]. The mortality from five leading malignancies for males and females aged 15–19 and 20–24 is summarized in Table 2. These statistics roughly correspond to the type of patients admitted for therapy to the Adolescent Unit at Roswell Park Memorial Institute, shown in Table 3. The local data, however, may be biased due to the pattern of referral and necessity of admission for certain disorders.

Table 3. Patients admitted to the Roswell Park Memorial Institute Adolescent/Young Adult Unit by disease category.

Disease category	Percentage of patients
Hodgkin's and non-Hodgkin's lymphoma	18.0
Testicular tumors	16.0
Leukemias	14.5
Soft tissue sarcomas	12.5
Ovarian, cervical and uterine tumors	9.0
Melanoma	7.5
Osteogenic and Ewing's sarcoma	7.0
CNS tumors	4.0
Miscellaneous	4.5
Benign tumors	7.0

GENERAL PRINCIPALS OF MANAGEMENT

Intensive multimodal treatment utilizing the concerted efforts of various medical, surgical, supportive care, rehabilitation and other disciplines allows prolonged survival or 'cure' for a large proportion of patients. As the success in treatment of cancer increases, the disease is viewed as a transient incident in life. With emphasis on the quality of life, many patients are capable of continuing their regular activities.

Diagnosis

The relative rarity of cancer in adolescents and young adults can result in procrastination on the part of the patient in seeking medical advice, delay by the physician in the initiation of proper therapy, and misdiagnosis of the disease. Often the treatment is directed to more common conditions which present with similar symptoms. The wide spectrum of neoplastic disorders can have a range of signs and symptoms, suggesting a variety of other diseases. As will be discussed later in this chapter, delay on the part of the patient in seeking medical help and physician delay in diagnosis and treatment, may leave the patient and family with a sense of guilt, animosity, disbelief, and suspicion toward medical providers. Furthermore, since as a rule, adolescent patients with cancer previously have been healthy, they may question the diagnosis.

Diagnostic procedures in patients suspected of cancer must be rapid and conclusive. It is not proper to discuss the malignancies under consideration with the patient and family until the diagnosis firmly is made. It is most important to be certain of the diagnosis and have concrete proof of the type of malignancy when discussing the disease and its treatment. If the initial impression of cancer proves to be incorrect, withdrawal or reversal of prior statements on the part of the physician seldom is sufficient to totally erase the possibility of cancer from the mind of the parents or the patient. Equally, changes in the type of diagnosed malignancy because the initial diagnosis was hastily made and pronounced, will cause confusion and a credibility gap just when patient trust is most needed. It is far more desirable to inform the parents and patient that the procedures required for a firm diagnosis are in the process of completion and request their patience rather than offer speculations. During the diagnosis-making process, it is also important to have a single spokesperson relating the information to the family and patient. Emphasis should be made that all those privy to information on the results of ongoing tests must avoid giving out conflicting reports. These 'leaks' from medical personnel can result in the patient and family receiving incomplete and misleading information and can produce an unnecessary and avoidable crisis.

Initial discussion of diagnosis

After all diagnostic procedures producing a conclusive result are completed, all the findings should be discussed in a meeting with the parents and the patient and their questions answered. Most physicians, justifiably, wish to meet with the patient and parents separately. If this is the case, identical information (as much as possible) should be given to the parents and the patient in their respective meetings. The physician responsible for the overall management and long-term care of the patient must be the principal in this meeting. Over the years, oncologists have found that in the initial meeting, when parents are informed of an unexpected diagnosis, the levels of emotion can be high. It is important that both parents be present in the meeting so they can be a source of comfort to each other. A very close relative can also be present. The meeting with the parent should not be attended by a large number of medical personnel. Parents generally do not want their feelings, which are invariably expressed upon hearing the diagnosis, to be witnessed by a group of total strangers. The expected expression of spontaneous emotions requires that the meeting place be quiet and free of disruptions. The shock of learning the diagnosis of cancer for the first time often prevents concentration even in the strongest-willed parents. Nevertheless, in such a meeting it is important to discuss the disease and its therapy, emphasizing that the information will be repeated and discussed with them again at a later date.

It is of utmost importance to indicate that the diagnosis is firm and certain and is based on conclusive facts. In the first meeting, when appropriate, parents should be told that the diagnosed cancer is not hereditary; that neither of them carry a gene which can transmit the same disease to their present or future children; and that they themselves would not have a substantially increased chance of having cancer. These reassurances, even though stastistically not correct in certain malignancies, are true enough in practice and can decrease parental apprehension. It can be mentioned that it is highly unusual, and indeed a rarity, to see two children of the same family afflicted with cancer during their childhood and adolescence. The point also should be made that cancer is not contagious nor is it transmitted by any type of contact. It is perfectly safe for others to share items with the patient without any fear of contagion. It is important to mention that the disease, to date, does not have a recognized mode of prevention, and the exact time of the beginning of the disease cannot be accurately established.

The possible guilt feeling of the parent for not having sought medical advice earlier for minor symptoms they may have noticed, should be diffused. For the same reason, a point should be made of the fact that past personal doings, geographic place of residence, possible prior illness and contacts have no proven direct connection with the diagnosis of cancer, and that the origin of this disease unfortunately remains enigmatic.

Information that the physician provides in the first meeting primarily must be volunteered without request on the part of the parents and the patient. They often are overwhelmed with the news of diagnosis, and some do not feel at ease or are too shy to ask questions. The information given can ease, to some extent, their minds and establish a line of communication.

Parents and patient should be told of the available options of therapy and the one which the physician recommends, along with prognosis for the disease with and without therapy. It is necessary that, along with the verbal description, they be given a correct spelling of the name of the disease, each drug used, the schedule of therapy, and a written summary of the expected benefits of each drug, their side effects and the timing of their development. They also should have the opportunity of taking notes on the pertinent materials. To avoid confusion, all descriptions must be simple, using non-medical terms, and tailored to the individual's degree of sophistication. It is important to demonstrate that the physician has kept current with new developments in the field, especially as it relates to new drugs and schedules, and that should there be any additional significant 'breakthroughs', the patient's therapy will be updated to include the best possible treatment available. It is also worthwhile to mention that patients have the option of consulting physicians in other institutions and that the information regarding the disease can be sent out without fear of reprisal.

The first meeting with the parents should also include a determination of prognosis. Estimates in response to the common question, 'how long has the patient to live' need not be overly exact. Such predictions are often meaningless and almost always incorrect. These can only frighten the patient and the family and eventually discredit the physician. When giving the prognosis, one must be optimistic and emphasize the positive without minimizing the gravity of the disease or eliminating the possibility of failure from the minds of all concerned. Mean values of survival or disease-free survival which are based on prior experiences, while a good guide for the physician, often are not well understood by patients and their families. Dates become fixed in their mind and they build expectations around them.

Parents are encouraged to have an open dialogue with their child to any extent possible. While the physician presents a young adolescent with a more optimistic picture, patients still should know the truth about the condition. Concealing the diagnosis and therapeutic information from patients should be highly discouraged. Such a practice often results in confusion and lack of communication and will affect the parents–patient–physician relationship. The resulting 'conspiracy of silence' soon is sensed by the patient, causing hostility, resentfulness and isolation. The concealment of diagnosis does not usually last. Since most patients are knowledgeable of their diagnosis, conversations between a newly diagnosed patient and an 'old hat' soon will provide the teenager with any withheld knowledge. Further inquiry such as a look at the encyclopedia or a visit to the local library, may reveal the facts and result in a total distrust of the physician and parents, and an uncooperative and antagonistic patient. Even in the unlikely event that the diagnosis remains a secret, something that in our society and times is highly unlikely, the rather extensive pre-clinical evaluations, invasive procedures and often toxic therapies employed will be viewed as ridiculous by the patient in light of the often simplistic false diagnosis he or she is provided with.

The physician must make it clear that effective therapy usually can produce remissions, but these should not be equated with cure. It should be emphasized that, despite even the seemingly total disappearance of the malignancy, therapy should be continued for the prescribed course, if the full benefits are to be gained. Parents and patient should be told to check with the oncologist before administration of any medications, including vitamins, and over-the-counter drugs of any nature. They also should be warned against the use of aspirin or products containing this agent because of its hemostatic side effects. Many parents do not consider non-prescription drugs as 'medications', a point that should be clarified. Since live viruses may produce a full-fledged disease in an immunosuppressed host, and response to other inoculation may not be complete [36–38], caution should be given against the use of any immunizations without checking with the oncologist. Due to the relative rarity of cancer in adolescents, private practitioners may not be fully aware of the effects prescriptions for non-cancer management may have on the therapy for cancer. Proper communication and joint decision making will minimize this problem. Provided that patient and parents are aware of the latter point, they can continue to recieve care from their referring physician for non-cancer related problems.

A few words of caution, when deemed necessary, must be added to deter patients from being taken advantage of by quacks offering unrealistic 'cures' [39–41]. In one pediatric study, 39% of those interviewed had tried, considered or received recommendations to try unapproved remedies [39]. It is advisable to ask parents and patient to share with the oncologist what they read, especially the news of discoveries (which are often dramatized by the popular press) in order to obtain more realistic medical views on the new developments. For most diseases, published booklets and sources of information written for parents are available. While the material content of these often is not identical with the information provided by the physician, and at times can be outdated, they can serve as a reading source for the patient. Excellent and regularly updated booklets for patients and parents addressing major malignancies of childhood and adolescents, such as that published by the Association for Research of Childhood Cancer (Buffalo, New York), are also available [42].

The importance of medical procedures, such as spinal taps, bone marrows, blood tests, etc., necessary for obtaining additional information and follow-up also should be emphasized. Patients' fear of the damages caused by these procedures can be minimized by explanation of the reason for their use and need. Furthermore, especially early after diagnosis, it is important to eliminate the unexpected by informing well in advance both patients and parents of the planned procedures as to when and how they are to be carried out. Most individuals accept various tests much easier if they are mentally prepared for it and are not caught by surprise.

The principal attending oncologist charged with the care of the patient should visit the patient very frequently during the first few days and reinforce what is discussed in the initial session, keeping in mind that patient and parents may not have acknowledged, fully comprehended, or retained previously given information.

During the initial discussion, parents and patients are encouraged not to conceal the diagnosis from relatives, friends and others. While this idea is not promoted by some [35], it appears to fend off the suspicion and rumors, which follow secrecy, and can result in patient and family isolation. Willingness of patients and family to reveal the nature of the disease and its implications will eliminate fears of contagion, which can be given a false credibility by a hesitancy to talk openly. Furthermore, this openness will decrease avoidance of the subject and provide for resolution of fright which often stems from lack of knowledge.

Siblings and other members of the family also should be briefed about the disease and their questions should be answered by the team caring for the patient. Parents should be asked not to pay exclusive attention and leniency to the patient to the depravation of their other children.

Depending on patients and parents beliefs, assistance of a clergyman familiar with the family may prove to be of great value and a source of reliance and hope.

During the initial meeting, the physician also must discuss finances, mainly to decrease parent and patient worries. The expenses imposed on the family of patients with cancer can be substantial and at times a source of concern second only to the disease itself. As will be discussed later in this chapter, parents often are not able to absorb substantial direct and hidden costs of cancer. At times, there is a gap in medical insurance coverage, where the parent's policy no longer provides coverage and the patient either does not have any or has inadequate insurance. As a young adult, many patients have been working only for a short time, and their frail budget cannot bear the burden of extra expenditures. A point should be made of the resources available which can provide assistance, and a mention be made that the physician and the social worker will assist the family in exploring these possibilities [43].

Finally, during the initial discussion with the patient and the parents, they should be provided with a list of services available in the hospital and the name, role, responsibilities and telephone numbers of the principal oncologist, other physicians, and members of the medical team providing care. Parents should be urged to write their questions and be offered the option of calling the physician on the phone.

Since, at least in the beginning, the family will relate to a greater extent to their local medical practitioner, he/she should receive the details of diagnosis, plans of therapy, and be encouraged to communicate with the family.

Supportive care

Sophisticated medical and surgical care which has prolonged survival has significantly increased the need for supportive care. Since present modalities of therapy are non-specific, their side effects can be substantial. Coupled with the disease and its complication, treatment effects can provide a challenge to the physician and the supportive team. Included in this category are gastrointestinal side effects; marrow suppression leading to anemia, increased chance of infection, and bleeding; disabilities caused by surgical resections or amputation; radiation or chemotherapy-induced pulmonary dysfunctions; hematuria; metabolic disorders such as hyperuricemia and hypo- or hypercalcemia; and long-term side effects including those affecting the reproductive and central nervous system, etc. The frequency, magnitude, and severity of these untoward effects depends on the extent and modality of therapy used and a variety of host factors. Early diagnosis and management of these complications requires prompt report by the patient, a high index of suspicion, and expeditious and aggressive therapy on the part of the physician.

Activities. It is not uncommon for some cancer patients to cease all activities they used to undertake [44]. Furthermore, in terminal patients, there is a tendency at times to withdraw from recreational activity. The problems with inactivity are several, including deterioration of skin condition, atrophy of the muscles due to disuse, etc. Prolonged periods of inactivity may produce a number of complications, the reversal of which are medically and psychologically difficult. Currently, at Roswell Park, exercise programs are an integral part of our patient care in the Adolescent Unit. Most patients can participate in varying degrees of exercise that minimize phlebitis and skin, muscle or bone deterioration. Passive and active range of motion is easily taught and can be performed by the patient or their family. It is a common observation that these activities boost the patient's and family's morale. Often the patients are underestimating their potential and are surprised to find that they are capable of performing many of their daily chores.

Attention also should be given to in-hospital provision of recreational activities suited to individual patients. These services include painting, arts

Table 4. Available activities for adolescents and their families on the Adolescent Oncology Unit at Roswell Park Memorial Institute.

Music therapy	Games and recreation facilities
Creative writing	Rap sessions
Family nights and dinners	Siblings care
Occupational therapy	Guidance counseling
In-patient field trips	Exercise for health
School outreach programs	Arts and crafts
Concert /movies	Videotape productions
Formal high school and college training	Bereavement follow-up

and crafts, crocheting, drawing, sculpture, sewing, writing, etc. Many patients find it possible to express themselves through the arts, and in the process decrease their stress and increase their sense of accomplishment. A list of programs used in the Adolescent Oncology Unit at Roswell Park is shown in Table 4.

School program. For the adolescent patient, attending school after diagnosis of cancer can be difficult [45–48]. Aside from the physical changes that stem from cancer and its treatment, the need for the clinic visits and treatments hampers regular attendance and participation in the school activities. Cancer patients may have difficulty with completion of school work, concentration, and may show a higher rate of learning disabilities and less energy [46]. Students with cancer may have a greater tendency not to reach out to others, initiate activities, or try new things [46]. They may try to protect themselves and to avoid expressing their feelings freely. This reaction is especially true in patients who are actively under treatment or are in relapse as compared to newly diagnosed patients or those individuals who are in a long-term remission. These problems are more evident in adolescence when body image is of great importance. Some studies have shown school phobia [45, 48], low concentration, and increased self-protectiveness in students who have cancer. While none of these problems are universal and many patients do fare well in school, school-related difficulties still remain an inherent problem. Many teachers become overly concerned about students with cancer and may overreact and become frightened by slight symptoms which in normal students surely would be ignored. Some educators consciously try to avoid discussing the subject at all costs, while others become sympathetic and extend extra favors to the student with cancer. In either case, the individual with cancer becomes an exception and can suffer adverse effects. It is the duty of the health care providers to discuss the matter with the patient and parents, and if desired, contact the school and provide education for teachers, school administrators and students. Through these interventions and recognition of a student's possible limitations, the school environment will be less threatening, thus providing an opportunity for students with cancer to continue their education without major interruptions or difficulties. Likewise, with a better understanding of patient problems, teachers will be able to handle questions from other students without feeling totally inadequate. It is important for students with cancer to participate in various school activities and not be left out by their peers.

Family planning. Several medical factors necessitate birth control in adolescent patients during periods of therapy for cancer. Amongst these conditions are malformation of fetus caused by chemotherapeutic agents or irradiation, premature delivery resulting in high fetal mortality and increased risk of malignancy in the offspring [49–51]. In the case of irradiation, it is suggested that pregnancy should be terminated if doses over ten rads reach the pelvis during the first trimester [52, 53].

Measures can be taken to preserve the fertility of adolescent patients. Among these steps are external shielding [54], temporary relocation of ovaries above and lateral to the pelvic rim [55], and sperm preservation prior to chemotherapy or radiation treatment.

Pregnancy itself does not appear to exacerbate malignancy in the mother. At least in the case of acute leukemia the development of the disease in the offspring is unusual [49, 56]. Only occasional cases of leukemia occurring in infants of leukemic mothers are reported [57]. Teenagers with cancer should be consulted regarding fertility and available birth control devices. In the adolescent male, sperm banking allows preservation of sperm prior to chemotherapy for a later use.

Care for siblings. Consideration of patient's siblings should be an integral part of care. This interaction may range from dealing with various concerns and fears to bereavement conferences. Siblings should be aware of the disease and its consequences and be able to communicate their feelings to any extent possible. The practice of relocating siblings among neighbors and relatives while parents stay in the hospital is not unusual. This step may result in confusion and can frighten the siblings, thus causing a substantial amount of psychological trauma [58]. This reaction, coupled with frequent pre-existent rivalry between siblings and the common belief that the hospitalized patient must get more attention than others, can lead to a major feud.

At times, the sibling is caught between feeling guilty about past aggressive wishes they may have had or the fact that their brother or sister has cancer and requires and receives more attention [59]. It is the responsibility of the medical care team to provide individual counseling as well as group meetings to discuss matters of concern for siblings of patients with cancer. Repeated reassurances, emotional contact with the patient, family talks, open discussion of the progress of the patients, and provision of information to the siblings can help to limit fantasies and maintain normal relations between the sibling and the patient.

The high cost of care

The financial expense imposed on the family of patients with cancer as noted previously, can be substantial and at times a source of concern second only to the disease itself. The cost of caring for a teenager with cancer is not limited to medical expenditures [62]. The list of expenses is long and includes: transportation, loss of work time, extra expense for food for the patient and family (dining outside the home, including in the hospital), change of dietary habits, adequate time for care, lodgings for those who live away from the medical center, parking fees, tolls, expenses for care of siblings when parents are away (baby-sitting), clothing purchased because of change in weight of the patient, wigs, gifts to bring to the hospital, telephone calls to the hospital and relatives, etc., to mention a few. Non-reimbursable medical costs also can be substantial [62]. Few insurance policies cover all medical expenses. The financial burdens on the family are even greater in cases of unemployment or poverty. In such a situation, at least during the early course of the disease and before provision of some financial assistance by various agencies is possible, extra expenses can place an extraordinary pressure on the family.

In one report, the loss of pay and the expenses for nearly half of the families of patients in a hospital during four consecutive weeks amounted to over $453.74 above covered expenses [62]. Another study indicates extra expenses of $39.70 or more per week for families with a child with cancer [62]. The largest catergories were transportation, followed by food and miscellaneous items. Expenses are influenced by the level of care, performance status, family size and distance from the hospital.

It is obvious that expenses are much higher for patients who are at the terminal stage of the disease. In most instances families of patients with cancer are likely to incur costs more than 15% of gross yearly family income [62]. This economic impact, added to the stress of disease, can be devastating for the family. Fortunately, there are a number of resources for absorbing a part of the cost. Nevertheless, some out of pocket costs rarely can be reimbursed.

Several financial studies done on a variety of chronic diseases, including cancer, have shown that the cost of home care can be substantially less than hospital care [63–68]. Examination of the cost effectiveness of home health care can be difficult [63]. The major obstacle in comparing home and institutional care is the fact that cost data for these two are not comparable [63]. Often institutional costs are expressed in per diem terms and include room, board and personal care, while home care expenses are expressed as the cost of health care services provided. Excluding expenses such as baby-sitters, taxis, meals, etc., some feel that there is a small or no reduction in home care costs compared to hospital costs [63]. However, in addition to the above exclusions, the lack of inclusion of patients in the terminal stage and those who live a greater distance from the hospital makes those data not directly applicable to cancer patients receiving care in highly specialized centers.

Recognizing that the cost of therapy for cancer can be overwhelming, a number of organizations provide assistance to these patients. A partial list of these sources are shown in Table 5.

Table 5. Available sources of support for cancer patients in the United States.

Assistance with medical expenses
Assistance with expenses
Nursing care
Assistance with expenses and medical equipment
Assistance with expenses and drugs
Social and emotional support, education, etc.
Referral and social support

Alternatives to hospital care of adolescents

Home care. In recent years, it has become exceedingly clear that provision of adequate medical care does not necessarily require a formal hospital setting [44, 70–81]. One of the advantages of home care, especially for the chronically ill, is the psychological benefit gained from an increased sense of participation and greater self-reliance [44]. Care at home often reinforces family and local ties, helps to reduce the need for travel to and from the hospital and has financial advantages directly to the patient and indirectly for the society [44, 70–72]. For the family, the opportunity and experience of caring for close ones can alleviate ill feelings, and in case of death, the warm memories may lessen the gravity of the loss.

Despite its numerous advantages, however, home care is not for everyone. Various factors, including the nature of the disease, the type and availability of various resources and services, and the degree of readiness and confidence of the patient and relatives play a role in the appropriateness of this care. This assessment requires extensive team evaluation, debate and a good deal of foundation work, expertise and experience. Furthermore, the factors are not static and are apt to change over a period of time. Several variables such as the patient's condition, the possibility of complication or the occurrence of emergency situations, the degree of education afforded the patient and the family by the medical team, and the desire for self-care should be taken into account prior to any decision. These aspects and numerous other considerations necessitate a high degree of individualization. In a number of situations, a patient seemingly 'unsuitable' for provision of home care may at some point become a prime candidate for such care. This variability underscores the need for continued patient education, constant health team re-evaluation and ongoing communication.

Home care for the terminally ill varies to some extent from that for patients undergoing active therapy with curative potential [60, 78–84]. The fundamentals of extended and terminal care are based on a multidisciplinary approach, without which the efforts are more often than not doomed to failure with possible medical and psychological consequences for the patients and their families [44, 70–78]. Even the seemingly easy task of patient discharge to the care of a relative may prove disastrous if the necessary preparations are overlooked and contingencies for the unexpected are not made. The plans for home care should originate early during hospitalization, building of patient's and relatives' confidence and knowledge of the disease and educating them by allowing in advance their participation in the patient's care [60]. The ingredients of successful family education are many and include: honest communication with the patient and relatives, provision of information about the disease and treatment including the degree and type of risk involved, rough estimation of the duration of care necessary, and the teaching of required skills with adequate supervision and plans for handling of possible complications [44].

Often, in opting for home or hospital care, patients are asked to choose between the comfort and familiar surroundings of the home, with care provided by a family with limited medical background, versus the 'safety', expertise and constant availability of medical personnel and facilities in an impersonal and unfamiliar setting of a hospital with limited comfort and privacy. However, in an ideal setting the choice should not be confined to these two arrangements. A combination of the two, i.e. provision of some services at the hospital and the availability of the same expert medical personnel to provide care at home after the acute phase of the disease, appears to be an alternative. In such a setting, the patient always can rely on a rapid response from the health providers and, if necessary, transfer to the hospital.

Home care for patients on active therapy. The goal of providing home care for cancer patients who are being treated with the ultimate goal of cure is to provide the patients with the best medical, psychological, nursing and rehabilitative care possible in the home environment. This effort, in turn, seeks to minimize the psychological trauma, discomforts and expense to the patient and his/her familiy. In other words, the aim is to provide adequate support so that the treatment for cancer is less of a burden upon the patient's established ways of life. In that context, arrangements are made to lessen the disturbance of family life by bringing the care to the patients rather than vice versa. It is obvious that in addition to home care, such patients require periodic hospital visits.

Home care for terminally ill patients. The aim of home care at the terminal stage is to maintain the patient's comfort and to provide an atmosphere in which the physical, emotional and social integrity of the patient and family is protected. Where terminal care at home is chosen, relieving pain, assisting the family in provision of care, and coping with the situation and expected death are of prime importance. The members of the health team do not have to be physically present at all times. The fact that they are available to the family on an around-the-clock basis will provide reassurance in the event that their services become necessary [60]. Most, if not all, parents have some degree of fear and feeling of inadequacy in facing death at home. No doubt siblings not previously exposed to a dying person may be fearful. This factor underscores the necessity of communication on the part of the health care team with the family of the dying person.

The advantages of home care for dying adolescents are many. The presence of siblings, parents, relatives and friends who may take part in providing care can be a great comfort to the patient [44, 60]. In the hospital, persons with terminal illness suffer isolation and may receive either overzealous treatment or neglect from medical personnel who are 'cure oriented'. At times, care providers fail to make frequent visits to the room of the terminally ill patient and neglect to talk directly to him. It is becoming increasingly evident that the dying patient's best interest is served when they are given the choice of their management [61].

Dying introduces a severe emotional situation for the family. Nevertheless, most parents and relatives want to be present at the time of death. Death itself is a highly personal matter and contrasts with the relatively impersonal and non-private situations which by nature exist even in the best of hospital settings [61]. When death is inevitable, the stress imposed on relatives either may or may not be better controlled and handled in the privacy of the home as compared to the hospital. During the terminal stage, many patients and families feel more at ease in expressing themselves and their feelings in the familiar surroundings. Some, however, do not want the final loss to occur at home and prefer to have such an event occur in the hospital, because among other concerns, home is a place for better memories. An adequate home care program should allow for both considerations.

Family of terminally ill adolescent. The emotional and psychological problems of the family of a dying patient can be overwhelming. While there is no universal reaction, most families show some degree of anger, resentment and bitterness, denial, grief and fear. On occasion, these feelings are projected toward the medical personnel providing care. This response requires a good degree of patience and sympathetic listening on the part of the medical staff. Home care provides an opportunity for the family to come to terms with these happenings and in time, to face the reality of the impending death and find ways to cope with it. Despite some reservations, it appears that for other children in the family, contacts with their seriously ill sibling throughout the last weeks of life are less damaging than a 'conspiracy' of silence and exclusion. Children appear to be more capable of withstanding the stress through a limited understanding of death rather than through mystery and lack of explanation regarding their exclusion. Many children unconsciously may be led to believe that their exclusion is in order to prevent them from acquiring the disease [88]. Transfer of the patient at the terminal stage of life to the hospital without adequate explanation to the siblings may accentuate this fear. The same fear can be experienced by the dying child who feels indignant and uncomfortable when isolated from the family.

Bereavement follow-up. Following the death of an adolescent, communication with the family expressing the continued caring and concern of the hospital is important. The continued commitment and support should be extended when needed and wanted. The family should be invited to return to the hospital whenever they would like to or need to come. Past experience shows that many parents return to the place and the people who took part in the care of their child and ask questions about the disease, especially the terminal phase and any autopsy findings. When necessary, the psychologist and family counselor should continue to see and work with the family of deceased adolescents if they need support and encouragement during the bereavement process. Group meetings of bereaved parents and siblings provide them a forum for expressing their feelings.

REFERENCES

1. Tebbi CK: Introduction. In: Major Topics in Pediatric and Adolescent Oncology, Tebbi CK (ed). Boston, GK Hall, 1982, pp 1–3.

2. Cameron N: Personality Development and Psychopathology. Boston, Houghton, Mifflin Co, 1963.
3. Maier HW: Adolescenthood. Social casework 46:3–9, 1965.
4. Fine LL: What is normal adolescence? Clin Pediat 12:1, 1973.
5. Hamburg BA: Coping in early adolescence. In: American Handbook of Psychiatry, Arieti S, Brody EB (eds). New York, Basic Books, 1974.
6. Leichtman SR, Friedman SB: Social and psychological development of adolescents and the relationship to chronic illness. Med Clin North Am 59:1319, 1975.
7. Kimball AJ, Cambell MM: Psychological aspects of adolescent patient health care. Clin Pediat 18:15, 1979.
8. Kolb LC: Disturbances of the body image. In: American Handbook of Psychiatry, Ariety S (ed). New York, Basic Books, 1975.
9. Hurlock EB: Adolescent Development. New York, McGraw-Hill, 1973.
10. Daniel WA: An approach to the adolescent patient. Med Clin North Am 59:1281, 1975.
11. Bloss P: Character formation in adolescence. Psychoanal Study Child 23:245, 1968.
12. Schonfeld WA: Body image in adolescence: a psychiatric concept for the pediatrician. Pediatrics 31:845, 1963.
13. Bloss P: The split parental image in adolescent social relations: an inquiry into groups psychology. Psychoanal Study Child 31:5, 1976.
14. Tanner JM: Growth at Adolescence. Oxford, Blackwell Scientific Publications, 1962.
15. Holton CP: The adolescent with malignancy. In: Medical Care of the Adolescent, 3rd ed, Gallagher JR, Heald F, Garell D (eds). New York, Appleton-Century-Crofts, 1976.
16. Kugelmas NI: Adolescent Medicine. Springfield, Illinois, Charles C Thomas Publishers, 1975.
17. Tull RM: Preferred Defense Mechanisms and Predominant Concerns of Adolescent Oncology Patients. Dissertation, State University of New York at Buffalo, May 1979.
18. Lazarus RS: Psychological stress and the coping process. In: Coping and the Process of Secondary Appraisal: Degree of Threat and Factors in the Stimulus Configuration. New York, McGraw-Hill Book Company, 1966, p 172.
19. Morris T, Geer HS, White P: Psychological and social adjustment to mastectomy. Cancer 40:2381, 1977.
20. Holland J: Coping with cancer. A challenge to the behavioral sciences. In: Cancer: The Behavioral Dimensions, Cullen JW, Fox BH, Isom RR (eds). New-York, Raven Press, 1976.
21. Mastrovito RC: Emotional considerations in cancer and stroke. NY J of Medicine i:2874, 1972.
22. Branter J: Life-threatening disease as a manageable crisis. Sem Oncol 1:153, 1974.
23. Falek A, Britton S: Phases of coping. The hypothesis and its implications. Soc Biol 21:1, 1974.
24. Chodoff P, Friedman SB, Hamburg DA: Stress, defenses, and coping behavior. Observation in parents of children with malignant disease. Am J Psychiatry 120:743, 1964.
25. Peck A: Emotional reactions to having cancer. Am J Roentgenol 114:591, 1972.
26. Maguire GP, Lee EC, Bevington et al.: Psychiatric problems in the first year after mastectomy. Br Med J 1:563, 1978.
27. Shands HC, Finesinger JE, Cobb S, Abrams RD: Psychological mechanism in patients with cancer. Cancer 4:1159, 1951.
28. Weisman AD: Coping with Cancer. New York, McGraw-Hill, 1979.
29. Boyle M, Tebbi CK, Mindell E, Mettlin C: Adolescent adjustment to amputation. Med & Ped Oncol 10:301–312, 1982.
30. Karon M: The physician and the adolescent with cancer. Ped Clin North Am 20:965, 1973.

31. Pruge DG et al.: A study of emotional reactions of children and families to hospitalization and illness. Am J Orthopsychiat 23:70, 1953.

32. Cancer Statistics. Ca 32:15-32, 1982.

33. Silverberg E: Cancer in young adults (ages 15-34). Cancer 32:32-42, 1982.

34. Segi M, Kurihara M: Cancer mortality for selected sites in twenty-four countries #6, 1966-1967, Japan Cancer Society, Nagoya, Japan, 1972, pp 12-15.

35. Steinherz PG, Miller DR: The adolescent with cancer. In: Adolescent Medicine Topics, Lopez RI (ed). New York, Spectrum Publications 1976, pp 209-249.

36. Smithson WA, Siem RA, Rilts RE: Responses to influenza versus vaccine in children receiving chemotherapy for malignancy. J Pediatr 93:632, 1978.

37. Gross PA, Lee H, Wolff JA, Hall CB, Minnefore AB, Lazicki ME: Influenza immunization in immunosuppressed children. J Pediatr 92:30, 1978.

38. Ganz PA, Shanley JD, Cherry D: Responses of patients with neoplastic diseases to influenza versus vaccine. Cancer 420:2244, 1978.

39. Faw C, Ballentine R, Ballentine L et al.: Unproved cancer remedies: a survey of use in pediatric outpatients. JAMA 238:1536, 1977.

40. Freireich EJ: Unproven remedies. In: Cancer chemotherapy. Fundamental Concepts, and Recent Advances. Chicago, Year Book Medical Publishers, 1975.

41. Unproven methods of cancer management: cancer quackery. Cancer 25:66, 1975.

42. Parent and Child Handbook. Buffalo, AROCC, 1982.

43. Smithson WA, Gelchrist GS, Burgert EO: Childhood acute leukemia. Cancer 30:174, 1980.

44. Rosenbaum EH, Rosenbaum IR: Principles of home care for the patient with advanced cancer. JAMA 244:1484, 1980.

45. Lansky SB, Lowman JT, Vata TS, Gyulay JE: School phobia in children with malignant neoplasma. Am J Dis Child 129:42, 1975.

46. Deasy-Spinetta P, Spinetta JJ: The child with cancer in school. Teachers' appraisal. Am J Ped Hemat-Oncol 2:89, 1980.

47. Katz ER, Kellerman J, Ryler D, Williams KO, Siegel SE: School intervention with pediatric cancer patients. J Pediatr Psychol 2:72, 1977.

48. Kaplan DM, Smith A, Grobstein R: School management of the seriously ill child. J School Health 44 (5):250, 1974.

49. Lingeman CH: Epidemiologic pathology of leukemias and lymphomas in man. National Cancer Institute Monograph 32, 1968.

50. Stewart A, Kneale WE: Radiation dose effects in relation to obstetric X-rays and childhood cancer. Lancet 1:1185, 1970.

51. MacMahon B: Prenatal X-ray exposure and childhood cancer. J Natl Cancer Inst 28:1173, 1962.

52. D'Angio GJ, Nisce LJ: Problems with the irradiation of children and pregnant patients. JAMA 223:171, 1973.

53. Becker MH, Hyman GA: Management of Hodgkin's disease: coexistent with pregnancy. Radiology 85:725, 1965.

54. Ray GR: Oophoropexy: a means of preserving ovarian function following pelvic megavoltage radiotherapy for Hodgkin's disease. Radiology 96:175, 1970.

55. Nahhas WA et al.: Lateral ovarian transposition: ovarian relocation in patients with Hodgkin's disease. Obstet Gynecol 38:785, 1971.

56. Harris LJ: Leukemia and pregnancy. Can Med Assoc J 68:234, 1953.

57. Cramblett HG, Friedman JL, Vajjar S: Leukemia in an infant of a mother with acute leukemia. New Engl J Med 259:727, 1958.

58. Adams MA: Helping the parents of children with malignancy. J Pediatr 93:734, 1978.

308

59. Fullerman EH, Hoffman I: Transient school phobia in leukemic child. J Am Acad Child Psychiatry 9:447, 1970.
60. Martinson IM: Home care for the child with cancer. In: Proceedings of the First National Conference for Parents of Children with Cancer, 'Maintaining a Normal Life'. Bethesda, MD, US Dept of HHS, Public Health Service, NIH, NCI, 1980, pp 255–256.
61. McNulty BJ: Out-patient and domiciliary management from a hospice in the management of terminal disease, Cicely M. Sanders (ed). London, Edward Arnold Publication, 1978, pp 154–165.
62. Black J: Cost of cancer. In: Proceedings of the First National Conference for parents of Children with Cancer, 'Maintaining a Normal Life'. Bethesda, MD, US Dept of HHS, Public Health Service, NIH, NCI, 1980, pp 227.
63. Widner G, Brill R, Schlosser A: Home health care: services and cost. Nursing Outlook 8:488, 1978.
64. Johnson RL: Cutting costs by controlling physicians. Hospital Progress 58:70, 1977.
65. Amado A, Cronk BA, Mileo R: Cost of care: home hospice vs hospital. Nursing Outlook 8:522, 1979.
66. Colt AM, Anderson N, Scott HD, Zimmerman H: Home health care is good economics. Nursing Outlook 10:632, 1977.
67. Kassakian MG, Bailey LR, Rinker M, Stewart CA, Yaks JW: The cost and quality of dying: a comparison of home and hospital. Nurse Practitioner 4:18, 1979.
68. Fine PR, Better SR, Ergstrand JL: The operation of a hospital based specialty home health team: activities and associated costs. ARN J 3:5, 1978.
69. LaVor J, Callerder M: Home health cost effectiveness: What are we measuring? Medical Care 14:866, 1976.
70. Stein REK: Pediatric home care: an ambulatory special care unit. J Pediatr 92:495, 1978.
71 Continuity of care for patients with malignant disease. Postgraduate Medical J 54:391, 1978.
72. Martinson IM: Home Care for the Dying Child. Professional and Family Perspective. New York, Appleton-Century-Crafts, 1976.
73. Tolkoff-Rubin NE, Fisher SL, O'Brien JT, Rubin RH: Coordinated home care. Medical Care 16:453, 1978.
74. Houghton L, Martin AE: Home vs hospital: a hospital-based home care program. Health and Social Work 1:89, 1976.
75. Cang S: An alternative to hospital. Lancet 2:742, 1977.
76. Brody SJ, Poulshock SW, Masciocchi CF: The family caring unit: a major consideration in the long-term support system. Gerontologist 18:556, 1978.
77. Maddox GL: The unrealized potential of an old idea. In: Care of the Elderly, Exton-Smith AN, Evans JG (eds). London, Academic Press, 1977, p 147.
78. Saunders CM (ed): The Management of Terminal Disease. London, Edward Arnold Publishers, 1978.
79. Fortunato RP, Komp DM: Death at home for children with acute lymphoblastic leukemia. Virginia Medical 106:124, 1979.
80. Martinson IM, Armstrong GD, Geis DP et al.: Home care for children dying of cancer. Pediatr for the Clinician 62:106, 1978.
81. Hinton J: Comparison of places and policies for terminal care. Lancet 2:29, 1979.
82. Sampson WI: Dying at home. JAMA 238:2405, 1977.
83. Thompson D: She died at home. Nursing Times 169, 1979.
84. O'Brien CR, Johnson JL, Schmink PD: Death education – What students want and need. Adolescence 13:729, 1978.

85. Clark I: Time to be home with the family. Nursing Mirror 36, 1979.
86. Lack SA: Hospice – a concept of care in the final stage of life. Connecticut Medicine 43:367, 1979.
87. Martinson IM, Geis D, Anglim MA et al.: When the patient is dying: home care for the child. Am J Nursing 1815, 1977.
88. Fifel H (ed): Contemporary America: New Meanings of Death. New York, McGraw-Hill, 1977.

14. The Care of the Terminal Patient

DONALD J. HIGBY

THE PROBLEM

Virtually every physician who cares for cancer patients faces a situation which seldom confronts his colleagues in other disciplines – the patient in whom death is statistically predictable within a relatively short time frame (weeks to months) and in which case nothing can be done to alter this inevitability. While it is true that the patient with severe coronary artery disease and Class IV heart failure may be in the same category, the life span of that patient is not defined in the same way as the patient with unresectable adenocarcinoma of the lung. Moreover, much can be done to maintain the former patient in some sort of equilibrium until the actual period of dying begins, which is usually of short duration. The patient with 'terminal' cancer, on the other hand, has a relatively long period of dying. Both the physician and the patient perceive that there is no realistic long-term hope, although at the moment the patient may be functional, communicating, and interacting with his environment.

Having to deal with such patients so commonly presents a special challenge to the oncologist and, unfortunately, this challenge is often met with inappropriate response. While it is appropriate for the physician to be oriented towards saving lives, it is also appropriate for him to assist the patient in dying so that his experience is not one of negation, but rather, affirmation.

As Noyes states, 'Of what value is the dying period? What contribution can the physician make to ease dying? Has he any special competence besides the administering of drugs to apply to this problem?' [1]. Unfortunately, modern medicine is not characterized by philosophical reflection. Furthermore, modern society, as has been pointed out repeatedly [2], is characterized by an almost pathologic avoidance of the fact of dying. It is almost impossible for a physician practicing in one of the developed coun-

Higby, DJ (ed), Supportive Care in Cancer Therapy. ISBN 0-89838-569-5.
© *1983, Martinus Nijhoff Publishers, Boston. Printed in The Netherlands.*

tries to relate to the views of dying held by most of the human race during most of its history. The reflections of various historical figures on their own deaths or those of loved ones sometimes seem morbid, alien, and almost psychotic when read today.

While the literature abounds with studies on the psychological processes experienced by dying patients [3, 4], the oncologist is in the unique position of having to deal with prolonged dying as an authority figure.

THE PHYSICIAN

Oncologists share with other physicians a self-image associated with their healing role. This self-image is oriented towards eliminating the disease of the patient or keeping it under control. Insofar as the physician's actions towards these ends are successful, he receives gratification. When they are not, the physician's view of himself is challenged, and for the oncologist several 'unsuccessful' cases occurring over a short time frame can lead to severe stress [5].

Also, by virtue of his education, the physician is oriented towards problem solving. The patient with a prolonged terminal illness has a problem that cannot be solved and the physician does not *a priori* have appropriate tools to deal with this 'mystery'.

Finally, the behavior of the physician towards the dying patient evolves with experience. However, unlike the evolution of other medical behavior, the possibility of feedback and modification of behavior is very limited. The house officer who repeatedly treats patients with diabetic ketoacidosis learns from his results and from more experienced individuals how to better treat the next patient. The process of helping the patient to die cannot be measured by examining end results. Furthermore, more senior physicians do not often verbalize their own experiences, and in fact, they may have developed defenses and evasive techniques so that they are not proper role models themselves.

The defenses and evasions used by physicians in caring for the terminal cancer patient are many. Physicians may successively offer new drug combinations or experimental drugs. While there is certainly a role for this sort of experimentation in patients, justification of this because 'there is always a small chance' or because 'it gives the patient hope' carries the danger of making both the physician and the patient turn their attention away from the fact of dying. As such, the patient is deprived of working through the process and the physician by continuing to behave in a problem-solving way does not learn from the experience [6].

Other times, the physician adopts avoidance behavior. Visits with the patient are perfunctory. If there is a housestaff, daily visits on in-patients may cease entirely. Visits may be characterized by short inquiries regarding current pain or discomfort, or discussions with family members rather than with the patient. Out-patient visits may become problem-solving sessions; adjusting pain medicines, ordering blood tests and X-rays, all important in themselves, but easily used as a substitute for dealing with the process of dying. Physicians tend to justify this sort of behavior by the assertion that their time could be best spent 'helping those who can be helped'. It is always easier to act in hopeful rather than hopeless situations. The attitude of the physician may be such that the patient is constrained from bringing up his real concerns. Non-verbal clues may suggest that the physician is in a hurry or that discussion of 'soft' issues like anxiety, depression, forebodings, etc. are not welcome. As a patient comes to accept the fact that his physician cannot 'save' his life, his attitude towards the physician changes and this new relationship, especially when substituted for the more traditional doctor–patient relationship, can induce a 'separation anxiety' in the physician which is often stress-producing. The physician may in fact react with some measure of unconscious anger towards the patient who ceases to view him as the one with all the answers, and justify his withdrawal from active involvement in the case by this understandable change in the relationship [7].

THE PATIENT

The psychological changes dying patients go through have been well described and while there is controversy regarding the universality or order of these adaptations, there is no doubt that the normal individual who learns that he will die within a real time frame becomes a different sort of person than he had previously been [3, 7].

What is it like to have gone through this 'grief' reaction and having reached the stage of acceptance? Some characteristics of this stage have been proposed.

a) The patient no longer behaves as though he has an 'indefinite' future as do the healthy [8].

b) As such, he becomes much more conscious of the 'now' time and his concerns are more immediate. His attention may be largely concentrated on his present comfort, or his orientation and effort may be directed to an occasion or event in the near future which becomes a 'goal' and as such, is invested with much more emotion than it would to be a healthy individual. A patient dying in a hospital may desperately desire to go out 'on pass' to do nothing more than lie on the sofa in his own home. To the physician and the nursing staff, this is not perceived as important and preparing the patient for such an excursion may be difficult and seen as an imposition on their time. To leave the hospital to attend a graduation, a wedding, or an important religious event is more understandable to the healthy, but at the same time, the importance of this to the patient is impossible for the healthy to understand [8].

c) As the patient is reclassified and reclassifies himself as 'dying', all social interactions change. Loneliness and withdrawal are common. Guilt feelings on the part of the patient for dying and on the part of his family and friends as they react to the stresses placed on their lives by the dying person (and wish for resolution of these stresses, i.e., for the patient to die), further exaggerate this reaction. Some patients may react to the altered relationship with the living by passive aggressive behavior, by exhibiting anger, and by inappropriate social behavior ('I'm dying so it doesn't matter what I say or do') which further strain the bonds that still exist [8].

d) Patients with terminal illnesses are often subjected to depersonalizing situations: conversations carried on in their presence which exclude them; routines in hospital which are obviously not geared towards their individuality; changes in the usual relationships with nurses, doctors, etc. Since depersonalization takes place, patients sometimes interiorize this disposition, which may reduce their anxiety. Their body as well as their malignant disease is seen as an unwelcome 'other'. Their physical and mental problems are the problems of the 'machine' which they disown [6, 7]. This reaction was carried so far in one patient that she was unable to refer to her bodily parts with the possessive. Instead of saying 'my head', she would say 'the head'. Even when this peculiar usage was pointed out to her, she continued to do this. Once cured of her disease which was a phenomenon of statistical rarity, she reverted to more conventional language.

e) In common with the aged, patients who have a terminal illness enter a consolidative phase, in effect, reflecting on life and summing up their experiences. As they look back, they cease to look forward. They begin to see their lives as a nearly completed whole, rather than a process [8]. 'I am ready to die' is an acceptable position for someone who is 90 years old to take, but for someone who is more of a peer in terms of age with the physician, it is discomforting because the physician cannot imagine himself as 'ready to die'. In the summing up, justification for actions past and present is often made. Lord Nelson, when offered last rites by a clergyman as he was dying, opined that the life he had led which had publically violated the moral conventions of the time, had held more good than bad. Deathbed statements of notorious 'sinners' have often seemed to reflect a less than serious attitude towards death. Deathbed 'conversions' are rare as pointed out in Chapter 15. These observations indicate that the new psychological balance achieved by the dying individual is not easily altered.

f) Osler observed and reported on a series of 500 dying patients. Of these, 18% suffered some pain and only 2% suffered mental apprehension [10].

g) The fact of terminal illness often results in the terminal patient dismissing as unimportant many of the concerns which have characterized his affective behavior. 'Forgiveness' of enemies, reconciliation with prodigal children, renewing the closeness of a marriage may all characterize this phase.

Obviously, the above are not manifest to the same extent in all dying patients and the degree to which some are accented and others diminished is related to the anxiety induced in the care providers and the family and friends [7, 8]. Death may induce both a sense of guilt or a sense of relief in those around the dying.

THE OBJECT OF DEATH: ONE PHYSICIAN'S PERSPECTIVE

The natural inclination of the healthy physician is to view death as an unwelcome competitor. When death is considered as beneficial at all, it is seen as an end to the process of suffering, but obviously, to end suffering by cure would be better. To view the process of dying as potentially positive and affirmative is difficult for the problem-solving mind set.

In an attempt to formulate the process of dying as a potentially positive experience, some look to a 'post-death' experience. Indeed, those who construe evidence for survival of the self from narratives given by resuscitated patients [11] or those advanced by less optimistic and more materialistic students which see death as an end to 'self' (the latter being an artificial construct rather than a reality [12], can be related rather easily to more traditional religious and philosophical perspectives of death. Whether death leads to an afterlife, results in dissolution of self into a universal whole, or is a final event in an uncaring universe, is not germane to this discussion, however, and regardless of 'evidence', what actually exists beyond the grave is outside the realm of scientific investigation, since without measurability, alternative explanations can be advanced for any phenomenon observed.

However, in order to view the process of dying as a positive experience, it is probably necessary for the physician to have a construct regarding dying to which he assents and on which he has meditated. Whatever this construct, the physician must, in order to best deal with the dying, face his own mortality and find potential meaning in his own death. Empathy with the patient is necessary for good medical practice in other aspects of medicine. In planning a patient's care, the physician should empathize with the pain, discomfort, and anxieties of the patient. Whereas this empathy is not difficult when the possibility of correction of the situation exists, it is exceedingly difficult to 'empathize' (as opposed to sympathize) with the fact of death. An excellent beginning is to read Toynbee's essay on the subject [13].

To 'identify' with the dying leads to an appreciation of 'right' death (euthanasia in the original sense). If the physician wishes to maximize the potential in dying, the approach can follow the lines of conventional medical intervention. From the physician's knowledge of the patient and from tactful, sympathetic questioning, he can learn of unresolved life conflicts; the degree to which the patient feels lonely, isolated, and depersonalized; the fears the patient has regarding his dying and his death; and the resources the patient has (religious, social, psychological) which will help him to cope with these issues. It is useful to construct a history, preferably written, outlining these issues. An example follows:

Mrs R.S. is a 68-year old widow with refractory multiple myeloma. Her anticipated survival is one to four months. Her physical problems include pathological and painful rib fractures, low back pain, and anemia. She has six children, all of whom are grown and with whom she enjoys a good relationship. Her family is very supportive. Her attitude towards death seems to be conditioned by her Catholic religion as well as her sense of her husband 'waiting for her'. She feels lonely, but understands and verbalizes that she has to die alone. She feels regret that she has not spoken to an estranged sister for the last ten years. Her oldest son is very unaccepting of her prognosis and wants her to have 'every chance' of prolonging her life.

Mrs R.S. seems to have reached the stage of acceptance and worries about future pain, although present pain is tolerable. She also expresses the hope that her family will understand why she doesn't want to 'fight' anymore. She is also concerned about 'being a burden' to her children.

After this, a diagnostic work-up regarding pain and other correctable physical problems is performed. Finally, a plan and a set of objectives are put forth. In the case of Mrs R.S., she was placed on intermittent transfusion therapy; intercostal nerve blocks were done which eliminated the pain of two severe pathologic fractures; and radiation was delivered to the low back, although the results of the latter were not as effective as desired. She was given oral morphine with instructions regarding dose titration and a back brace relieved her lumbosacral instability so that she could continue to ambulate.

The objectives formulated were:

1. *Conference with children*

   Object: to transmit mother's feelings regarding her approaching death and desire not to receive further therapy directed at controlling disease.

Object: to help family to deal with mother's desire 'not to be a burden'.

Object: to see if some reconciliation with her sister could be achieved using one of the children as a mediator.

2. *Conference with patient*

Object: to assure her that her symptoms and physical problems could be dealt with and that her physician would continue to keep her comfortable and would respect her wishes if she were unable to communicate them.

Object: to discuss with the patient that her children did not see 'being a burden' as she did, but rather, that her children looked forward to making her last days as comfortable as possible and that it was important to them to feel that they could in some way repay her for what she had done for them.

In this particular patient's case, relatively little 'extra time' was spent in this exercise and much was accomplished. After her death, her family expressed their feelings that her death had been positive and meaningful and that in their estimation, the approach had been ideal.

Thus, the physician who is 'sensitive' to what death may mean to an individual and has formulated in his own mind what death *should* mean, can strive using familiar tools and a limited problem-solving approach to maximizing the *positive* aspects inherent in dying for his patients while minimizing the negative aspects. Obviously, the process of dying is unavoidably associated with grief, loss, and other painful emotional experiences. Despite the best that can be offered, a 'good' death will not be available to all. On the other hand, it should be obvious that optimization of the dying experience is within the realm of most physicians to provide for most patients.

SUMMARY

The process of dying produces unusual stresses on the physician. The dying patient enters a state in which he is psychologically different from the healthy. Through introspection and identification with the dying, the physician can overcome rather than avoid, his own fears concerning mortality. After this, he can, by understanding the differences between the dying and the healthy, formulate a plan for the individual patient to optimize the process of dying. The achievement of formulated goals for the dying person can be considered 'successful therapy', and when seen as the object of the physician's intervention, can be as rewarding as 'curing' the patient.

318

REFERENCES

1. Noyes R: The art of dying. Perspectives in Biology & Medicine, Spring, 1971.
2. Aries P: Western Attitudes Toward Death: From the Middle Ages to the Present. Baltimore, Johns Hopkins University Press, 1973.
3. Kubler-Ross E: On Death and Dying. New York, MacMillan Publishing Company, 1969.
4. Grisez G, Boyle J: An alternative to 'death with dignity'. Human Life Review, Winter, 1978.
5. Epstein FH: Responsibility of the physician in the preservation of life. Arch Intern Med 139:919–920, 1979.
6. Cassem NH: Being honest when technology fails. Harvard Med School Alumni Bulletin 53:23–27, 1978.
7. Glaser B, Strauss A: Awareness of Dying. Chicago, Aldine Publishing Company, 1965.
8. Feifel H: Perception of death. Ann NY Acad Sci 164:669–677, 1969.
9. Verwoerdt A: Communication with The Fatally Ill. Springfield, Illinois, Thomas, 1966.
10. Osler W: Science and Immortality in the Student Life and Other Essays. Boston, Houghton-Mifflin, 1931.
11. Moody RA: Life After Life. Atlanta, Mockingbird Books, 1975.
12. Gifford S: Some psychoanalytic theories about death: a selective historical review. Ann NY Acad Sci 164:638–666, 1969.
13. Toynbee A: Various ways in which human beings have sought to reconcile themselves to the fact of death. In: Death: Current Prospectives, Schneidman ES (ed). Palo Alto, California, Mayfield Publishing Co, 1976.

15. Religion as Supportive Care

JEROME W. YATES

INTRODUCTION

Religion may be considered a complex construct, consisting of two components: practice (church affiliation, attendance and work usually within a specified organization) and religiosity (individual attitudes, thoughts, feelings, and faith). Though the two overlap, practice often requires group meetings or participation in group approved rituals by the individual, while religiosity represents individual activity. Although conflicting information is available, church attendance as a measure of practice appears to decline in the elderly as death approaches while religiosity increases [1]. This seems reasonable if churches are viewed as social organizations, deriving their participatory support from working adults. Just as the elderly leave the work force so do patients with advancing cancer, and both approach death. Insights from studies of the elderly with regard to religious practices and religiosity can supplant the meager information relevant to religion in the cancer literature.

Social commentaries would suggest that there is an increase in individual participation in religion as the risk of death increases. Bible reading by the elderly has been described as 'cramming for finals', ritual participation by the sick viewed as 'getting their house in order', and instant religion for the battlefield soldier reported as 'there are no atheists in foxholes'.

Ancedotal dissemination of these views are commonplace. It has only been in the last few decades that serious descriptive and analytic attempts to develop a better understanding of religious practices and their relation to other life events have become available.

Cross-sectional (surveys collecting items of interest at one point in time) and descriptive (demographic characterization) studies provide a snapshot look at religion. Retrospective cohort studies have been done, but the reliability of the information collected is suspect because of recall biases. This

Higby, DJ (ed), Supportive Care in Cancer Therapy. ISBN 0-89838-569-5.
© *1983, Martinus Nijhoff Publishers, Boston. Printed in The Netherlands.*

wide ranging group of studies has generally found greater religiosity in the elderly, women, and those from the lowest socio-economic classes [2].

Although these studies provide important information, they avoid the individual fluctuations known to occur in religiosity. Practical considerations, time, expense, and access to a study group, make longitudinal observation more difficult and expensive but concomitantly more informative. Longitudinal study of battlefield soldiers is impractical, and for the dying cancer patient sometimes intrusive, but studies of the elderly are possible. Information derived from each of these environments may not be generalizable but cautious interpretation of some cross-situational observations may be informative.

The Duke Longitudinal Study of Aging provides a period of 20 years for follow-up, looking at changes in religion [3]. Womens' religiosity and practices consistently surpassed men, but both demonstrated decreases in religious activity (primarily practice) with advancing age. Other measures collected from the elderly indicated happiness, personal adjustment, and feelings of usefulness were associated with indicators for religion. Other associations reported have included measures of religiosity with personal adjustment and church-related activities with satisfaction with life [1, 4]. The decrease in religious activity among the elderly without measurable decreases in religiosity may reflect the stability of the latter and/or the sensitivity of the former to increasing debility and decreasing mobility.

For patients with advanced cancer, time becomes a precious commodity. The relative physical stability seen in the elderly without cancer provides time for adjustment and adaptation. With progressive cancer, death becomes a real threat, suffering common, and disability almost universal. Measures of physical performance consistently diminish as death approaches [5]. If this is rapid, rationalization and denial are inadequate individual resources for coping, making both physical and psycho-social adaptation difficult. Religion may offer a socially acceptable framework through which the individual may negotiate an acceptable understanding of his deteriorating situation while avoiding the paralysis of paranoia, guilt, and withdrawal. The dearth of studies and abundance of testimonials related to the role of religion in the patients with advanced cancer, stimulated the systematic effort reported earlier and summarized below [6].

VERMONT STUDY

As part of a larger study, a selected group of patients with cancer having a predicted survival of greater than three months but less than one year were followed [7]. Observer and self-rated scales were used at least monthly to

Table 1. Variables studied.

1. Measures of religious belief or religiosity religious belief index (RBI).
   Sum of ten items (shown below) 'agree completely' codes as 2, 'not sure' codes as 1, and 'disagree' codes as 0. (Range of RBI is thus 0 to 20.)

(1). Meaning:	There is meaning and purpose in everyone's life, no matter what he is like or what he does.
(2). Think about life:	I think seriously about my life and what it means.
(3). Afterlife:	I believe in some kind of afterlife.
(4). Power:	I believe there is a power greater than man.
(5). God as personal being:	I believe in God as a personal being with whom I can talk.
(6). God as taught by church:	I believe in God as taught by my church.
(7). God exists:	I feel sure that God exists.
(8). Heaven:	I believe in some kind of heaven.
(9). Hell:	I believe in some kind of hell.
(10). Prayer:	Prayer is helpful to me.

2. Measures of religious practices (activity and connections).
   Affiliated with church –
   Are you active in or affiliated with any particular church or religion? (Yes/No)
   Importance of church –
   How important is your church or religion in your life? Would you say it is very important, somewhat important, not too important, or not at all important?
   Attended services –
   In the past month, have you attended services at your church? (Yes/No)
   Close to God or Nature –
   Did you ever feel especially close to God or Nature in the past few weeks? (Yes/No)

3. Measure of survival days before death
   (For those patients who died in the 12–18-month period following the data collection.)

4. Measures of pain presence of pain
   Have you been having any pain in the past few days? (Yes/No)
   Pain level –
   If 0 is no pain and 100 is more pain than you can stand, what is your present level of pain?

   ```
   [- - - - - - - - - - - - - - - - - - - - - - - -]
   0                                              100
   ```

5. Measures of well-being
   Satisfaction with life –
   Here are some faces expressing various feelings. Above each is a letter. Which face comes closest to expressing how you feel about life as a whole? (Seven faces, labeled from 'delighted' to 'terrible') [8]
   How happy –
   Taken all together, how would you say things are these days; would you say that you are very happy, pretty happy, or not too happy? [9]
   Positive affect –
   Sum of five positive items on Bradburn's Affect Balance Scale, slightly modified [9].
   Negative affect –
   Sum of five negative items on Bradburn's Affect Balance Scale [9].

collect information related to: 1) religious activity and church connections (practice); 2) religious belief (religiosity); 3) overall well-being (physical performance status, satisfaction, and happiness); and 4) pain. Survival data was analyzed with these other factors for 36 deaths among the 71 patients studied.

The study group consisted of 43 women and 28 men with a mean age of 59 ranging from 28 to 85. Of the 28 Roman Catholics, 32 Protestants, 2 Jewish, and 9 undeclared, only slightly more than one half were church affiliated and only 37% reported attending a religious service in the month prior to their entering the study. Two thirds of the patients reported 'feeling close to God or Nature' in the two weeks before study entry, while only one half reported their 'religion was very important' in their lives. The dimensions of religiosity and practice assessed at several intervals prior to death for the 71 patients are seen in Table 1.

For each measure taken from patients at the same time, an analysis of the religious belief index (RBI) showed a positive correlation with satisfaction with life (see Table 2). Happiness and affect variables generally did not correlate with religious belief.

Table 2. Pearson correlation coefficients $(63 < N < 70)$.

	Satisfaction with life	How happy	Positive affect	Negative affect
Belief				
RBI	0.406 [c]	0.154	0.175	−0.080
Activity and connections				
affiliated with church	0.246 [a]	0.230 [a]	0.056	−0.070
Importance of church	0.310 [c]	0.064	0.244 [a]	0.018
Attended services	0.352 [c]	0.336 [c]	0.318 [c]	−0.160
Close to God or Nature	0.328 [c]	0.219 [a]	0.433 [c]	−0.030

[a] $= p < 0.05$.
[b] $= p < 0.01$.
[c] $= p < 0.005$.

Satisfaction with life showed a significant correlation with activity and church connection variables. Those attending religious services were happier as measured in this study than those who did not. Both the religious belief and activity variables were significantly and negatively correlated with individual patient's level of pain (see Table 3).

There was no association between the measures of religiosity or practices and individual patient survival.

Table 3. Pearson correlation coefficients.

	Pain level	Presence of pain	Pain level for those with pain (n = 31)
Belief			
RBI	−0.293 [b]	−0.139	−0.368 [a]
Activity and connections			
affiliated with church	−0.221 [a]	−0.135	−0.145
Importance of church	−0.327 [c]	−0.170	−0.374 [a]
Attended services	−0.238 [a]	−0.080	−0.346 [a]
Close to God or Nature	−0.251 [a]	−0.287 [b]	−0.173

[a] $= p<0.05$.
[b] $= p<0.01$.
[c] $= p<0.005$.

There was little variability for the same individuals in the RBI taken at different times suggesting these measures are either not very sensitive or that religiosity is a trait and not a state. This may explain why patients do not express greater interest in religion as they approach death. Stability of the RBI mirrored the direct interview experience of the clergyman involved in the research. During the final few weeks or days of life when it was commonly not possible to collect patient data, the clergyman observed a general decrease in the patients' interest in religion, which paralleled their withdrawal from other social interactions. Metabolic encephalopathic changes, increasing pain customarily treated with narcotics and depression, mix to blunt the patients' interest and responsiveness to their environment.

DISCUSSION

Our study supports the contention that religious activity and church connections are associated with both satisfaction and happiness. These results agree with those from studies in the elderly [10–12]. Happiness has been related to interaction with one's environment and these results imply religious participation may promote happiness, or possibly those with religious interests represent a selected happier cohort [9].

Consistent negative correlations between measures of religious practice and religiosity with reported pain levels were found. Many studies have demonstrated a direct relationship between anxiety and pain perception. The link between anxiety and religion is weak but tranquility and confidence induced through suggestion, as well as purposeful behavior, are known to increase pain tolerance. The athlete playing the latter half of a football game unaware of pain from a broken bone, or the soldier with a severe battlefield wound demonstrating extraordinary pain tolerance, are documented examples of environmental influences on pain perception [13]. Religious support may augment endurance in distressing situations by providing an acceptable explanation for both pain and suffering, thus reducing individual anxiety.

Nowhere is suffering of the innocent more poignantly presented than in the book of Job [14]. Suffering is depicted not as retribution but rather as a test of faith. After the unwarranted loss of family, finances, and health, Job remains faithful to earn God's restoration of family, wealth, and a life of 140 years. This poetic presentation of the inexplicable can offer understanding and hope for the faithful. This Judeo-Christian classic facilitates intellectualization and provides faith in the face of severe adversity.

An analysis of survey data from voluntary participants, consisting of American women readers of a popular magazine, showed that the very religious and anti-religious were most likely to report greater happiness and also fewer symptoms of illness [15]. Confidence in belief, regardless of its characteristics, is likely to be associated with happiness and an absence of tension. Reported results of associations from cross-sectional studies such as this have the characteristics of being unable to prove causal relationships. Covariation may occur as a result of selection or reporting bias limiting our ability to dissect which comes first.

SUMMARY

Religion as support for the patient with cancer is an important consideration when planning and collecting other subjective observations and responses. The relationship between pain response, satisfaction, happiness, and measures of religion should be explored in future longitudinal studies. Religion should not be ignored because of its importance in the lives of many individuals.

Regardless of the beliefs and practices of the caregiver, minimizing dissonance for those patients with religious inclinations holds promise for reducing anxiety and improving adjustment. Where appropriate, cooperation with the clergy should be sought. Religious connections may provide a practical social support structure, the ritual an opportunity to allay guilt and suffering, and the belief system some hope for the future. In patients destined to die of their disease, last-minute changes in their religious beliefs are unlikely. For those with strong religious convictions, significant benefit from the security of their religion may provide a good source of support.

REFERENCES

1. Moberg DO: Religiosity in old age. The Gerontologist 5:78–87, 1965.
2. Gallop G, Jr: Religion in America, 1977–78. Gallup Opinion Index, Report No 145, Princeton, New Jersey, 1978.
3. Blazer D, Palmone E: Religion and aging in a longitudinal panel. The Gerontologist 16: 82–85, 1976.
4. Edwards JM, Klemmack L: Correlates of life satisfaction: a reexamination. Journal of Gerontology 28:297–302, 1973.
5. Yates JW, Chalmer B, McKegney FP: Evaluation of patients with advanced cancer using the Karnofsky performance status. Cancer 45:228–232, 1980.
6. Yates JW, Chalmer B, St. James P, Follansbee M, McKegney FP: Religion in patients with advanced cancer. Med Pediatr Oncol 9:121–128, 1981.
7. Yates JW, McKegney FP, Kun LE: A comparative study of home nursing care of patients with advanced cancer. Proc of the Third National Conference on Human Values and Cancer. New York, American Cancer Society, 1981.
8. Campbell A, Converse PE, Rodgers WL: The Quality of American Life. New York, Russell Sage Foundation, 1976.
9. Bradburn NM: The Structure of Psychological Well-Being. Chicago, Aldine Publishing Company, 1969.
10. Blazer D, Palmore E: Religion and aging in a longitudinal panel. Gerontologist 16:82–85, 1976.
11. Riley MW, Foner A: Aging & Society, Volume I: An Inventory of Research Findings. New York, Russell Sage Foundation, 1968.
12. Moberg DO: Social indicators of spiritual well-being. In: Spiritual Well-Being of the Elderly, Thorsen JA, Cork TC (eds). Springfield, Illinois, Charles C Thomas, 1980.
13. Beecher HK: Relationship of significance of wound to pain experienced. JAMA 101:1609–1613, 1956.
14. The Bible: Job.
15. Shaver P, Lanauer M, Sadd S: Religiousness, conversion, and subjective well-being: The healthy-minded religion of modern American women. Am J Psychiatry 137:1563–1568, 1980.

INDEX